THE
FIBRE
FUELLED
COOKBOOK

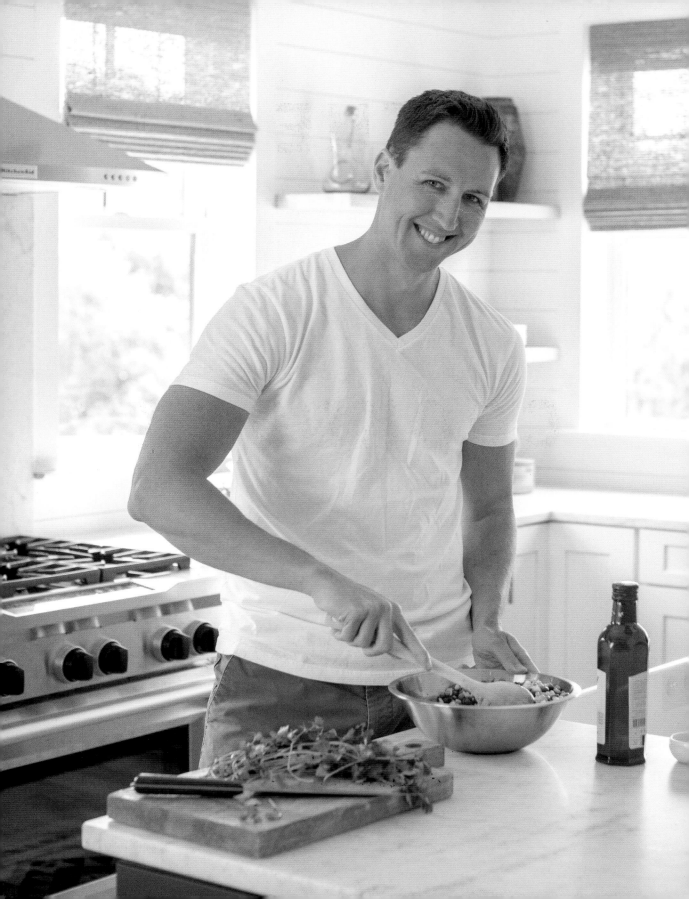

THE
FIBRE
FUELLED
COOKBOOK

Inspiring Plant-Based Recipes
to *Turbocharge Your Health*

Dr Will Bulsiewicz

Recipes by Alexandra Caspero

Vermilion

1

Vermilion, an imprint of Ebury Publishing,
20 Vauxhall Bridge Road,
London SW1V 2SA

Vermilion is part of the Penguin Random House group of companies whose
addresses can be found at global.penguinrandomhouse.com

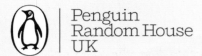

Penguin
Random House
UK

Photographs by Ashley McLaughlin
Photographs on pp. 2, 6, 11, 14, 24, 34, 46, 57, 122, 194, 204, 216, 224, 304,
315, 319, 344, and 360 by Margaret Wright
Bristol stool chart on p. 30 copyright © 2000 by Rome Foundation, Inc.
Food diary illustration on p. 31 copyright © Ana Bartel
Figure of man on p. 125 copyright © shutterstock/Toxa2x2

Book design by Ashley Tucker

First published in 2022 in Great Britain by Vermilion
First published in 2022 in the United States by Avery, an imprint
of Penguin Random House LLC, New York

www.penguin.co.uk

A CIP catalogue record for this book is available from the British Library

ISBN 9781785044175

Printed and bound in in Germany by Firmengruppe APPL, aprinta druck,
Wemding

The authorised representative in the EEA is Penguin Random House
Ireland, Morrison Chambers, 32 Nassau Street, Dublin D02 YH68.

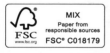

Penguin Random House is committed to a sustainable
future for our business, our readers and our planet.
This book is made from Forest Stewardship Council®
certified paper.

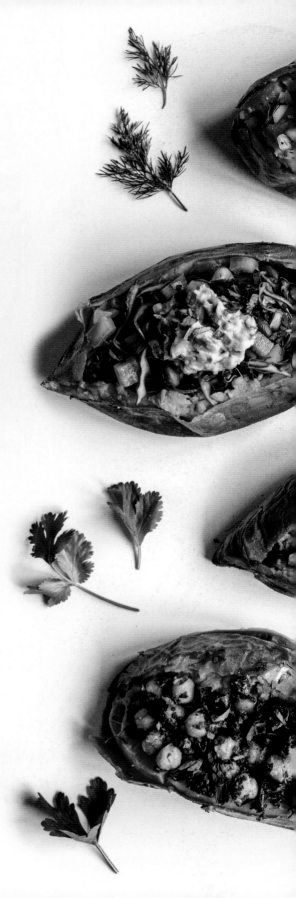

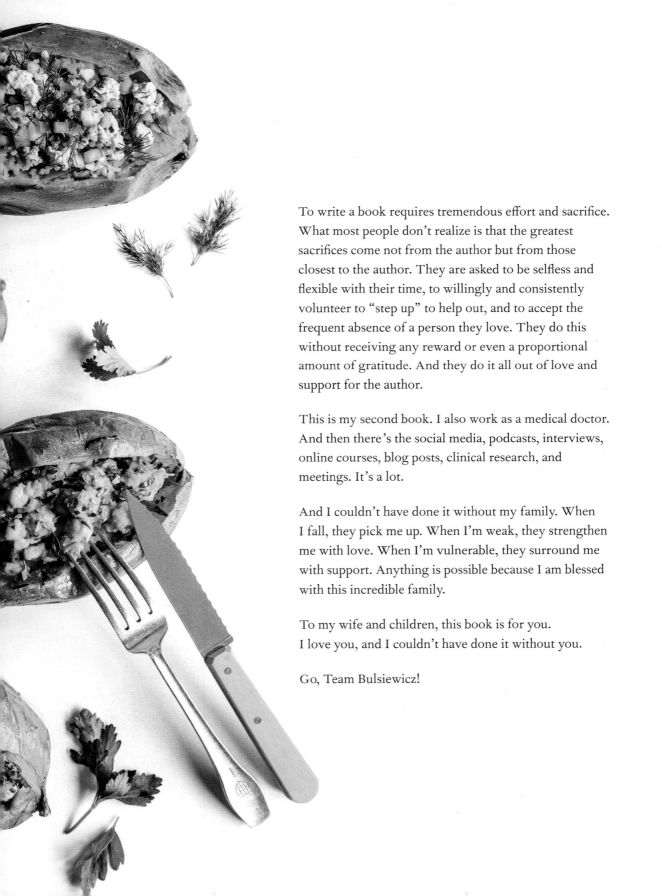

To write a book requires tremendous effort and sacrifice. What most people don't realize is that the greatest sacrifices come not from the author but from those closest to the author. They are asked to be selfless and flexible with their time, to willingly and consistently volunteer to "step up" to help out, and to accept the frequent absence of a person they love. They do this without receiving any reward or even a proportional amount of gratitude. And they do it all out of love and support for the author.

This is my second book. I also work as a medical doctor. And then there's the social media, podcasts, interviews, online courses, blog posts, clinical research, and meetings. It's a lot.

And I couldn't have done it without my family. When I fall, they pick me up. When I'm weak, they strengthen me with love. When I'm vulnerable, they surround me with support. Anything is possible because I am blessed with this incredible family.

To my wife and children, this book is for you.
I love you, and I couldn't have done it without you.

Go, Team Bulsiewicz!

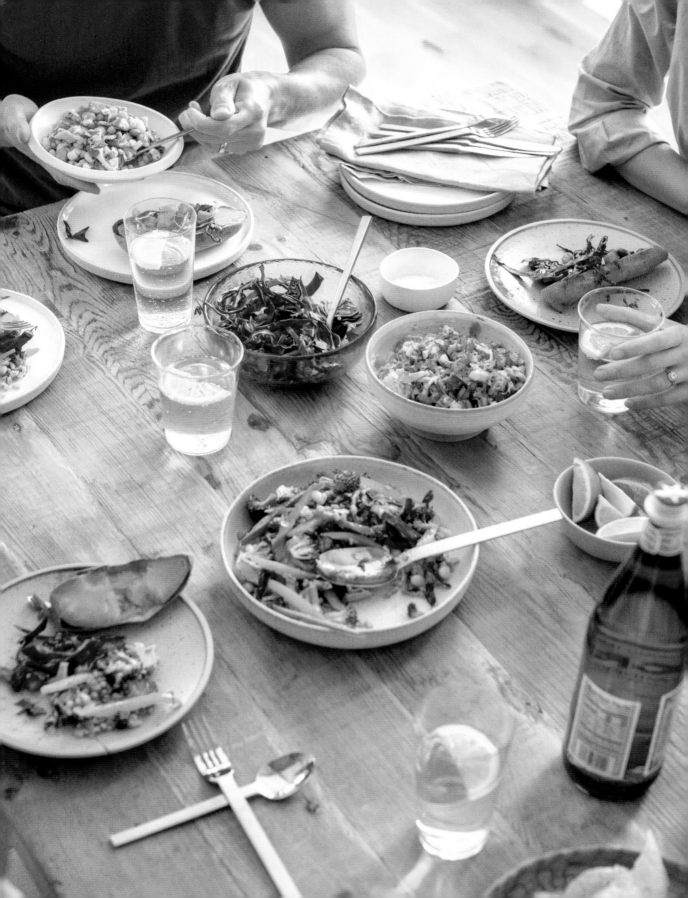

CONTENTS

HOW TO USE THIS BOOK

With humility, I have learned during my career as a gastroenterologist that no two people are created the same. We all have unique qualities, and a biology that is distinctly ours. We also have a distinct gut microbiome. On a planet with eight billion souls, no two of us have the same gut microbes. With our individuality in mind, I expect you to make this book your own. You can think of it as a sort of Choose Your Own Adventure for gut health.

If you're looking for delicious recipes and are plant-based or freshly plant curious and exploring, I'm glad you're here. This book is definitely for you. If you have no digestive issues, then you can jump right in and enjoy the recipes from all sections of this book (look for the "FF Unleashed" boxes in the recipes in the food sensitivity protocol chapters, Chapters 4 and 5). Keep track of your Plant Points as a fun way to challenge yourself (for more on Plant Points and becoming a "plant-based rock star," see Chapter 9). Or, challenge your friends!

If you're here with gut issues and food sensitivities and your goal is to feel better, I'm glad you're here, too. This book is also a practical guide that will lead you to better health. If you follow these strategies, you will be on a healing path to restore function to your gut. Over time, you'll be able to enjoy foods you didn't think you could eat, have more flavour and variety in your life, amp up your nutrition, and get back to feeling like yourself again—alive, optimistic, and thriving. It's all possible, and we will get there.

This book offers a step-by-step programme to support your journey to better digestive function. If that's the goal you have in mind, start from the beginning. Every chapter builds upon the one before it, so I'd encourage you to read all of the chapters before you step into the kitchen. There are two protocols included in this book—low FODMAP and low histamine. They are intended to help you understand your personal gut function and your own strengths and weaknesses. By reading each chapter before starting the protocols, you will have all the tools you need for an optimal experience and success.

If you are suffering from complex chronic health issues, getting to the root of the problem and getting it fixed can feel like trying to untie a complex knot. It requires patience and persistence to make progress. I want you to know that you are not alone. I am here to support you, and our online community is here to help you, too (visit theplantfedgut.com and my social media—@theguthealthmd). I also suggest reaching out to a qualified health professional who lives in your community for added support.

No matter who you are and what goals you have in mind, I hope you feel at home in this book and that you make it your own, refer to it often, and share it with a friend. I encourage you to try something new and push yourself to a higher level. Don't forget to tag me in your food pictures and message me with your progress!

Welcome to the Fibre Fuelled Life

"Can't we just do a blood draw, and it'll tell me what to eat?"

Sitting in front of me in my clinic is Maria. She's a forty-two-year-old mother of three who has been struggling her way through the healthcare system for the better part of thirty years. All she's asking for is a solution to her chronic digestive symptoms.

She has wind day and night, regardless of what she eats, and a bloated, distended belly after lunch. It's annoying, she says, but at this point she's too tired to care. She has zero energy, enthusiasm, or motivation. The brain fog doesn't help. She often feels queasy; she knows she's not going to throw up, but she wishes that she could.

She doesn't take a lot of joy from eating, and she hides out in the loo with gut-wrenching, fold-you-over abdominal pain instead of enjoying time with friends and family. She feels like a subservient victim to what she calls "the food monster."

"Maria," I tell her, "I can relate to everything you're describing."

It wasn't that long ago that I was living with a food monster of my own. I was in my early thirties, though I felt much older, and although I was doing my gastroenterology fellowship, I had a slew of my own digestive issues. A few spoonfuls of beans, for example, would set off waves of crippling abdominal pain, wind, and bloating. One bowl of wholewheat pasta would make me feel like my insides were a distended balloon, causing me to sneak around corners or step into the loo to discreetly vent some of the wind for about thirty seconds of relief. I'd toss and turn at night with stomach pains, feeling hungover the next day from lost sleep.

Back in those days, my solution was to avoid the issue. I didn't want to acknowledge that my food monster even existed. There were too many Philly cheesesteaks and Italian salami subs to inhale for me to miss the beans and wholegrains. They certainly weren't required for my tater tots.

I also hated the way I looked in the mirror. I was 23 kilos overweight with a saggy gut hanging over my belt. It was sobering. This was not the person I remembered from years past. I'd always thought of myself as an athlete, but the blood pressure pills sitting on the sink were a harsh reminder of how much had changed.

Psychologically, I was in even more pain. I was anxious and depressed. I had low self-esteem and low energy. It didn't matter if the outside world saw everything going well for me. I wasn't feeling that way. I hated how I felt, and I didn't love myself.

The one thing that made me feel better—if only for a fleeting moment—was junk food. It was quick, accessible, low effort, and it tasted good. With my rigorous work schedule, I wanted convenience, and junk food reliably delivered it. During my medical residency in Chicago, it was Portillo's for an Italian beef sandwich (add the mozzarella), chilli cheese dog, and cheese fries. I would offset the damage by drinking a Diet Coke instead of regular. That was what I knew about nutrition at the time.

There was no Portillo's in Chapel Hill, where I did my gastroenterology fellowship, so I had to find a new dealer to feed my addiction. There was good ole Merritt's Grill for the extra-bacon BLT or the Carolina dog (chilli dog topped with coleslaw). Or I'd head over to Bojangles for the spicy Cajun biscuit and ask them to add the egg and cheese on top. That's not even on the menu, but they would do it for me.

I was addicted to unhealthy food. It was on my mind between meals; my appetite for it was insatiable. I always wanted more. And I would make myself miserable with it, lying on the couch groaning and exhausted, only to roll off and walk out the door like a zombie so I could go find another fix.

Funnily enough, recent research has shown us that our gut bugs may be the driving force behind what I was experiencing. The invisible critters in our colon have the ability to produce chemical compounds called indole metabolites that activate specific parts of our brain associated with compulsive eating behaviour and even food addiction. It's fascinating to consider in retrospect that it was my gut bugs behind those cravings. But at the time I was completely unaware of the importance of our gut microbes, and this research that I'm describing was still years away from being published. Even more important, I was in denial that the food I had been raised on—that my family routinely ate *and enjoyed*—was the problem.

It was embarrassing. Here I was, a celebrated doctor with degrees from Vanderbilt, Georgetown, and Northwestern who was chief medical resident and the top award recipient at Northwestern on a grant from the NIH. But I didn't know how to fix myself. I had elite training from elite institutions, but the pills and procedures in my toolbox weren't going to correct the problem I was facing.

What I didn't understand at the time, the irony of all ironies, was that I (the gastroenterologist) needed to fix my gut if I wanted to fix my problems. And when I did fix my gut, I not only felt better,

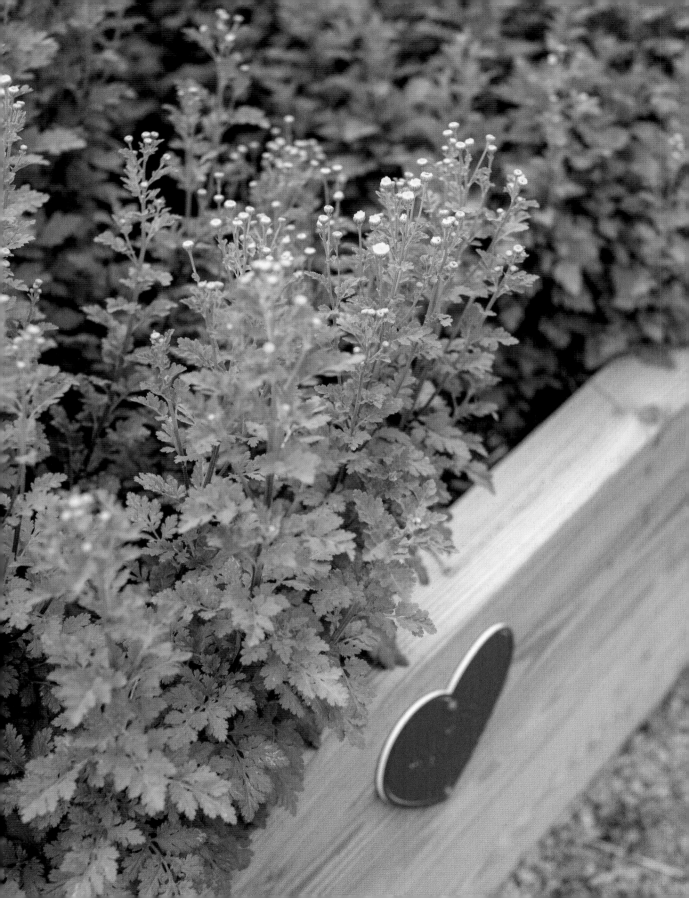

but I was actually able to restore function. Not only could I eat a few scoops of beans or a bowl of wholewheat pasta without having waves of pain, but I actually became capable of eating them without restriction. I no longer had to fear my food. By fixing my gut bugs, I had banished the food monster inside of me.

I felt like William Wallace from *Braveheart*, triumphantly raising the sword while riding atop a powerful warhorse.

"You can take my life, but you'll never take . . . my food freedom!!!"

◆

Perhaps you've read my first book, *Fibre Fuelled*. I'm incredibly proud of that book. It's the consummation of my life's work, and I'm blown away by the messages of healing that I receive on a daily basis from people who have chosen a *Fibre Fuelled* lifestyle.

But there's unfinished business to address. For some of you, the Fibre Fuelled 4 Weeks meal plan isn't enough. You need a methodology that offers more precision to identify the root of your food sensitivity. This book goes beyond *Fibre Fuelled* and dives deeper into FODMAPs, histamine intolerance, and other causes of food intolerances.

For others, the eighty recipes found in *Fibre Fuelled* were a great start, but that was just the beginning! There are so many delicious flavours from around the world to be celebrated, and in this book you'll find creative and exciting recipes like Sweet and Spicy Peanut Tempeh Wraps (page 106), Paella (page 261), Tuscan Flatbread (page 281), Sweet Potato and Okra Bowl (page 277) . . . I could keep going, but you're about to see in just a few pages.

There are three basic steps for gut healing that I've taken from my own experience and learned from working with many patients, including Maria. First, we restore hope. Healing is possible; we can do this together. Second, we need to find the root of the problem. You can't truly heal until you know what you're trying to fix. We need to identify the source of the problem in order to find the solution. And third, once we have the underlying problem identified and addressed, we can work towards healing the gut, restoring function, and making it stronger than ever before.

Maybe you can relate to Maria's struggles. Maybe you've been there yourself or are there right now. If so, this book is for you. I want to be your partner on a path that heals. This book contains all three phases of healing food sensitivities—hope, root cause understanding, and a plan for healing. I said this to Maria, and now I'm saying it to you—

This isn't always going to be easy, but I have a plan that can heal you.
If you stick with me and we commit to working through this together,
I am 100 per cent sure that we can get you better.

But this is also more than a blueprint for those suffering from food sensitivities. It's a cookbook for those searching for delicious, gut-nourishing, plant-based meals. We have designed these scrumptious recipes using cutting-edge science to make sure they are helping your trillions of gut microbes to produce the postbiotics that enhance health throughout your entire body. And, we've made sure they are easy for you to enjoy in your everyday life.

This book is a celebration of plants. The colours. The flavours. The healing properties. The way they are designed by nature to feed our gut microbes, reduce inflammation, protect us from disease, and extend our life expectancy.

Being *Fibre Fuelled* isn't a diet or a fad. It's a lifestyle that heals. It all starts with plant diversity, emphasizes our foundational foods, and honours progress over perfection. It's a path that heals from the inside out, and it is built on a foundation of rock-solid science. I'm here to help you see how exciting and effortless the *Fibre Fuelled* lifestyle can truly be—come join me on this delicious journey and let's be *Fibre Fuelled together*!

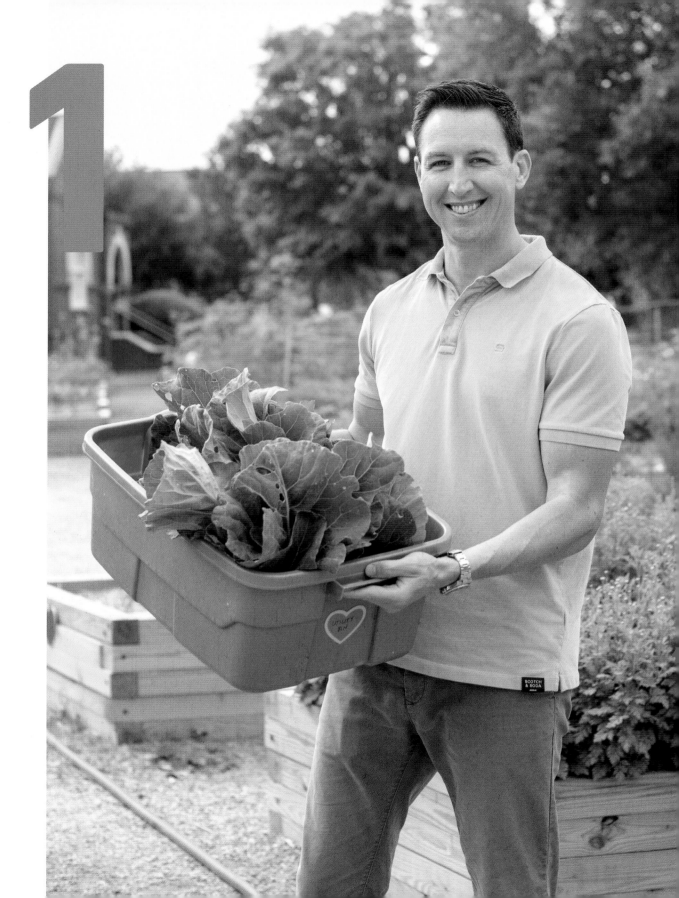

The Fibre Paradox

What seems like the problem is actually the solution

Imagine discovering a new human organ in the twenty-first century. Seems impossible, right? We all recognize that the depths of the ocean and outer space are mostly unexplored, but eighty million CT scans are done in the United States per year. How could you find a new organ?

Now, imagine that this new organ may be the missing puzzle piece that explains several mysteries of human health—it's deeply intertwined with digestion and access to nutrients, our metabolism, immune system, hormonal balance, mood and brain health, and even the expression of our genetics. Imagine that this new organ—the centrepiece of human health—isn't even human; it's mostly bacteria, fungi, archaea, and in some cases parasites that are actually outside your body.

This isn't hypothetical. It's completely real. It's called your *microbiome*. For decades, the scientific community knew there were a whole bunch of invisible microbes living inside us, but we lacked the tools needed to really study them. We didn't lose sleep over it—after all, these are the lowly bugs that produce fart smells and poo. Why would we need to know anything about our waste? How could those microbes possibly compete with the human mind or genetics?

Our view of these microbes changed dramatically in the early twenty-first century. Laboratory testing became less expensive and our computers became powerful enough to shed light on what turns out to be an absurd amount of essential information that is contained in poo. Suddenly, we had the tools we needed to start studying these microbes, and what we discovered continues to revolutionize what we know about health.

From the top of our heads to the tip of our toes, we are covered in an overwhelming number of invisible microbes. Not millions. Not billions. *Trillions of them.* They cover all external-facing structures, like your skin, mouth, and nose. Your thumb alone contains as many microbes as there are people in the UK. Seems like a lot, but that's nothing compared to what you'll find inside your gut, specifically your large intestine. That's where they're most concentrated, about thirty-eight trillion of them.

Your colon is an external-facing surface, too. Because your intestine is a continuous, unbroken tube beginning at the mouth and ending at the anus, everything running through your intestine is actually outside your body, just like your skin. Therefore, your intestinal microbes and the food you had for dinner last night are both technically outside your body, even when they are sitting in the depths of your bowels. Fascinating, right?

These microbes outnumber our human cells. If we look at just the classic eukaryotic cells that have a nucleus, mitochondria, etc., you would find that we have ten microbes for every one of these types of cells. That makes you less than 10 per cent human!

These microbes aren't passive—and very few of them are parasitic. They are symbionts existing in our superorganism ecosystem, and they are there with a purpose. They are deeply connected, and arguably at the centre of human health and biological processes. We actually rely on their presence and competence in order to be healthy. When they fail, we fail. Damage to the gut microbiota—termed "dysbiosis"—has been associated with the development of a variety of diseases: Crohn's disease, ulcerative colitis, irritable bowel syndrome, obesity, diabetes (both type 1 and type 2), eczema, asthma, coronary artery disease, colon cancer, breast cancer, endometriosis, female infertility, rheumatoid arthritis, Alzheimer's, Parkinson's, erectile dysfunction, and even depression. Is your head spinning? That's actually only a partial list. I include a more complete version in Chapter 1 of *Fibre Fuelled*.

The job of these trillions of important microscopic workers inside your colon is to process and unpack your food. They do this so you have access to nutrients; optimize your immune system so it can eliminate real threats without being trigger happy or attacking false threats; maintain your metabolism to keep your blood sugar and lipids in check; balance hormones and other endocrine signalling molecules; support and protect your brain so it remains sharp, focused, and upbeat; and flip the switches on your genetics to turn the right ones on and the wrong ones off. In other words, you need strong, empowered microbes that are thriving, fully functioning, and capable of supporting all of your many needs as the superorganism. How do you help your microbes thrive? By feeding them their preferred food: FIBRE!

The Fibre Solution

I know, I know. When I say "fibre," all you see is Grandma stirring her orange fibre drink so she could poo. But what I see is a sexy, gut health game changer. I want you to see what I see. To convince you, let me tell you about my favourite fibre study of all time, published by Dr. Andrew Reynolds in *The Lancet* on 2 February, 2019. In the hierarchy of scientific evidence, the most powerful conclusions come from systematic reviews and meta-analyses, randomized controlled trials, and large prospective population studies. That's what we're dealing with here: the strongest evidence possible. In this study, Dr. Reynolds analysed 185 prospective cohort studies encompassing 135 million person-years of data. I'll say it again—135 million person-years of data. Folks, the entirety of human existence is only three million years. We are looking at more than forty times the entire history of humanity here! I should mention that the study also included fifty-eight randomized controlled trials. Again, this is the highest-quality study done to date in order to examine the effects of dietary fibre on human health.

So what were the effects? Those who consumed more dietary fibre:

- Lived longer.
- Were less likely to have a heart attack.
- Were less likely to die of heart disease, our number one killer.
- Were less likely to be diagnosed with colon, oesophageal, or breast cancer.
- Were less likely to die of cancer, our number two killer.
- Were less likely to have a stroke, our number five killer.
- Were less likely to be diagnosed with type 2 diabetes, our number seven killer.
- Lost weight during clinical trials.
- Reduced their blood pressure during clinical trials.
- Lowered their cholesterol levels during clinical trials.

Mic drop! I'm out! Just kidding, there's more. Adding additional power to the study were linear dose-response relationships between dietary fibre intake and health benefits. In other words, the protection conferred was proportional to the amount of fibre consumed. More fibre means fewer problems. Taken together with the consistency of the findings, it's nearly impossible for any honest person to deny that fibre is massively beneficial to human health.

But why? If you think fibre simply goes in the mouth, sweeps through the intestines, and then launches out the other end like a torpedo, my friends, you have been sold a boring story about something incredibly exciting.

While it is true that as humans we lack the enzymes to digest fibre, not all fibre comes out the other end. That's where your microbes come in. They have the specialized enzymes that we humans lack. Their presence in your colon turns you into a superhuman with the ability to deconstruct your fibre.

In doing so, they create powerful anti-inflammatory molecules—short-chain fatty acids (SCFAs) acetate, propionate, and butyrate.

These SCFAs are the medicine our bodies crave. They immediately get to work right there in the colon. They enhance the growth of the good-guy bacteria like *Lactobacilli*, *Bifidobacteria*, and *Prevotella*. They directly suppress bad-guy bacteria like *E. coli* and *Salmonella*. Butyrate serves as the principal source of energy for healthy colon cells. They increase the expression of tight junction proteins lining the colon, reducing intestinal permeability and effectively reversing "leaky gut." An absence of short-chain fatty acids has been described in the setting of colorectal cancer, our second most deadly cancer. On closer inspection, we find that cancer cells are actually hypersensitive to SCFAs and will programme themselves for destruction in a process called apoptosis when met with SCFAs. The SCFAs act like a targeted missile for colon cancer prevention. Baroom!

Beyond the colon, SCFAs inhibit inflammatory signalling molecules and activate regulatory T cells to optimize the immune system. They reduce blood pressure, lower cholesterol, enhance insulin sensitivity, and activate satiety hormones to let us know when we are full. Patients with symptomatic coronary artery disease have been found to have depleted levels of butyrate-producing gut bacteria. SCFAs alter breast cancer cells and appear to make them less invasive. Basically, these last two paragraphs lay out how getting more SCFAs from dietary fibre explains the most powerful findings from Dr. Reynolds's study on page 17. Fibre is getting sexier by the moment here.

If you dig into the medical literature, as I have, you will start feeling like SCFAs are popping up everywhere—not just gut health but studies involving the immune system, too. For example, one of the burning questions of the COVID-19 pandemic was why one person can carry the virus symptom-free while another crashes into the ICU with cardiopulmonary failure. Given the strong connection between the gut and the immune system—70 per cent of the immune system lines the intestine—I had my suspicion that the gut was once again in play.

The answer came in January 2021 in the journal *Gut* when they compared the gut microbiome of those with COVID-19 to healthy controls. They found that people with COVID-19 were harbouring more inflammatory microbes and missing anti-inflammatory microbes. These changes became more pronounced as COVID-19 severity got worse, correlated with inflammation in the body, and persisted even after the infection cleared. Basically, the disturbed microbial pattern was creating inflammation, and that inflammation was behind the severe manifestations of COVID-19.

Upon closer examination of the microbes that were missing in severe COVID-19, it all starts to make sense. The microbes missing in severe COVID-19—*Faecalibacterium prausnitzii*, *Eubacterium rectale*, and *Bifidobacteria*—all increase butyrate production. More recently, an exciting new study connects long COVID—complications and symptoms that persist for months after initial COVID-19 infection—to the gut microbiome. The missing microbes in long COVID yet again enhance butyrate production—*Faecalibacterium prausnitzii*, *Bifidobacterium pseudocatenulatum*, and *Roseburia hominis*. Could butyrate be the linchpin in COVID-19 severity? Laboratory research has given us a reason to believe so.

In another study of dietary fibre, scientists were absolutely shocked when mice fed a high-fibre diet lived longer, had less severe symptoms, and had better lung function after a respiratory virus infection. They thought that because fibre is anti-inflammatory it would suppress the immune system, allowing the virus to have a free-for-all. Instead, they found that dietary fibre activated gut microbes to produce SCFAs that optimized the immune system to fight the virus. In other words, butyrate boosted antiviral immunity in the right spots while simultaneously tempering any excess inflammation. Short-chain fatty acids were shaping the immune system in the fight against the virus like a skilled general commanding the army.

So fibre *should* help protect us from COVID-19. But does it? A June 2021 study of frontline healthcare workers in six countries found a 73 per cent reduced odds of having moderate to severe COVID-19 among those eating a plant-based diet. Meanwhile, there was a 48 per cent greater chance of severe COVID-19 in those consuming a low-carbohydrate, high-protein diet. The low-carb consumers were nearly four times more likely to have moderate to severe COVID-19 compared to the plant-based crowd! Analysis of 592,571 participants in the ZOE COVID-19 Symptom Study revealed similar findings—a 41 per cent reduced odds of severe COVID-19 in those following a plant-predominant diet. See the pattern? What I have just shown you is multiple layers of evidence pointing in the same direction—the importance of dietary fibre for optimal immune function in the fight against viruses like COVID-19.

In case it's not obvious yet, these SCFAs have far-reaching effects and are incredibly powerful. At this point, the science is overwhelming and undeniable. Healthy humans have adequate amounts of SCFAs in their lives. Since we get SCFAs from consuming fibre, this must also mean that healthy humans have adequate amounts of fibre.

But this is not just a matter of cranking up the fibre supplements and calling it a day. That wouldn't be very exciting, and I promised excitement! We need to dive deeper into our relationship with fibre.

Fibre isn't just fibre. It's not all the same. That would be like saying all protein is the same. It's not. Both protein and fibre are just categories of nutrients. There's a lot of nuance and variation within the categories. Fibre is incredibly biochemically complex, making it difficult for even a biochemist to describe unique forms of fibre.

Despite the complexity, there are some simple rules. Fibre exists in all plants—fruits, vegetables, wholegrains, seeds, nuts, and legumes. To keep it straightforward, we describe fibre as either soluble (dissolves in water) or insoluble (doesn't dissolve). Most soluble fibre is prebiotic, which means that it is food for our gut microbes and leads to health benefits. Each plant has its own unique mix of both soluble and insoluble types of fibre. Those unique forms of fibre have unique properties and also feed unique families of microbes.

You see, these microbes are just like us. They have their own personalities. Some are friendly, some are grumpy. They also have their own unique skill sets. Some create butyrate; others help us process our fats. And they have their own dietary preferences. Some prefer black beans; others prefer avocados.

Although it's hard to imagine, these are living creatures. They need sustenance to survive. Because they live in our colon, our food is their food. The ones that get fed grow stronger and are more well represented. The ones who aren't fed begin to starve, become weaker, at some point become incapable of doing their job, and eventually die off.

We're in the driver's seat with our dietary choices. Every bite we eat determines the rise and fall of families of microbes inside us. And what we ultimately want in our gut is biodiversity. This is a measure of health.

Our gut is an ecosystem, in the same way that the Amazon rain forest and the Great Barrier Reef are ecosystems. What we find in all ecosystems is that biodiversity equates to strength. A diverse ecosystem is resilient and adaptable. You can punch it in the face, but all life in that ecosystem helps to absorb that punch, shake it off, and give you the "That's all you got?" look.

On the flip side, I don't like snakes or sharks, but if you remove them from the ecosystem, you will create a void that the other creatures aren't designed to fill. We humans may selfishly not like them (can you imagine what they think of us!), but even the most hated animals are an important part of that ecosystem. Eliminating diversity results in a ripple effect of instability throughout the system. Now the ecosystem isn't ready to take that proverbial punch to the face.

The same goes for our gut microbiota. We want a biodiverse ecosystem for maximum stability because each microbe has its own skills. When there is a loss of diversity, there is instability within the system.

But as we now understand, these microbes also have unique dietary preferences, so if we consume a biodiverse, fibre-rich diet, we help nourish as many of these microbes as possible. This is more than just "Dr. B's theory on gut microbial health." This is actually scientifically validated. As the American Gut Project found, the single most powerful predictor of a biodiverse gut microbiota was the diversity of plants in the diet.

Specifically, they found an advantage when thirty or more different plants were consumed per week. It's not that thirty is a magical number. I'd take thirty over twenty-nine, but heck, give me thirty-five or forty. Why not? The bottom line is that we should make plant diversity the centrepiece of our dietary philosophy. It's simple, but maximally effective for your health, which is why I call it the Golden Rule. Forget all the squabbling and diet wars on YouTube. Here is your one Golden Rule—diversity of plants.

But to be clear, your microbiome isn't simply the product of plant-based diversity. It is also powerfully attached to your overall dietary pattern. If you eat a meat-heavy diet but sneak in a whole bunch of small portions of different plants, you won't have the healthy microbiome that you *could* have by making plants the foundation of your diet. If you make plant diversity the centrepiece of your dietary philosophy, make sure that plants also make up the majority of your calories. Ideally, you want to be 90 per cent or more plant-based. When you go heavy on the plants, you tip the scale of health in your favour by drowning out and replacing the unhealthy stuff with the best stuff—fibre-rich plants.

As you can see, the science is clear: A diverse, plant-centred diet is the optimal diet for micro-biome health. It's also the optimal diet for human health, in large part because our gut bugs are so critical to our physiology. Once you realize how vital the Golden Rule is for our health, it's time to put it into action. Let your shopping trolley, your kitchen, and your plate all be a technicolour expression of plant diversity. Challenge yourself at every meal. Share it with your friends. Shout it from the rooftops. The entire world needs to hear this healing message—

Diversity of Plants, Diversity of Plants, Diversity of Plants!

Bridging the Gap from Fibre Starved to *Fibre Fuelled*

It sounds simple enough—make plants and plant-based diversity the centrepiece of your diet—but it's easier said than done. For starters, 95 per cent of us are not even getting the *minimum* recommended amount of fibre in our diets. The average daily adult fibre intake is 15.6 grams in women and 18.6 grams in men while the minimum recommended amount is 25 grams per day for women and 38 grams for men. We are the most fibre-deprived society of the modern era, and there are no signs of that letting up.

If you're searching for the root of our issues, look no further than the standard American diet. According to US Department of Agriculture estimates, 32 per cent of our calories come from animal foods; 57 per cent from processed plant foods; and only 11 per cent from wholegrains, beans, fruits, vegetables, and nuts. Among that 11 per cent, the number one item is potatoes from french fries and chips. The United States also has the highest meat consumption in the world—about 100 kilos of meat per person per year. Considering that the average American weighs 82 kilos, we are consuming the equivalent of our own body weight plus a five-year-old child in meat on a yearly basis. And yet, our most popular fad diets are encouraging us to double and triple down. Meanwhile, a plant-based diet *seems* increasingly popular and we are repeatedly warned about the risks of meat consumption for human and planetary health, yet our meat intake is actually increasing.

In the most recent dietary guidelines, the US Department of Health and Human Services (HHS) and the US Department of Agriculture (USDA) jointly laid out governmental recommendations for healthy dietary choices and how we're performing relative to those recommendations. It's a national report card for our diet, and the results summarize our woeful, disease-inducing diet. We're encouraged to limit added sugars, saturated fats, and sodium, yet at least 62 per cent, 71 per cent, and 84 per cent of us are overdoing it on each of these, respectively. Meanwhile 80 per cent of us are inadequately consuming fruits, 90 per cent are inadequately consuming vegetables, and 98 per cent fall below recommendations for wholegrains. We're good at eating the bad stuff, and bad at eating the good stuff.

And now here we are: 74 per cent of adults and 40 per cent of children are overweight or obese; 45 per cent of adults have hypertension and 46 per cent have prediabetes or diabetes; 18 million have coronary artery disease, our number one killer; 150,000 will be diagnosed with colon cancer and 280,000 with breast cancer this year (and the story in the UK is much the same). It's no coincidence that these are the exact same conditions that Dr. Reynolds powerfully showed are reduced when we increase our dietary fibre intake. We're not consuming fibre, and our epidemic diseases reflect that. It is our most pressing, most important nutrient deficiency.

Simply put, we need more plants in our diet. This cookbook aims to help you with that, and, for some of you, that's why you're here. More inspiring, gorgeous, simple, and delicious ways to add more plant diversity (i.e. fibre) into your diet. Don't worry. *fist bump* I got you. You're going to love these recipes.

But for many of you, there's another issue, and that is your gut needs a little help to add all that fibre. Perhaps you even suspect you have a food intolerance. I want you to love this fibre-rich diet, too, and this book is the bridge that's going to take you there.

Unlike a food allergy, which is an immune system response to a food, a food intolerance is a response to food that does not involve the activation of your immune system. There are a number of different mechanisms that can cause food intolerances, ranging from enzyme deficiencies (lactose intolerance is a classic), to pharmacologic (such as monosodium glutamate, or MSG), or your digestive system struggling to keep up with the demands of your diet or other factors of digestive and gastrointestinal function. Symptoms may not occur for several hours after the food ingestion and can last for hours or even days. An individual can be sensitive to multiple foods or food groups, making it difficult to isolate what is what. It's complicated! We estimate that 20 per cent of the population has a food intolerance but, given these complexities, it's really hard to know.

What's the Deal with Food Intolerance Testing?

I totally understand why food intolerance tests are so attractive. When you're struggling, you just want to be told what to eat and what not to eat. Antibody-based food intolerance tests make it seem like the answer could be so simple. But if a test uses antibodies to diagnose food intolerance, it assumes that the immune system is causing the food intolerance, which it is not. I've had hundreds of patients waste their money on these tests, only to be confused by the results or, worse yet, sent down an inappropriate path of dietary restriction. Sometimes the antibody test tells them that they are intolerant of a food that they've never had any symptoms with. Other times, the test will say that they aren't intolerant of something that they know for a fact triggers their symptoms. Sadly, these antibody food intolerance tests are unreliable and a waste of time and money. Instead, focus on identifying the specific foods that trigger your symptoms. This is the tried-and-true "gold standard" strategy. It definitely works, it's backed by science, and it is what you will find in this book.

I see the consequences of a fibre-starved gut microbiota in my clinic on a daily basis. My patients manifest the corollaries of dysbiosis—irritable bowel syndrome, chronic constipation, coeliac disease, and food intolerances. I also frequently see the consequences of unaddressed food intolerances and the challenges of trying to increase your plant diversity with a gut that needs healing. My patients, and perhaps many of you, are suffering and miserable, with a myriad of digestive and other symptoms that feel overwhelming. You deserve a solution. That solution, quite simply, is to reconstruct the gut microbiota, restore the healthy gut microbes to power, and repair the broken tight junctions. Once repaired, put that machine for human health to work by fuelling it with its preferred fuel—fibre!

I'll provide you with a path that will allow you to rekindle your relationship with food so that you can stop fearing it and get back to loving it. Through education, you'll be able to understand and properly interpret what's happening with your body, identify the root of the issue, and generate solutions. It's a powerful, life-changing method designed to heal your digestive issues, restore function to your digestive mechanism, and allow you to thrive on a diet that celebrates plants in abundance and diversity.

If your gut is feeling good and ready for exciting new flavours, feel free to skip to Chapter 9 (though please enjoy the recipes in any of these chapters!). Otherwise, keep reading for my fresh approach to digestive healing.

>> *To view the 49 scientific references cited in this chapter, please visit theplantfedgut.com/cookbook.*

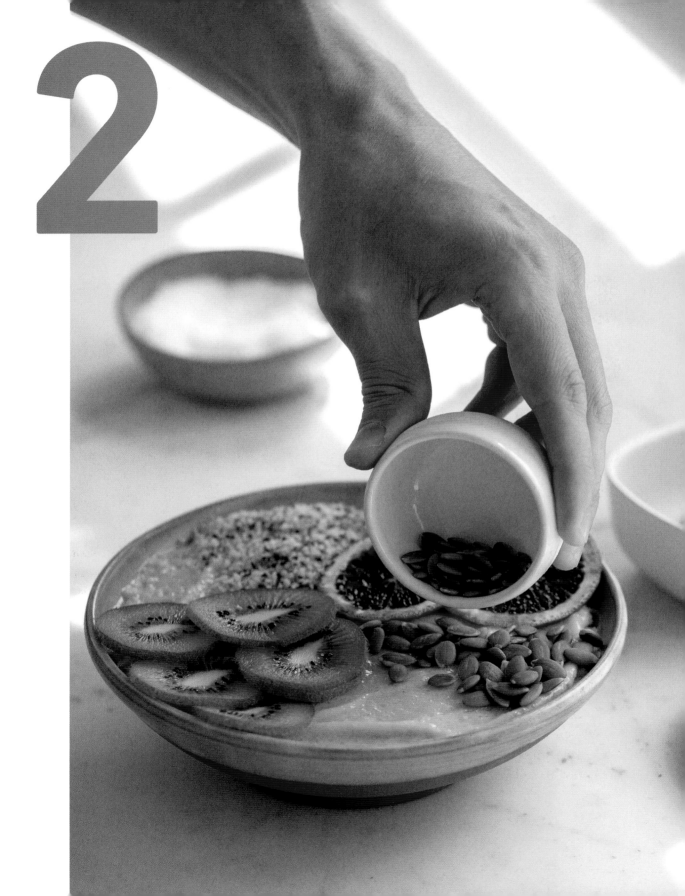

The GROWTH Strategy:

GROW Beyond Your Food Intolerances

Our method to identify
your personal food intolerances

Allow me to introduce you to the protocol I've created to help you have the gut health of your dreams and to enjoy the biodiverse, plant-centred diet I've been heralding. I've packaged it into an easy-to-remember acronym that just so happens to also embody our mindset when it comes to the direction we're moving with our diet. It's called the GROWTH strategy:

GROWTH

G Genesis
R Restrict
O Observe
W Work it back in
T Train your gut
H Holistic healing

G: Genesis

Step one in our GROWTH strategy is to understand the genesis of your symptoms. If you're experiencing wind, bloating, nausea, or upper abdominal pain that is brought on by food, we want to understand the root of your discomfort. This is always my first step in my clinic. In order to properly treat something, we need to know what we're treating.

In simple terms, food sensitivity is when you manifest symptoms because your body is reacting to some component of your food. It could be your immune system reacting, making it a food allergy. It could also be your digestive system struggling to keep up with the demands of your diet, leading to food intolerances. This is the how, and it helps us to understand the mechanism at the root of our problem. Now, there are some root causes of digestive symptoms that cannot be treated with the GROWTH strategy—including things like coeliac disease and altered gallbladder function. You need directed therapy if that's what you're suffering from. So part of the "G" is ruling out what I call the Big Three of Food Sensitivity. In Chapter 3, I will give you an expanded look at the Big Three as well as several other potential causes of food intolerance.

The GROWTH strategy is, however, designed to address food intolerances in a person with a damaged gut microbiome. Chapters 4, 5, and 6 take a deep dive into the kinds of food intolerances I most often see, particularly FODMAPs and histamine intolerance. Irritable bowel syndrome, inflammatory bowel disease, small intestine bacterial overgrowth (SIBO), acid reflux, and chronic constipation are just a few of the conditions associated with a damaged gut microbiome. In fact, the vast majority of digestive disorders are associated with a damaged gut microbiome, or dysbiosis. So while it's a requisite first step to understand better the genesis of your symptoms, the vast majority of you are here because part of the problem that you face is a damaged gut microbiome. The GROWTH strategy is the solution for the wind, bloating, and discomfort after meals and restoring function to your digestive system. You can be healed. That's what we're here to do.

Regardless of your symptoms or what you perceive to be the problem, though, you should seek the assistance of a qualified health professional to identify the genesis of your symptoms. That evaluation becomes more urgent if you have any of these red flag symptoms: severe pain, intractable vomiting, unintended weight loss, unexplained anaemia, blood in the stool or vomit, fever, neurologic symptoms, or chronic diarrhoea.

I know that food intolerances can be complicated. It's quite possible you've been struggling with symptoms and no concrete answers or solutions for some time. There's no proven blood test to figure out what's bothering you, since food intolerances don't activate your immune system; if only it could be that simple. And because digestive ability varies from person to person, you may have a genetic enzyme deficiency without knowing it. Our gut microbiome is completely personal and definitely plays a role in digestion, but we haven't figured out how to explain food intolerance through microbiome testing. (We're working on it!) And, just to make matters even more complicated, our diet changes meal to meal, altering our exposure to different proteins, fat, carbohydrates, fibre, and other micronutrients, not to mention the preservatives, flavours, emulsifiers, thickeners, humectants, firming agents, and flavour enhancers added to ultra-processed foods. But while the biochemistry of food intolerance may be complicated, our GROWTH strategy has the ability to simplify it and still give you the rock-solid results you seek. It's a series of steps you follow, repeated as needed, to help you identify the food intolerances that are uniquely yours. This is the 1, 2, 3 of food sensitivity:

R Restrict
O Observe
W Work it back in

Pick a food, any food . . . Sorry, gluten is not a food. It's a protein. But we can roll with wheat. Say you're wondering if you have a food intolerance to wheat (or if wheat is the genesis of your symptoms). Cool. If we do the 1, 2, 3 of food sensitivity and restrict wheat, observe what happens, then work it back in, we will be able to isolate our response to wheat and know whether or not you have a food intolerance.

Knowledge is power. Once we know exactly where your issues lie, you'll be empowered to make smarter food choices as you move forward. The 1, 2, 3 of food sensitivity becomes your tool that allows you to simply and systematically identify your problems. We will be coming back to this technique time and again. It's time to master the art of food intolerance detection.

R: Restrict

"Hold up, Dr. B! I thought we weren't supposed to restrict our foods. The single greatest predictor of a healthy gut microbiome is the diversity of plants in your diet—remember?" Yes, our goal is absolutely a diet where we thrive on abundance. No question about that. GROWTH is more than an acronym; it's our motto for gut health and our mindset for life. When Fibre Fuellers hear the word GROWTH, we tap our heart three times to acknowledge our shared commitment to everything this beloved word embodies. But, for people who are suffering with food intolerances who aren't sure exactly which foods are the issue, restriction is a temporary step on our journey to achieve an unrestricted diet.

Consider the rosebush for a moment. You can leave it to its own devices, and there will be flowers, but they will grow straggly and unattractive. Or you can prune the rosebush, which encourages vigorous growth. The old shoots support the structure of the plant, while the new shoots stimulated by pruning produce the largest, most attractive flowers. Pruning is a step on the path to floral abundance.

Taking one step backwards so that we can take two steps forwards is necessary because temporary restriction is our way of isolating individual foods that we want to put to the test. For every single food, there is a threshold when food intolerances kick in. If you eat less than that threshold, you won't suffer the negative symptoms. For example, a person with the worst lactose intolerance on the planet can handle a drop of milk on their tongue. But the minute that person increases their intake beyond their threshold, symptoms show up—and those symptoms will continue to exist as long as their intake exceeds that threshold. On the other hand, I don't have lactose intolerance (and I don't drink milk), but I could make myself sick if I drank enough of it. It's like the saying "all good things in moderation," but in this case what defines moderation is personal, and for some of us that threshold is less than the amount we would consider moderation. Hence why we call it a food "intolerance"—it's the limit at which you can no longer tolerate that food.

As a part of our GROWTH strategy, our first step is to identify the genesis of our symptoms. We need to rule out the Big Three and consider other diagnoses that could be driving our food sensitivity. But we also want to identify which specific foods you are sensitive to. Through ROW—Restrict, Observe, Work It Back In—we have a method to put individual foods or food groups to the test, figure out whether or not you have an intolerance, and even identify your threshold for those foods.

Perhaps you already suspect which foods you want to test. That's great—you can follow the advice in this chapter. Lactose is a perfect example and a great place to start. If you're not sure what to test, I have two powerful food intolerance protocols for you in Chapters 4 and 5. It will take some time, but if you complete those two protocols, you will know so much more about the strengths and weaknesses of your gut and be empowered in your choices.

Restriction with a History of Disordered Eating

The idea of dietary restriction may not come easily to you, especially if you've had fear, anxiety, or loss of control with food. I hear you and I see you. Your safety and healing are my priority. I want to emphasize that the restriction here is temporary and it is done as part of a deliberate process intended to identify which foods we are intolerant of so that we can add them back in appropriate moderation. With that said, trust your instincts. If your gut says that restriction doesn't feel right, then let's step away from the restriction for a moment and focus on healing our relationship with food first, potentially with the help of a therapist or eating disorder specialist. Then, when you feel ready, this GROWTH strategy is there for you, done with the support of your health professionals. The topic of food fear and nurturing a healthy relationship with our food is very important to me, so we will continue this conversation in Chapter 8.

O: Observe

Observation isn't something we spend much time discussing, so I want to shine a spotlight on it for a moment. This is a fundamental part of human experience. It's how we learn! Observation is when we apply thought to our experiences and link them together so that moving forwards, in our minds, they are now connected to one another. Creating these connections allows us to understand the world around us.

While I needed something linear to make the acronym work, in truth, Restrict and Observe are more like partners in a dance than sequential letters in a word. Observation is a critical part of this process and it should start before you restrict *and* continue after you work it back in.

Sherlock Holmes is the most famous fictional detective of all time. Perhaps you've seen him in the movies or on television? We're going to turn you into the Sherlock Holmes of food intolerances. Holmes's formal method is called inductive reasoning. When he entered a crime scene, he spent time observing it, looking for patterns. He took his time and did not rush. These observations allowed him to form hypotheses and eventually a complete theory. Inductive reasoning is how we are going to form our theory on which foods specifically are causing trouble. We want to start making observations and connections that explain our symptoms.

In order to do this, you'll need to collect the proper information so that we can identify a pattern. Before even considering restriction, you can first use inductive reasoning with your usual diet to try to identify potential food triggers by spending a few days keeping a food diary. A food diary is a record of what you eat, when you eat, and how you feel. It captures the information you need to make connections between your overall well-being and problematic foods. The result will culminate in a greater consciousness for how our choices influence how you feel.

This is more than just food. There are many aspects of our daily life that can have an effect on how we experience our food. Here's what we want to pay attention to:

- Meals, Snacks, and Beverages: Make sure to include the time, location, and how long you devote to eating. There's a difference between inhaling a doughnut while you drive to work and sitting down at the kitchen table for a slow-paced breakfast. Don't forget to keep track of beverages, too. Dairy, sweeteners, caffeine, and alcohol are all common causes of digestive symptoms.

- Signs and Symptoms: Technically speaking, food intolerances may be delayed by up to forty-eight hours. Thankfully, the vast majority of symptoms begin about a half hour after eating and occur within the first six hours after eating. So try to focus on that period of time with your food.

- Hydration: Sometimes our bodies get confused and will signal fatigue or even hunger when in fact they're thirsty! Water is a requisite part of human physiology, including digestion. The

Institute of Medicine recommends 3.9 litres for men and 2.8 litres for women per day. Bear in mind that the water you eat counts, too. Fruits and vegetables can be a great contributor. But make it a point of emphasis to get enough good old fashioned H_2O.

• Medications/Vitamins/Supplements: One of my mentors at the University of North Carolina, Dr. Henry Lesesne, was famous for encouraging us to pay attention to medication side effects. "Step 1: Make sure it's not the meds. Step 2: Double-check it's not the meds." These days meds can include vitamins and supplements. Every single one has the potential to alter digestive function.

• Sleep: Research has shown that sleep and your gut microbiota are intertwined. A damaged gut negatively affects sleep. Sleep deprivation negatively affects your gut. It can either work for us or against us. Either way, it's important to keep track of the correlation between sleep and digestive symptoms because just two nights of poor sleep have been connected to alterations in the gut microbiota.

• Mood/stress/emotional state: Modern times are stressful! Unfortunately, your emotional state or mood can throw your digestive rhythm out of whack. This isn't a small factor, it's a big factor. Here's my one-sentence summary of the effects of stress on gut health: Studies have shown that stress alters gut permeability, absorption, mucus and stomach acid secretion, electrolyte and water balance, and appetite; increases our response to inflammation; slows stomach emptying; activates inflammatory pathways in the gut; accelerates colon motility; increases sensitivity of the nerves in the gut; negatively affects blood flow to the gastrointestinal (GI) tract; activates mast cells that release histamine; and alters the gut microbiota. So perhaps it would be helpful for us to monitor our stress levels in the context of digestive function, eh?

Bristol Stool Scale

TYPE 1		Separate hard lumps, like nuts (hard to pass)
TYPE 2		Sausage-shaped but lumpy
TYPE 3		Like a sausage but with cracks on the surface
TYPE 4		Like a sausage or snake, smooth and soft
TYPE 5		Soft blobs with clear-cut edges (passed easily)
TYPE 6		Fluffy pieces with ragged edges, a mushy stool
TYPE 7		Watery, non solid pieces. Entirely liquid.

• Bowel movements: I think bowel movements should be the fifth vital sign after temperature, blood pressure, pulse, and breathing rate. Sixty per cent of the weight of your stool is gut microbes. Recent research indicates that the form of your stool provides information about what's happening with your gut microbiota. If you believe that the gut microbiome is relevant at all to your health (which I suspect you do since you're reading this book), then we should be closely monitoring our best (and least expensive) window into the health of these microbes. Our digestion thrives on rhythm. When we are in rhythm, it's amazing how so many issues will just disappear. When our bowel movements are out of rhythm, we should expect our digestion to be out of sorts as well. The best way to understand the information encoded in your stool is to look at the typical forms and shapes of stool using the Bristol Stool Scale. The scale varies from type 1 to type 7, with type 1 being constipation and type 7 being diarrhoea.

Ideally, we want to settle into a glorious, doves-flying-in-slow-motion-and-angels-trumpeting type 4 bowel movement.

To help facilitate our Sherlock Holmes food intolerance investigation, you'll need to create a proper food diary. If you grab yourself a bound notebook, you can set up each page like I have here. Or, if you like, you can come to my website (www.theplantfed-gut.com/cookbook) and register to receive my *Fibre Fuelled Cookbook* resources and I'll send you a printable version that you can put into a binder.

Let me break down the value of a good food diary before we move on. This isn't just about finding foods you are sensitive to. This is about understanding your relationship with food. We need to get to the genesis of your symptoms if we really want to heal. But this goes beyond a biochemical misfire in digestion. We have a

Date

Sleep

Hours: Quality:

Exercise

Bowel Movements

Time: Type: Symptoms:

Meal 1

Time/ Location/Mood	Foods	Symptoms/ Reactions

Plant Points

Meal 2

Time/ Location/Mood	Foods	Symptoms/ Reactions

Plant Points

relationship with our food that is dynamic and ever evolving. The better that we understand that relationship, the better we will be able to fully comprehend our food intolerances, recognize our limits, and know exactly how to nourish our body. A food diary organizes and describes that relationship. It is a powerful tool that should not be overlooked or underestimated.

W: Work It Back In

Inductive reason and observation allow us to understand potential food intolerances, and now we need to bring clarity to our relationship with these foods. The way we do this is using the Restrict—Observe—Work It Back In method. By having an intentional pattern of include—exclude—include again, we can create shifts in our diet that allow us to isolate the effect of the food on our symptoms. This means you may not feel so hot at baseline when you eat a food, but there's a noticeable improvement when the food is restricted, and then there's a noticeable return of symptoms when you work it back in.

Let me warn you about a banana peel on the floor because I don't want you to slip on it. When we Work It Back In, we're not just here to identify *what* foods we are sensitive to. That's beginner information. We want to be *Fibre Fuelled*, so we need the full knowledge. Knowledge is power! We need to make sure that we learn *how much* we can tolerate.

Food intolerances aren't yes or no propositions, like food allergies. The *how much* of food intolerance is the critical question. As I've explained, there is a threshold at which any food will initiate symptoms for all of us. If I eat 3 kilos of kale, I'm pretty sure I'm not going to be feeling so great. Our goal here is to understand where that threshold lies for the foods that we are intolerant of.

If we stay below our threshold, then we can enjoy those foods in appropriate moderation without triggering the symptoms. Make no mistake, that threshold may be really, really low. That's okay! As long as we know that it's really, really low, then we can adjust your intake accordingly.

T: Train Your Gut

If you're sitting there wondering, "Why take my chances with a food that I can barely tolerate?" I want you to know that this isn't the EXCLUDE strategy. This is the GROWTH strategy. You are not locked into perpetual suffering and a limited diet. Instead, you have a gut that's adaptable and, when properly challenged, it will rise to the occasion, grow stronger, and overcome your current limitations. You absolutely can restore function and not just eat but get back to enjoying the foods you've been missing. In Chapter 7, I'll teach you how to train your gut like you would any muscle.

H: Holistic Healing

Your gut is not simply a machine for digesting food that works in isolation. It is a part of the greater whole that ultimately is uniquely "you" and includes your personality, mood, body, and the different organ systems. It's all interconnected. When we talk about healing your gut, we have to look beyond the gut microbes or the dietary choices and zoom out to take a look at this amazing human being that you are and how certain aspects of your life—both past and present—may be affecting your digestive function. The last step of the GROWTH strategy is to focus on healing the whole person in the interest of rising the tide on human health and simultaneously lifting up your gut health. We will do this in Chapter 8.

Y'all ready to get started? Okay, let's do this thing! In the next chapter, I'll discuss the Big Three of Food Sensitivity and then share the two protocols—FODMAP and histamine intolerance—for you to apply the Restrict—Observe—Work It Back In technique when you feel ready.

>> *To view the 13 scientific references cited in this chapter, please visit theplantfedgut.com/cookbook.*

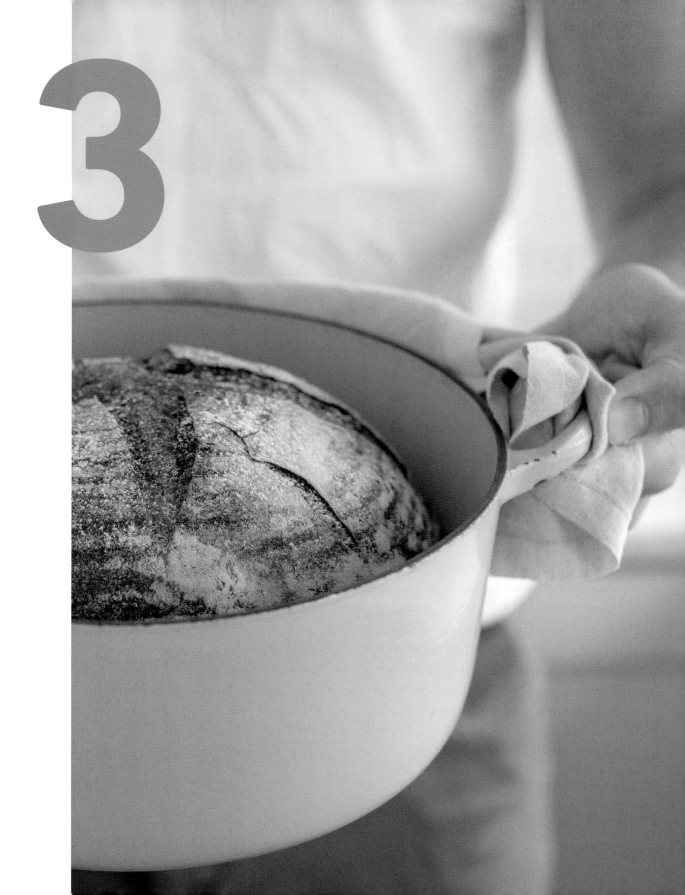

3

Ruling Out the Big Three of Food Sensitivity

Let's find the root cause of your symptoms

Let's take a brief time out from the GROWTH strategy and the march towards testing it out through delicious food, which we will be doing shortly. Before we go there, I want to focus on what I consider to be the Big Three of Food Sensitivity—constipation, coeliac disease, and gallbladder dysfunction. If you suspect you have one of the Big Three, your treatment needs to address that issue first. Even though IBS is the most common cause of food sensitivity, I consider these the Big Three because they are frequent causes of food intolerances, they're highly treatable, and once you treat them, you'll find that your food intolerances will improve dramatically. The last thing that I want is for you to be facing headwinds and struggling to correct your food intolerances if there's an identifiable root cause that can be swiftly remedied and will dramatically improve your digestive capacity. So with that in mind, let's dig into the Big Three and some of the other causes of food intolerance that I'd like you to be conscious of.

Constipation

The number one cause of wind, bloating, and food sensitivities in my clinic is constipation. It's incredible how many people have constipation as the genesis of their problem and don't even realize they're constipated. If you poo every day or even several times a day with diarrhoea, you might be tempted to skip this section—but believe it or not, you could still be constipated! Constipation isn't defined by the frequency of bowel movements. Instead, it's the manifestation of symptoms or digestive disruption caused by inadequate evacuation of stool.

Inadequate evacuation of stool comes in many forms. Some people don't poo for an entire week. Others go more often, potentially every day, but struggle to get it out. They strain to have a small little turd or weird shapes, have multiple small bowel movements, go once and then have to go again thirty minutes later, or feel like they didn't get it all out. These are the many faces of constipation. This is how you could poo every day and still be constipated.

Then there's what we call "overflow diarrhoea" or loose, watery stool several times per day. If you experience this, you or your healthcare practitioner may assume you have diarrhoea and that you need to slow down your motility with anti-diarrhoeal medicine, which only makes things worse. That's because the problem isn't diarrhoea, it's constipation manifesting as diarrhoea. How is this possible? Basically, there's a solid column of stool inside the colon that's stuck and not moving. For lack of a better expression, you have a logjam. So the solid stuff backs up, but the liquid stuff is able to sneak through the cracks and crevices and descend down to the bottom, where it explodes out as diarrhoea. Anti-diarrhoeals exacerbate the problem. The paradoxical solution to overflow diarrhoea is to make that person poo, which I usually do with a quick little bowel flush.

Virtually 100 per cent of patients with constipation have gas and bloating. It's the most common manifestation of inadequate evacuation. But there are a number of other symptoms that are quite common with constipation: abdominal pain virtually anywhere in the abdomen, nausea or queasiness, getting full quickly after a meal, loss of appetite or food aversion, even acid reflux. There's often fatigue and sometimes brain fog. Many of my patients will show me a photo of themselves at 7:00 a.m. with a flat stomach, and then a second photo at 10:00 a.m. showing a protuberant, pregnancy-like belly. That's almost always constipation behind that.

To know whether you have constipation, the best test is to get imaging. You can do either an abdominal X-ray or a CT scan. In either case, it helps if you ask the radiologist specifically to answer whether there is constipation. The problem is that the radiologist reads dozens of studies per day; hasn't heard your story, let alone met you; and tends to not focus on the poo. As a result, radiology studies are often read as "normal," but closer inspection reveals constipation that correlates with and explains the symptoms. It's for this reason that I review all imaging studies myself, so that I can connect what I'm seeing with my own eyes to the story that my patient is describing for me.

Nearly everyone with constipation will also experience food sensitivities. These sensitivities are typically pretty non-specific, meaning that they are sensitive to many different foods and also there doesn't seem to be a reproducible pattern to the symptoms. The problem in this case is the constipation and generally not the food itself.

These food sensitivities will improve, and many times completely disappear, when the constipation is adequately treated.

The solution is to establish rhythm. Your body thrives on rhythm. When we are constipated, we are out of rhythm, out of balance. We need to get things moving once more and get into that flow state where bowel movements are effortless, complete, and, frankly, enjoyable. I am being totally serious—having a good, healthy bowel movement absolutely should be one of the highlights of your day! You should look forward to it, and feel satisfied afterwards. If you don't, we have work to do.

I don't recommend making dietary changes while you're constipated, because constipation amplifies and fuels food sensitivities. If you start adding more plants to your diet, you'll often feel gassy and bloated and have worsening abdominal pain. Instead, focus first on restoring rhythm. Once you are in a rhythm, having good regular and complete evacuations, you will feel SO much better and also be in the best position to start adding back foods without food sensitivity standing in the way.

In order to restore rhythm, you must first understand that there are two main contributors to constipation. First is motility. People with slow motility struggle to adequately empty their bowels. This often manifests with a hard, lumpy, bumpy stool that has cracks and crevices in it, or comes out like a golf ball. The solution here is to help move things along, which we can often accomplish through natural means:

- Drink at least 6 (ideally 8) glasses of water per day. Your poo is a log. We need to float that log down the river. Don't let it get dried up on the rocks.

- Ramp up your physical activity. When you move, your colon moves to expel both poo and wind. That's what we're trying to accomplish, right?

- Slowly increase your fibre intake. Increased fibre intake can often help get the bowels moving. Consider introducing prunes, oats, ground flax, or chia seeds and slowly increasing over time.

- Consider a fibre supplement. I'm a big believer and have had tremendous success with them in my clinic. Some of the options include wheat dextrin, acacia powder, psyllium husk, partially hydrolyzed guar gum, and glucomannan. Always start low and go slow. If you feel like it's making things worse, back off.

- Add magnesium before bedtime. Magnesium is great for sleep, anxiety, headaches, and also constipation. Generally you want to opt for magnesium oxide, magnesium citrate, or magnesium sulfate. The dosing depends on the formulation, and your magnesium level should be checked before starting and once you reach a steady dose.

Is There Such a Thing as Too Much Fibre?

People often ask me if there's such a thing as too much fibre. Of course there is. Literally anything can be consumed to excess and become problematic. While we should all strive to increase our fibre consumption and enjoy the health benefits that follow, sometimes the time isn't right or it can be more than you can handle at that moment. Constipation can be one of those moments. Many people start pouring fibre in when they're constipated, and they feel worse. The reason this happens is that if you remain constipated, then the fibre just sits there and gets fermented to produce even more wind. Believe it or not, methane gas slows motility. We end up in a vicious cycle where constipation causes wind, leading to more constipation. The solution is to focus on restoring a healthy rhythm before you ramp up your fibre intake. You break the cycle if you get the bowels moving. Fibre is fantastic for keeping the bowels moving when they're already moving, but fibre can cause trouble for some if their gut is in gridlock. Get the bowels moving first, then eat more fibre to keep them moving.

As recently as a few years ago, we only really thought of constipation in terms of motility. Unfortunately, we were missing something very important. Motility is important, but it's impossible to poo if you can't relax your butt muscles. I don't mean the glutes/booty/bum. I'm referring to your anal canal and four additional muscles that comprise the pelvic floor. They're there to prevent incontinence, and thankfully, they usually work pretty well. That barrier is designed to keep our underwear fresh until we're hovering over a commode and consciously choose to initiate a sequence of synchronized pelvic muscle relaxations that clear a path for a microbial torpedo to launch. Unfortunately, many of us take for granted that when we want to poo, these pelvic muscles will behave the way we're asking them to. That's not the reality for many of my patients and perhaps some of you.

There's a condition called pelvic dyssynergia where the muscles fail to relax when they're supposed to, and in some cases, they actually contract. This results in a scenario where the only way to poo is to strain and push, often to have a small little nugget slip out. Or, people experience weird poo shapes or feel like they can never completely empty. Another symptom is going once, then returning to the loo forty-five minutes later to go again. All of these point to pelvic dyssynergia.

For many, treatment requires working with a pelvic therapist, which is effectively a physical therapist who specializes in pelvic floor issues—both bowel and urinary. However, one thing you can try first is to simply orient your pelvic muscles in a proper position on the toilet. Here's how you do it:

- sit with your knees higher than your hips (use a footstool or other flat, stable object if necessary)
- lean forward and put your elbows on your knees
- relax and bulge out your stomach
- straighten your spine.

In some cases, constipation does not respond to first-line interventions. Further testing with anorectal manometry and efecography are warranted at this point. It's important to work with a qualified health practitioner from the beginning to make sure that your plan is properly fitted to your needs.

Coeliac Disease

Coeliac disease is an inflammatory, immune-mediated condition in which the immune system becomes activated when you consume gluten. In nature, gluten is a protein found in wheat, barley, and rye. But in the real world (where most people don't really eat wholegrains), gluten is, well, everywhere: most processed foods, deli meats, soy sauce, make-up, and many prescription drugs. Potatoes are inherently gluten-free, but if your restaurant serves up fries prepared in oil that's touched gluten, then they're contaminated.

Over the past few years, the relationship between gluten and coeliac disease has motivated an entire generation of fearmongering influencers, books, and products. Gluten isn't the food monster that they've made it out to be, and I will discuss that more fully in Chapter 4. But let me be totally clear—if you have coeliac disease, we need to know, because if so, then you need to be gluten-free for the rest of your life; no ifs, ands, or buts.

Coeliac disease can manifest in a number of different ways. Classically there's diarrhoea, bloating, wind, and abdominal pain after a meal, but it can also present with constipation. Weight loss happens with malabsorption. Iron deficiency anaemia can set in and cause fatigue. Outside the intestine, coeliac can present with arthritis, dental enamel defects, osteoporosis, elevated liver tests, neurological symptoms, and even infertility. Lastly, I've diagnosed coeliac disease in people who are completely free of symptoms but have a first-degree family member with coeliac disease. The most important thing is to consider coeliac disease as a possibility for the symptoms. Open your mind to whether it's possible. If it is a possibility, then you must be appropriately tested for it.

Coeliac disease is a genetically motivated condition, meaning that if you don't have the gene then you can't have the condition. So, one option is to have the genetic test performed. It's a non-invasive blood test, and if the test shows the gene to be absent, then you have proven to not have coeliac. If, however, the gene is present (which it is in about 1 in 3 Caucasians), then all that we have proven is that coeliac is possible. In fact, there's a 97 per cent chance that you don't have coeliac disease despite having the gene. But if you are genetically positive, additional testing is necessary to determine whether it's present.

Many healthcare practitioners will order a non-invasive antibody blood test called tissue transglutaminase to determine if coeliac disease is present. The traditional teaching through the years was that this is a good test and could help us rule out coeliac. Unfortunately, that has been proven untrue. Most cases of coeliac disease that I diagnose have a negative antibody test because the changes occurring in the intestine haven't yet matured to the point of actually activating the antibody. Make no mistake, though. These patients are suffering with just as many symptoms, and they improve in a powerful way after the coeliac is diagnosed and the gluten-free diet is implemented.

The gold standard test for coeliac disease is upper endoscopy with multiple biopsies of the small intestine. In order to do this properly, you have to consume gluten prior to the exam—one slice of gluten-containing bread per day for at least two weeks. The biopsies obtained during endoscopy will definitively answer the question of whether coeliac disease is causing your symptoms. Ultimately, that's the question we're trying to answer.

If You're Completely Convinced That You Have Coeliac Disease, Why Not Just Go Gluten-Free?

You may think you have coeliac disease and you'd rather change your diet and skip the testing. But why isn't this a good idea? I'll give you three reasons. First, whether you have coeliac disease may have implications for your family, since it is passed on genetically, and so it's good to have a complete family history. Second, it may have other implications for you. People with coeliac disease are at increased risk for thyroid disease (particularly Hashimoto's autoimmune thyroid), pancreatitis, and liver disease—among others. Third, having coeliac disease means you need to have a higher standard of gluten-free diet than others. You need to be hyper-rigorous. If you do not have coeliac, you can occasionally cheat and have that biscuit you've had your eye on. That's not an option with coeliac disease. You need to be strictly gluten-free if you have coeliac, and if you are not, then you increase your risk of heart disease and cancer.

Gallbladder Dysfunction

Most medical school textbooks say that people with gallbladder issues present with right upper quadrant abdominal pain that radiates to the back thirty to sixty minutes after a meal. Okay, take that textbook and throw it over your shoulder and let me bring you up to speed on the real deal with the gallbladder.

The gallbladder is a small little sac that sits under your liver in your right upper quadrant. Its job is to store liver juice called bile, which helps us to digest fat in our diet. When we eat a meal, particularly a high-fat meal, our gallbladder squeezes to release this digestive juice down a series of tubes, almost like a water slide, called the bile ducts. The bile splashes down into the small intestine, just after the stomach, where it mixes with food and goes to work.

Here's the issue: There are a million and one ways that the gallbladder can cause symptoms. The classic textbook example of right upper quadrant pain radiating to the back is maybe 20 per cent of them, which is why we're going beyond the medical textbook. The gallbladder can cause pain in the middle upper abdomen, right upper or right lower quadrant, or the back on the right side. I've even seen it cause chest pain, similar to acid reflux. Naturally, if you have chest pain, you need to make sure your heart is safe first. The gallbladder will not cause left-sided pain, whether front or back. So if the pain is on the left side, it ain't your gallbladder!

Dr. B's Advice

One of the key questions I ask when evaluating the gallbladder is whether the pain wakes them up from sleep. People can have the most rip-roaring, out-of-control irritable bowel syndrome—but it rests when they rest. The gallbladder doesn't rest. It doesn't care that it's three in the morning and you have a huge day tomorrow. Gallbladder pain can occur at any time, and nocturnal symptoms is a major clue I look for.

The gallbladder isn't just about pain, though. In fact, sometimes there's no pain at all. It can also cause chronic nausea, wind and bloating, and discomfort after meals. It's for this reason that I've got the gallbladder on my mind as a possibility for anyone suffering with food intolerances or who has upper GI issues.

My job is to determine whether the gallbladder is in fact the genesis of the issue. My approach involves three steps:

1. Gallbladder imaging such as ultrasound or CT scan to make sure there is no gallbladder inflammation (called cholecystitis) and no gallstones (cholelithiasis) that would explain the symptoms.

2. HIDA scan to assess gallbladder function. The gallbladder squeezes the juice out after a meal. With a HIDA scan, we can quantify how much of the juice the gallbladder squeezes out, and it should be more than 35 per cent. If it's less, it means that gallbladder motility is diminished, and this may be the cause of the symptoms. This is where I discover most gallbladder issues, so it's important to have both imaging and HIDA.

3. Make sure there's no other explanation for the symptoms.

There's one foolproof way to determine whether the gallbladder is the cause—to remove it. But the foolproof way feels awfully foolish if it proves to be an unnecessary gallbladder removal and the symptoms persist. Therefore, the best approach when it comes to making decisions on the gallbladder is a cautious one where you collect all of the available information before making a fully informed choice. Ultimately, getting good advice from a qualified health professional is important.

There's no silver bullet that will fix gallbladder problems, but evidence suggests that a wholefood, plant-centred diet rich in fibre, plant protein, and unsaturated fats reduces our likelihood of having gallbladder dysfunction. Coffee has also been found to be protective, which I personally celebrate. On the flip side, gallbladder disease is more common with increased intake of saturated fat and dietary cholesterol from red and processed meats and eggs or sugar and other ultra-processed grains.

Beyond the Big Three

The Big Three of Food Sensitivity are not actually the three most common causes of food sensitivity, but they are the three that I *always* make sure we rule out in a person with food sensitivity, because, if present, they can be quickly fixed and food sensitivity will improve dramatically when that is the case.

But there is so much more that is possible, so I want to go rapid fire and touch on a few of the other conditions that could be the genesis of your symptoms.

- **Acid-related issues:** Otherwise known as acid-peptic disorders among gastroenterologists, these can include ulcers in the stomach or small intestine, irritation of the stomach lining called gastritis, or gastro-oesophageal reflux disease. They occur when there is an imbalance between stomach acid secretion and the stomach lining's defence mechanisms. Upper endoscopy can diagnose some but not all cases, and at the end of the day, the test of choice is really to reduce stomach acid using high-dose medication for four to six weeks and then see if symptoms resolve.

- **Pancreatic insufficiency:** This means that the pancreas is not able to pump out enough digestive enzymes to allow you to properly digest your food. This can occur in people with damage to the pancreas (pancreatitis) or who have had part of their pancreas removed. But it can also occur naturally as we age or in conjunction with diabetes, coeliac disease, tobacco use, or in people who have had part of their stomach removed. It tends to be triggered by fat in the diet, because this is the macronutrient that our pancreas struggles to keep up with the most. Testing can be done to look for excess fat in the stool, a marker called faecal elastase, or a trial of pancreatic enzyme replacement.

  Dr. B's Advice
  The digestive enzymes that are available over the counter (OTC) are not the same as those produced by your pancreas. OTC enzymes are derived from plants and therefore

do not have the same biological function as your pancreatic enzymes. If you have pan-creatic insufficiency, you'll need a prescription pancreatic replacement therapy.

- **Inflammatory bowel disease (IBD):** This includes Crohn's disease and ulcerative colitis. They are immune-mediated inflammatory conditions where the immune system goes on the attack, and as a result the intestine becomes inflamed. Ulcerative colitis is, by definition, limited to the colon. Crohn's disease, on the other hand, can manifest anywhere from the lips to the bottom, but is most common in the colon and the last part of the small intestine, called the terminal ileum. Both conditions can also manifest symptoms outside the gut like mouth ulcers, joint or back pain, rashes, liver or eye issues, and blood clots. A colonoscopy will rule out ulcerative colitis and identify most cases of Crohn's disease. Persistence and a complete evaluation are sometimes needed to find Crohn's, so if it is possible, further testing may be required.

  Dr. B's Advice
  If you have a colonoscopy for chronic diarrhoea, make absolutely sure that your doctor takes biopsies for something called microscopic colitis. The colon will appear normal, but the biopsies will reveal the condition. It's generally not hard to treat, but you need to know that it's there before you can fix it.

- **Bile acid malabsorption (BAM!):** Bile is released from the liver to help us absorb fat, but in the case of BAM, an excess of bile acids actually irritates the lining of the intestine and causes diarrhoea. It's often found in people who have had their gallbladder removed, had surgery on the last part of their small intestine (called the terminal ileum), or who have Crohn's disease. It's easily treated with a bile salt binding agent.

- **Irritable bowel syndrome (IBS):** I left perhaps the most common cause of food intolerances for last. Why not put it in the Big Three of Food Sensitivity? The reason is that my GROWTH strategy is really about treating the person with food intolerances due to IBS or another disorder of digestive function. The Big Three are the conditions that I want to make sure are not present, because if they are, then you need to correct them first and get them out of the way. But if they're not, you may ultimately land on a diagnosis of irritable bowel syndrome. It presents with abdominal pain and a change in bowel habits. Symptoms improve when you have a bowel movement. There's no test to prove that you have IBS, so it's generally diagnosed if you have the pattern of symptoms and you've ruled out everything else.

Doc, What's Your Take on SIBO?

Small intestine bacterial overgrowth, or SIBO, is the hottest of health topics on the internet. Yet, you haven't seen me say much about it, for good reason. The reason is that the science isn't clear. Does SIBO exist? Yes. Do we have reliable tests for SIBO? Absolutely not.

Non-invasive breath tests are generally used to diagnose SIBO, both in the clinic and for research purposes. But there's a problem: The breath tests are highly imperfect, fraught with an unacceptably high rate of false positives *and* false negatives. The gold standard test is to take a sterile culture from the small intestine during an endoscopy. Unfortunately, this is a flawed test, too. Bacterial overgrowth may be patchy, confined to other parts of the intestine that are not being sampled during the test, leading to false negative results.

In a recent study published in *Nature Communications*, they showed that our "gold standard" test generally does not correlate with patient symptoms and often reflects dietary preferences. A high-fibre diet caused false positive results when using small bowel culture! But on the flip side, microbiome analysis using 16S rRNA technology revealed that many patients with symptoms had dysbiosis and a loss of diversity in their small intestine. What this means is that we have a testing problem when even our gold standard test isn't accurate.

If you can't properly test, how can you know who to treat? And how can we trust research studies that rely on severely flawed tests? I do expect that better tests will be available for both research and clinical purposes in the future, but we're not there now. For what it's worth, my approach to those with a positive SIBO test or who believe they have SIBO is to first evaluate for other causes of their symptoms. Most of the time, I find an alternative explanation, and I will treat that. If not, I usually start with a dietary approach aimed at healing their dysbiosis. In fact, in the *Nature Communications* study, they found that two major risk factors for small bowel dysbiosis were reducing fibre intake and also recent treatment with antibiotics. In a pilot study, they showed that reducing fibre intake and increasing sugar intake made intestinal dysbiosis worse and elicited symptoms. Conventional therapy for SIBO often involves reducing fibre intake and taking an antibiotic on a recurrent basis. There are also the herbal antimicrobial protocols, which people often perceive to be different because they're not a pharmaceutical, only they are doing the same thing as an antibiotic but without the studies to support efficacy or define risks. This worries me, as the relapse rate using our current treatments is extremely high. These treatments have the potential for long-term collateral harm to the gut microbiome and may contribute to the increasing rates of antibiotic resistance. As you can see, I have my concerns that we don't adequately understand this condition, and until we have better studies and better testing, I will continue to treat my patients as if they have dysbiosis and use the techniques described in this book to help them heal.

What If All My Tests Are Negative?

I routinely have patients who are tired of being sick and incredibly frustrated to the point that they just want to be diagnosed with something, anything. I totally understand where they are coming from, but you're always better off knowing that you don't have colon cancer or Crohn's disease. What I want you to know is that there's something causing your symptoms and every single test moves us closer to figuring it out. A normal test may not identify the specific cause by itself, but it often allows you to cross multiple different possibilities off the list. You are narrowing it down and bringing the truth into focus.

Also, bear in mind that many of the most frequent causes of food sensitivity do not have a test to prove that they exist—irritable bowel syndrome, a damaged gut microbiome, a disordered relationship with food. There is no blood or stool test to tell you that these are the cause of your food sensitivity. They are diagnosed by ruling out alternative possibilities and by having a commensurate medical history.

But here's the good news: The GROWTH strategy is designed specifically for people with these conditions. So the key here is to work with a qualified health professional who can help guide you to make sure that you properly understand the genesis of your symptoms. If you're looking for added support and to be empowered with the knowledge to understand this on a deeper level, join me in The Plant Fed Gut Masterclass.

Once we have properly identified the genesis of our problems and created a plan to address them, we're now ready to move to the next phase in our GROWTH strategy—to identify our specific food intolerances using the Restrict—Observe—Work It Back In approach.

>> *To view the 49 scientific references cited in this chapter, please visit www.theplantfedgut.com/cookbook.*

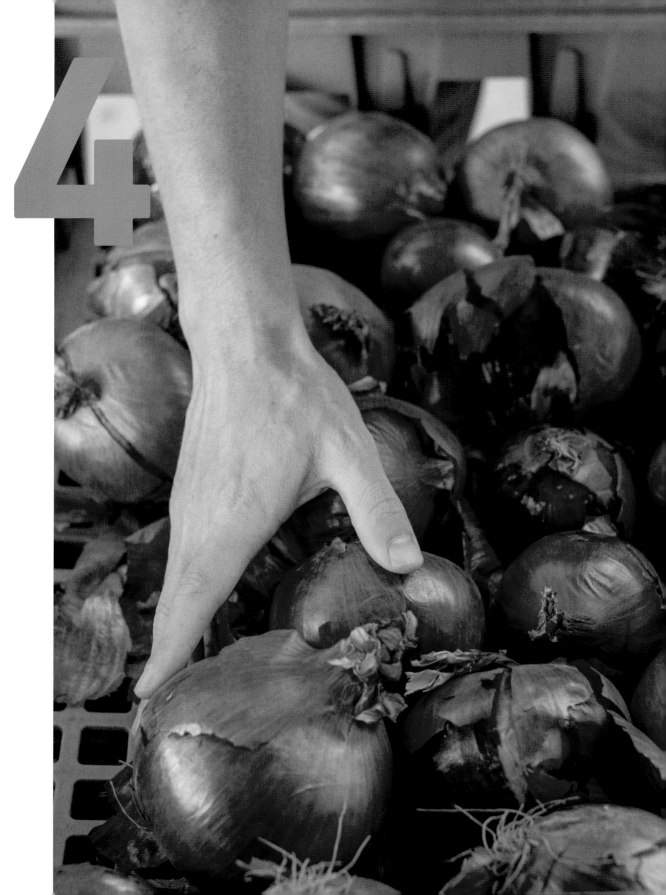

FODMAPs Can Be Our Friends!

The recipes and strategy you need to master and enjoy FODMAPs

I've discovered in my work as a gastroenterologist that there are two primary groups of food intolerances: FODMAPs and histamine. We'll tackle FODMAPs in this chapter and histamine in Chapter 5.

You may have heard of FODMAPs before, especially if you've ever sought help for digestive symptoms. The two most common foods that get called out when someone has a sensitive gut are dairy (lactose) and gluten. They both fall under the umbrella of FODMAPs, and we'll be taking them and more on in a moment. FODMAP is an acronym that stands for fermentable oligosaccharides, disaccharides, monosaccharides, and polyols. Really, what we're talking about are simple sugars, sugar alcohols, or short chains of sugars (two to ten of them) that are linked together. We group them together because they behave similarly in the intestine.

FODMAPs are generally not well absorbed, so they pull water into the intestine. This is how they can cause diarrhoea. They are also fermentable by our gut microbes, which results in the production of wind—methane, carbon dioxide, and hydrogen. As we learned in Chapter 3, methane actually slows gut motility, promoting constipation. So FODMAPs can cause the intestine to become distended from a combination of solids, liquids, and gases. Distention triggers pain, the sensation of bloating, and the pregnancy-like belly (even in a guy). And it causes a tug-of-war—the increased water in our bowels causes diarrhoea, while methane gas slams on the motility brakes to cause constipation. Who will win out? Only time will tell, but the one thing you can be sure of is that it's a sloppy mess in there.

It's no wonder that elimination of FODMAPs has been associated with improvement of digestive symptoms. Developed by a research team at Monash University in Melbourne, Australia, the low FODMAP diet has been shown to improve irritable bowel syndrome symptoms in randomized controlled trials. Specifically, abdominal pain, bloating, and overall symptoms improve.

It may seem like the obvious thing to do to end your miserable digestive symptoms would be to avoid FODMAPs forever, but we're going to use the GROWTH method to Restrict, Observe, and Work It Back In rather than just eliminate them. Let me show you why.

There are five FODMAPs. They are:

O—Oligosaccharides Three to ten sugars bound together	· **Fructans:** Combinations of fructose chained together that require gut microbes to be digested. You'll find fructans in garlic, onions, wheat, asparagus, artichokes. Food additives FOS and inulin are also fructans. · **Galactans (or GOS):** Combinations of galactose chained together that require gut microbes to be digested. You'll find them predominantly in legumes—peas, lentils, and beans.
D—Disaccharides Two sugars bound together	· **Lactose:** Naturally occurs in milk and most dairy products. It requires lactase, a digestive enzyme in the small intestine, for absorption. Unabsorbed lactose may be processed by the colonic microbiota.
M—Monosaccarides One sugar	· **Fructose:** It is found in most fruits, some vegetables, and honey. Mangoes are unique because they have fructose and no other FODMAPs. Fructose has also been bastardized to artificially produce high-fructose corn syrup.
P—Polyols Sugar alcohols with names that typically end with "-ol."	· **Polyols:** Mannitol, sorbitol, xylitol, and erythritol are naturally occurring polyols that you'll find in various vegetables, fruits, mushrooms, and some fermented foods. And then there are all of the artificial sweeteners: lactitol, maltitol, and isomalt. About one-third of polyols are absorbed in the small intestine, and the rest come into contact with our gut microbes.

Notice anything about the table? A theme perhaps? Four of the five FODMAPs are plant-based *Fibre Fuelled* foods. That means they contain fibre, which we already know is good for our gut microbes. But these foods have even more goodness for our gut microbes—fructans, galactans, and polyols. Surprise! The FODMAPs, which have been vilified, are actually prebiotic. According to the prebiotic concept, these carbohydrates that escape digestion in the small intestine can have health benefits through their effects on the gut microbes. They increase the representation of healthy microbes like *Bifidobacteriaceae* and *Lactobacillaceae*, and can be metabolized in a series of steps to create short-chain fatty acids. Fibre isn't the only prebiotic. Now you know that FODMAPs are, too.

If this prebiotic theory of FODMAPs is true, then we should see differential effects between a low and high FODMAP diet. Well, that's exactly what we see. *Bifidobacteria* are healthy microbes known to help produce short-chain fatty acids, they suppress unhealthy microbes, and they optimize our immune system. You'll also find low levels of *Bifidobacteria* in people suffering with abdominal pain. By contrast, *Bilophila wadsworthia* is an unhealthy microbe that thrives with the consumption of saturated fat in animal-based diets. It promotes inflammation, intestinal barrier dysfunction, and bile acid dysmetabolism, and as a result has been associated with inflammatory bowel disease, colorectal cancer, fatty liver, and diabetes. So ideally we'd like to have more *Bifidobacteria* and less *Bilophila wadsworthia*, right? Well a low FODMAP diet has been associated with *less Bifidobacteria*, and *more Bilophila wadsworthia*. Eek! Yet the high FODMAP diet delivered our desired effect—more *Bifidobacteria*, less *Bilophila wadsworthia*. I told you FODMAPs can be your friends.

Should I Consume Lactose for Its Prebiotic Effects?

No, you should not. Literally the first thing I will do when addressing a person with food sensitivities, bloating, flatulence, or diarrhoea is to eliminate dairy products and artificial sweeteners. These are the two most common dietary culprits that should be dropped. As for the prebiotic benefits of lactose, it's important to understand that it's a conditional prebiotic, meaning that lactose is only prebiotic if it escapes digestion in the small intestine. For many, this means they receive no prebiotic benefits from the lactose in their diet. There is some evidence that dairy may be beneficial for the gut microbiota, but the authors of a recent systematic review acknowledge that the effect is likely negligible and that we are currently lacking adequate quality studies to draw clear conclusions. And … the study was sponsored by the dairy industry. It is all too common that dairy studies are being funded by the industry that stands to profit from a positive result if they can find/create one. Unfortunately, the evidence that industry-funded research is problematic is stronger than the evidence to support the consumption of dairy. In a recent review of the health effects of dairy in the highly respected *New England Journal of Medicine*, dairy consumption was tied to increased risk of bone fractures, prostate cancer, endometrial cancer, asthma, eczema, and food allergies, not to mention that it contributes to greenhouse gas production and climate change, water use and pollution, and antibiotic resistance. Got milk? Not me.

So yes, the FODMAPs in our diet are food for our gut microbes. But nutrition isn't exclusively about feeding the gut microbiota in the interest of human health. Obviously, there are aspects of our nutrition that are more complicated than that or that do not involve the gut microbiota. This is why we look at outcomes research. Quite simply, I want to know what happens when you eat an apple or beans. Or what happens when you substitute wholegrain wheat for refined wheat.

Every plant, including the high FODMAP ones, has a story about how it can benefit your health that goes beyond the individual components. It gets even better when you combine multiple different plants, otherwise known as a diversity of plants, and get the benefits from all of them. Let's look at how a few high FODMAP foods have been shown to be beneficial to your health.

Fructose	Mangoes	Daily mango consumption was more effective at relieving chronic constipation than a supplement containing a similar amount of soluble fibre.
Fructose	Apples	Over 10 weeks, consuming 3 apples daily led to weight loss, while eating 3 oat biscuits with the same fibre content and calorie count did not.
Polyols (Sorbitol)	Avocado	Adding avocado to either salad or salsa can increase the absorption of health-promoting antioxidants dramatically (2.6- to 15-fold).
Polyols (Mannitol)	Watermelon	Eating fresh watermelon daily for 4 weeks led to lower hunger, lower body weight, lower systolic blood pressure, and higher antioxidant levels in the blood when compared to eating low-fat biscuits with the same number of calories.
Galactans	Pinto beans	Compared to placebo, pinto bean consumption significantly reduced triglyceride and LDL cholesterol levels.
Galactans	Kidney beans, black beans, and pinto beans	Blood glucose levels were significantly lower in people with diabetes when eating a meal including beans and rice rather than rice alone, even though the number of carbohydrates was the same.
Fructans	Garlic	A systematic review and meta-analysis of randomized, placebo-controlled trials showed that garlic significantly reduces both systolic and diastolic blood pressure.
Fructans	Wheat	Using wholegrain wheat instead of refined wheat altered the gut microbiome and led to reduced measures of inflammation.

Dr. B, Is Gluten Triggering My Symptoms?

Many of you have probably tried a gluten-free diet or at least heard that a gluten-free diet can improve your digestive symptoms. The rumours are true, but it may not have anything to do with the gluten. Quick refresher: Gluten is a protein found in wheat, barley, and rye. It has developed a bad reputation because in people who have coeliac disease, it activates their immune system to tear into their intestine and wreak havoc throughout the body. In Chapter 3, we defined coeliac disease as one of the Big Three of Food Sensitivity that you absolutely need to take off the table. So it's my expectation that you will determine whether you have coeliac disease, and if you do, you need to go gluten-free for the rest of your life, no exceptions. A wheat allergy, which is different from coeliac disease, is also grounds to permanently eliminate wheat.

But is gluten the source of problems in non-coeliac wheat sensitivity? The evidence would suggest it's not. In a double-blind, placebo-controlled trial of people with non-coeliac wheat sensitivity, there was no evidence that gluten worsened symptoms. In fact, people actually had *fewer* overall symptoms, bloating, and flatulence but *BETTER* stool consistency on a high-gluten diet compared to low-gluten or placebo. There was also no evidence of increased intestinal inflammation with low- or high-gluten diets when compared to placebo. Notably, people in the study did feel better on a low FODMAP diet, though. And in one of my favourite studies of all time, another double-blind, placebo-controlled trial of people with non-coeliac wheat sensitivity, a concealed gluten-containing breakfast actually caused *FEWER* symptoms than a placebo. Read that again. What did trigger symptoms? The fructans did. Wheat, barley, and rye contain gluten, but they also contain fructans. If you have a non-coeliac wheat sensitivity that improves on a gluten-free diet, the evidence would suggest it's the elimination of fructans that's making you feel better.

This is more than "Dr. B's theory that FODMAPs are important." Evidence continues to emerge indicating that it is absolutely necessary to reintroduce the FODMAP foods that you temporarily eliminate for optimal digestive health. In a recent year-long study, they found that by reintroducing FODMAP foods after a brief period of restriction, they were able to substantially improve digestive symptoms while simultaneously maintaining high levels of the gut-healing *Bifidobacteria*. Reintroduction allows you to support your gut microbes while reducing your symptoms.

But you need to personalize your diet to make this work. FODMAPs are good foods for our gut microbes, but if you consume more of them than your digestive system can handle, they can wreak havoc. This isn't the first time we've heard that too much of a good thing can be bad for us. You need oxygen and water to live, right? But if you breathe pure oxygen for too long, you can get oxygen toxicity. If you drink too much water, you get water intoxication. With all good things in life, there's an ideal amount and there are boundaries that define inadequacy or excess. In biology we call that a tolerance range, but in the real world we call it the sweet spot. How do we find the sweet spot, where we reap the benefits without crossing the trip wire to get the negatives? You use the GROWTH strategy. That's what we're here for, and now we're going to use it to find our sweet spot with FODMAPs.

Implementing the GROWTH Strategy to Identify Your FODMAP Sensitivity Thresholds

Step 1—Restrict

You need to reduce your FODMAP intake for a minimum of two weeks. You should see an improvement in your symptoms if you have a FODMAP intolerance. Our goal is to establish a baseline where you're feeling good before we move towards working anything back in. If you feel like you're making progress but not yet ready to reintroduce, it's okay to extend the temporary restriction for a week or two. This is a very restrictive diet, however, so I don't want you to go beyond four weeks in this phase.

You're probably wondering what you're going to eat. Good news! We're making it easy for you. All of the recipes that you'll find in this chapter are low in FODMAPs. So, you have the freedom to use these recipes, in any pattern and in any order, during this restriction phase. Also, if you have a copy of my first book, *Fibre Fuelled*, you will find that all of the recipes in Week 1 of the Fibre Fuelled 4 Weeks are low FODMAP and therefore also in play during this time.

Step 2—Observe

Throughout the restriction period, you want to document how you feel using your food sensitivity journal we discussed in Chapter 3. Start recording for a week before initiating the low FODMAP diet. Make sure to document improvement in your symptoms during the restriction phase, and as we start to work the foods back in, it will be imperative to keep tabs on what food causes you to experience symptoms and in what amounts.

Step 3—Work It Back In

Once your symptoms are stable, you're going to systematically work each FODMAP back into your diet, one by one, in escalating doses to identify your food intolerance thresholds. You may be surprised to find that you can tolerate several of them. We will use the method taught by Monash University to test individual foods, which should give us a good idea of which FODMAPs you are sensitive to and in what amount. Bear in mind that throughout this period you will continue to be on a low FODMAP diet.

You'll begin eating each FODMAP again over three days. You only need to test one food for each category. Using the suggested serving sizes, you will move from a small portion to a full portion of the food consumed at one meal. You may have symptoms during this time. Some wind and bloating is to be expected, even in those with a healthy gut. But if the symptoms are severe, then you should

10 FODMAP Challenges

Adapted from Tuck and Barrett, Journal of Gastroenterology and Hepatology *(2017) and* Re-challenging and Reintroducing FODMAPs *by Lee Martin, MSc RD*

FODMAP	Food	Day 1	Day 2	Day 3
Galactans	Almonds	15 nuts	20 nuts	25 nuts
	Canned chickpeas (rinsed)	2 tablespoons	4 tablespoons	6 tablespoons
	Green peas	2 tablespoons	4 tablespoons	6 tablespoons
Fructans—grains	Wheat pasta	100 g	200 g	300 g
	Bread (wheat/white)	1 slice	2 slices	3 slices
Fructans—garlic	Garlic	¼ clove	½ clove	1 clove
Fructans—onions	Onion (any)	1 ring	¼ onion	½ onion
Fructans—vegetables	Cabbage (savoy)	35 g	70 g	105 g
	Okra	8 pods	12 pods	16 pods
Fructans—fruits	Pomegranate	½ small	1 small	2 small
	Raisins	1 tablespoon	2 tablespoons	4 tablespoons
Fructose	Asparagus	1 spear	2 spears	4 spears
	Honey	1 teaspoon	2 teaspoons	1 tablespoon
	Mango	¼ mango	½ mango	1 mango
Polyols—mannitol	Cauliflower	2 small florets	4 small florets	8 small florets
	Celery	¼ large stick	½ large stick	1 large stick
	Sweet potato	165 g	130 g	195 g
Polyols—sorbitol	Apricot	½ small	1 small	2 small
	Avocado	¼ small	½ small	¾ medium
	Blackberries	2-3 berries	5 berries	10 berries
Lactose (optional)	Cow's milk	60 ml	120 ml	240 ml
	Soured cream	2 tablespoons	60 ml	120 ml
	Yoghurt (plain)	70 ml	160 ml	240 ml

stop reintroducing this particular FODMAP group and document the amount that triggered your intolerance in your food journal.

In Chapter 7, we will learn about training your gut. If you're not able to tolerate something now, it doesn't mean that you're locked in to be this way in perpetuity. But for the time being, at least you know where the weakness in your gut exists and you can work towards restoring function to your gut in the future.

After you are done testing one FODMAP category, you can repeat this entire process to test another FODMAP category. You need to wait until you are symptom-free again before starting a new test. That means a minimum of one day in between. During this time, you continue to remain on the low FODMAP diet.

There's quite a bit of work to do here, isn't there? We have ten total FODMAP categories, including five fructans and two polyols. In case you're wondering, it's because fructans and polyols are broad categories of FODMAPs with many different varieties, so we're testing the different varieties here to be more specific in our understanding. Nonetheless, I want to take a quick TIME OUT to acknowledge that testing ten different FODMAP categories is a heavy lift. It definitely can feel a bit overwhelming. I hear you and see you out there! It's time we had a pep talk.

You may have been bruised or beaten down by your food. You may feel desperate for solutions. Correcting multifaceted health issues is like trying to untie a complex knot. You don't want to do it because you know it's not going to be easy. It requires patience and persistence. But if you make the investment and stick to the method that works, you will eventually get it unravelled.

This is a process, and it is admittedly time-consuming and involved. But it is also the best approach out there for identifying food sensitivities. Every single step in this process provides you with new information, and it's information that's trustworthy. Track it in your food journal. It moves you closer to your goal. It feels good to know that you can trust what you are doing here. That if you do it, it won't fail you.

I want to be very direct and say this to you—following the process that I lay out in this book is not meant to cause you stress. I totally see where it could. Growth/GROWTH is never easy. We only grow when we face challenges. It's a process that requires effort, persistence, and resilience. Admittedly, it's not easy; we do it because victory exists on the other side. But we need to be explicitly aware that stress can enter into what we're doing here, and it's not welcome at this plant party! We need to have a plan for stress management to not allow it to happen.

Please go at your own pace. Take a break if you need to. Maybe you do it in chunks, with just a few at a time and then step away from it for a little while. If you find a FODMAP that you're able to tolerate, feel free to reintroduce it. Provided your symptoms are stable, you are free to keep moving forwards with testing. Don't hesitate to ask for the assistance of a registered qualified dietitian to help guide your journey. I strongly recommend it! And for additional support, check out the Monash

Uni Low FODMAP Diet App, which has specific FODMAP amounts in common foods, and *Rechallenging and Reintroducing FODMAPs* by Lee Martin, MSc RD.

Don't forget, you are a part of the Fibre Family. There are literally hundreds of thousands of us in our online community on Instagram (@theguthealthmd), on Facebook (@theguthealthmd), on my email list, and in my online courses. We are all here to support one another because at the end of the day, we all share one common goal—to heal and optimize our guts. We become so powerful when we are all pulling the rope in the same direction—TOGETHER. One team. United.

What About Doing a Breath Test Instead?

Perhaps you've heard that they have breath testing available for several food intolerances—lactose, fructose, or sorbitol. Unfortunately, the breath tests for fructose and sorbitol do not correlate with symptoms and therefore are potentially misleading. It's best to use our low FODMAP GROWTH strategy for fructose and sorbitol to reliably determine whether they cause symptoms. The lactose breath test performs well enough to be considered, but bear in mind that false positives and false negatives are still possible, and ultimately it is your symptomatic response to lactose exposure that determines the presence or absence of lactose intolerance.

In the pages that follow, you will find a collection of low FODMAP recipes. They are here to be enjoyed by anyone, whether you are doing a low FODMAP protocol as a part of your GROWTH strategy or not. This is inclusive nutrition! Sprinkled in with the recipes is a healthy dose of Pro Tips to enhance your culinary experience. We also have some ingredients listed that you can add or substitute when you're ready to break free from the low FODMAP diet. Our goal with FODMAPs is to understand the strengths and weaknesses of your gut. With that knowledge in hand, we will be ready to apply it to training your gut in Chapter 7, restoring function, strengthening it, and getting to a place where what once was your enemy has become your new friend!

Low FODMAP Breakfasts

Cocoa 'Nana Smoothie Bowl

The Trinity Overnight Oats

Vanilla Berry Overnight Oats

Ancient Grain Porridge with Berries

Veggie Scramble and Sourdough Toast

Crunchy Maple Peanut Granola

Simple Sourdough Sammy and Chia Jam

Low FODMAP Salads, Soups & Sandwiches

Creamy Aubergine Sandwich

Roasted Aubergine Dip

Edamame Kale Salad

Lemon Lentil Salad

Ginger Broccoli Pasta Salad

Great Greek Grain Salad

Homemade Tofu Feta

Low FODMAP Biome Stock

Weeknight Minestrone Soup

Healing Miso Soup

Cheesy Broccoli and Potato Soup

Low FODMAP Hearty Mains

Coconut Curry Bowl

Edamame Pesto Pasta (with quinoa pasta/ gluten-free pasta)

Zippy Coriander Bowl

SP&L Burger Patties

Quinoa Fried Rice

Sweet and Spicy Peanut Tempeh Wraps

Chickpea Glow Bowl

"I Can't Believe This Is FODMAP Friendly" Pasta Sauce

Rosemary Smashed Potatoes

Tempeh Stir-Fry with Saffron Rice

Crispy Tempeh Rice Bowls with Steamed Greens

Aubergine Hummus Buddha Bowl

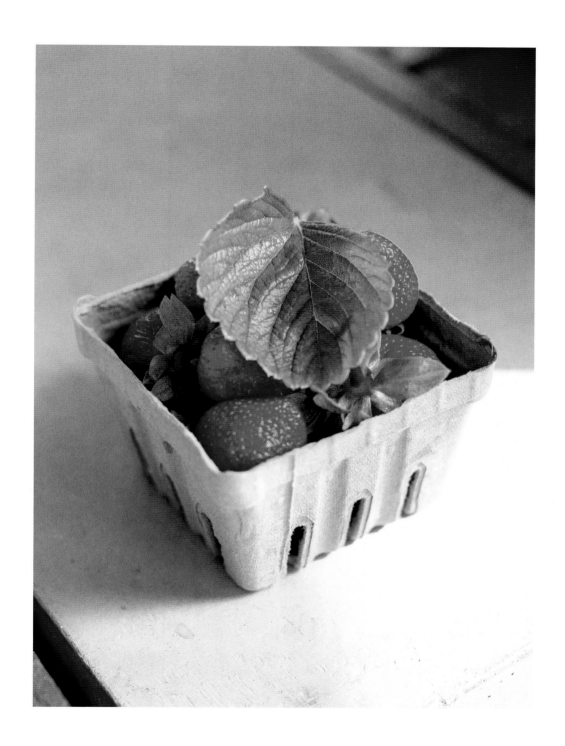

COCOA 'NANA SMOOTHIE BOWL

4+ Plant Points

Makes 2 smoothie bowls

In case you haven't noticed, I'm obsessed with smoothie bowls. It's all about the toppings for me: Simply pour the smoothie into your bowl and create your artwork on top. I like to sprinkle toppings in a pattern like slices of a pie. It's fun, delicious, and shares well on Instagram. Tag me if you do it.

FODMAP note: A third of a ripe banana is low FODMAP. One whole unripe banana is low FODMAP per serving. A third of a date per serving is considered low FODMAP.

240 ml almond milk

⅔ frozen banana

2 tablespoons cocoa powder

2 tablespoons peanut butter

½ teaspoon ground cinnamon

¼ teaspoon vanilla extract

1 tablespoon hemp seeds

½ of 1 date

4 or 5 large ice cubes

Supercharge it! (optional toppings):

17 g shredded coconut

30 g pumpkin seeds

2 tablespoons chia seeds

28 g Crunchy Maple Peanut Granola (page 69)

Peanut butter drizzle

Place the almond milk, banana, cocoa powder, peanut butter, cinnamon, vanilla, hemp seeds, date, and ice cubes in the base of a blender and purée until creamy and smooth. Add the toppings of your choice.

PRO TIP:

Freezing your banana is the key to creating a thick, ice cream–like consistency. If you keep your banana at room temperature, then your smoothie ends up much thinner. Alternatively, you could use 360 ml to 480 ml almond milk to thin the smoothie.

FF UNLEASHED:

If you are not following a low FODMAP approach, increase the bananas and dates for added sweetness.

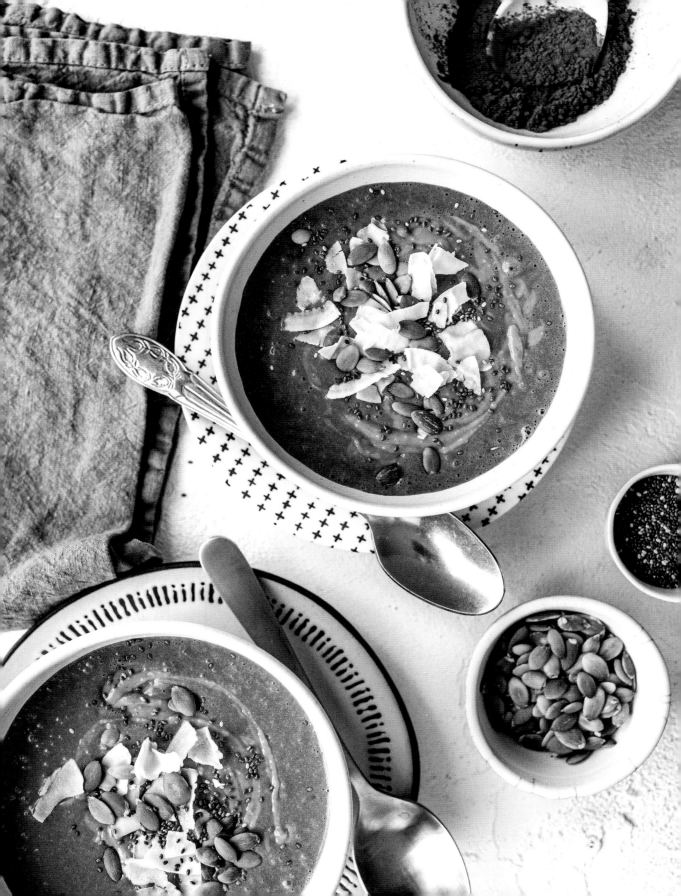

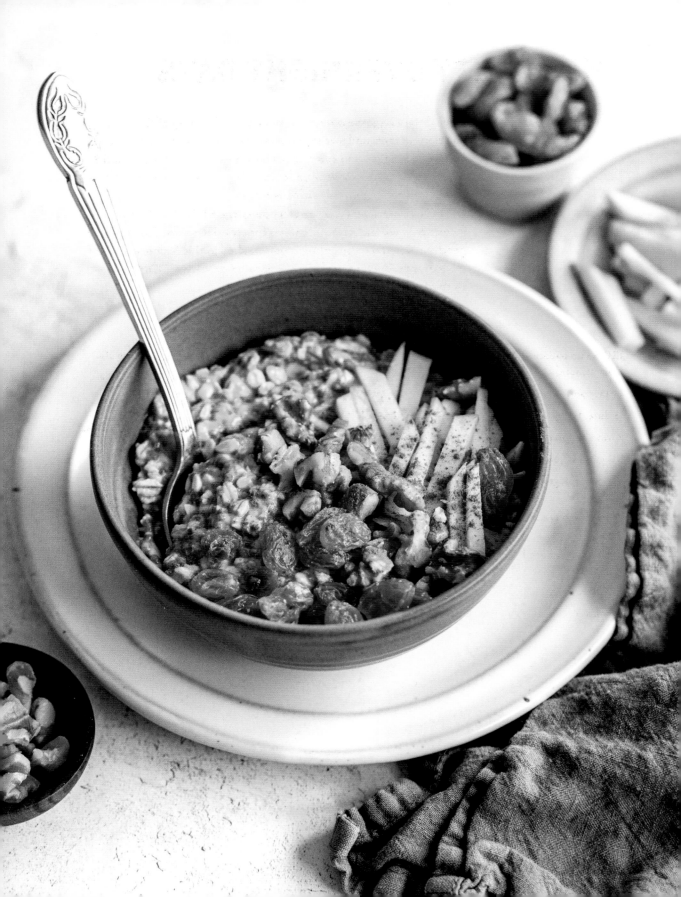

THE TRINITY OVERNIGHT OATS

4+ Plant Points

Serves 1

Chef Emeril Lagasse always spoke of the holy trinity of Cajun cuisine as celery, onions, and sweet peppers. Well, my holy trinity of spices is turmeric, ginger, and cinnamon. I have been loving this combo in my morning coffee for years, and now it's part of this overnight oats recipe. You can't go wrong with spices!

FODMAP note: As a banana ripens, the FODMAP content increases while the resistant starch content decreases. That said, we need the banana to be soft and get mashed in this recipe. A third of a banana per serving is generally tolerated on a low FODMAP diet. A third of a date is FODMAP friendly.

120 ml unsweetened plain almond milk

1 teaspoon chia seeds

⅓ date, finely chopped

⅓ ripe banana, mashed

50 g jumbo oats

½ teaspoon ground turmeric

½ teaspoon ground ginger

¼ teaspoon ground cinnamon

Pinch nutmeg

Pinch salt

Supercharge it! (optional toppings):

1 tablespoon golden raisins

1 teaspoon chopped Granny Smith apple

2 tablespoons roughly chopped walnuts

Dash ground cinnamon

1. In a jar or small bowl with a lid, add the almond milk, chia seeds, date, and banana. Stir with a spoon to combine.

2. Add the oats, turmeric, ginger, cinnamon, nutmeg, and salt and stir to combine. Cover with the lid and place in the fridge overnight, or until the oats have thickened (about 6 hours).

3. In the morning, open the jar/bowl and top as desired with suggested toppings. If the oat mixture is too thick, you can add a little more almond milk to your preference.

FF UNLEASHED:

If you are not following a low FODMAP approach, you can use 1 teaspoon maple syrup instead of the date or 1 whole date per serving.

VANILLA BERRY OVERNIGHT OATS

3+ Plant Points

Serves 2

Overnight oats are the product of slow cooking, much like fermentation. Rather than transforming our food with a burst of flames, we instead apply a heavy dose of self-restraint by walking away and nothing more. When we return, we discover that nature has rewarded our patience with a bowl of magical goodness.

1 small or medium ripe banana

100 g jumbo oats

3 tablespoons chia seeds

360 ml unsweetened almond milk

½ teaspoon vanilla extract

Toppings: sliced ripe banana, 10 medium strawberries, 45 g blueberries, 30 raspberries, or 1 blackberry, hemp seeds, chia seeds, coconut flakes, chopped pitted dates, Cacao Drizzle Topping (see below)

1. Slice the banana and place in a bowl or a wide-mouth kilner jar. Using a fork or the back of a spoon, gently mash together until a smooth paste forms. Add in the rest of the ingredients, mix well, and let sit for 15 minutes.

2. Remix well, then put it in the refrigerator overnight, or for at least 8 hours.

3. Enjoy as is, or garnish with toppings of choice.

CACAO DRIZZLE TOPPING:
Blend together 1 to 2 tablespoons maple syrup, 2 tablespoons cacao or cocoa powder, and enough warm water until just smooth.

FF UNLEASHED:
If you are not following a low FODMAP diet, you can use unlimited fruit for topping, and sub 4 pitted dates for maple syrup and use 7 tablespoons warm water to create the Cacao Drizzle.

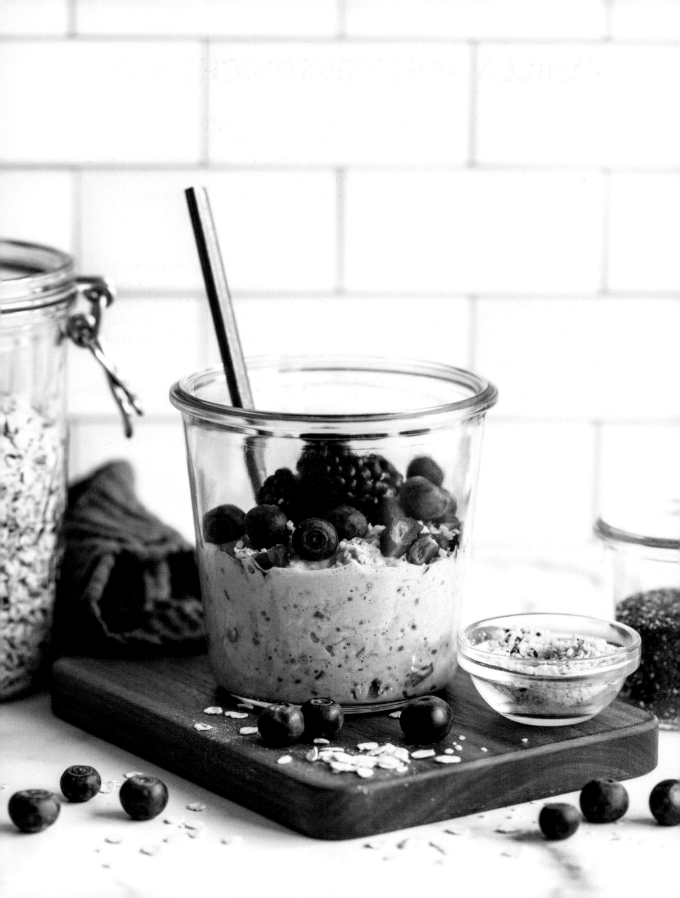

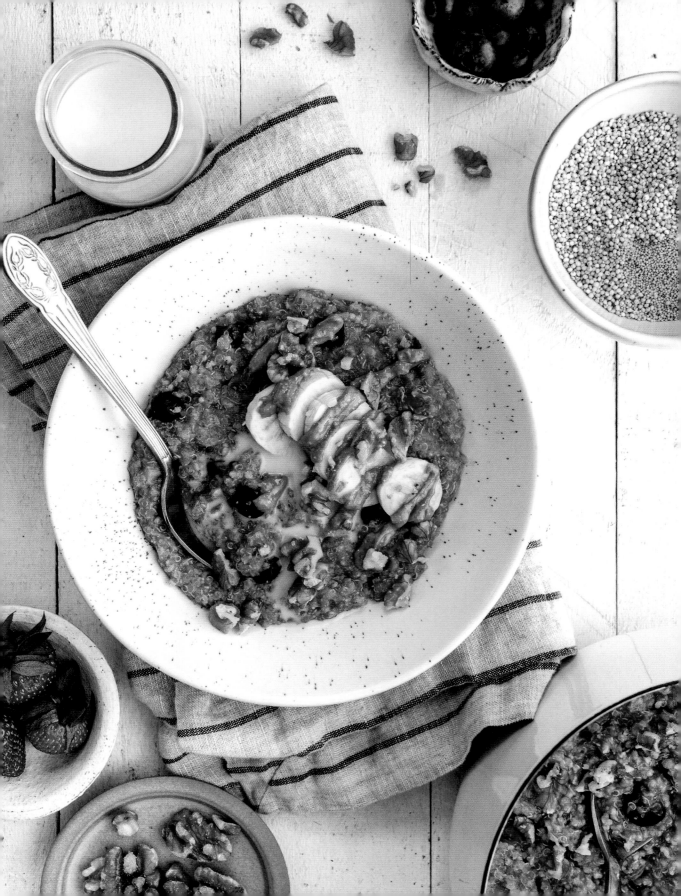

ANCIENT GRAIN PORRIDGE
with Berries

3+ Plant Points

Makes 4 servings

Millet, quinoa, and amaranth are all gluten-free and are considered ancient grains. This means that they have their origins in early society and are largely unchanged over the last several hundred years. They are also an excellent source of dietary magnesium, which is involved in more than six hundred chemical reactions in the body and contributes to mood, sleep, metabolism, and healthy bowel movements. Note that it's best to soak the millet, quinoa, and amaranth overnight before making this porridge.

FODMAP note: Low FODMAP servings of berries include 10 medium strawberries, 45 g blueberries, 30 raspberries, or 1 blackberry.

85 g rinsed millet

90 g rinsed quinoa

50 g rinsed amaranth

240 ml almond milk

¼ teaspoon salt

1 teaspoon ground cinnamon

¼ teaspoon vanilla extract

190 to 380 g berries of choice (see FODMAP note)

2 teaspoons tahini (optional)

Supercharge it! (optional toppings):

Sliced banana (⅓ banana per serving)

Peanut butter

Chopped walnuts or pecans

1. The night before serving, place 1 litre of water in a medium pan and bring to the boil. Add the millet, quinoa, and amaranth and stir to combine. Cover with a tight-fitting lid and turn off the heat. Allow the grains to sit overnight.

2. In the morning, mix in the almond milk, salt, cinnamon, vanilla, and berries. Over medium-high heat, bring the mixture to the boil. Cover the pan with a tight-fitting lid and reduce the heat to low, allowing the mixture to simmer for about 10 minutes, or until thickened.

3. For extra-creamy porridge, stir in the tahini right before serving. Add supercharged toppings, if desired.

FF UNLEASHED:

If you are not following a low FODMAP approach, add berries liberally.

VEGGIE SCRAMBLE AND SOURDOUGH TOAST

5+ Plant Points

Serves 4

You're going to love the spice blend here, and there's a little kitchen chemistry happening behind the scenes. Turmeric has dominant earthy notes. Adding cumin warms up the earthiness while paprika brings toasted, smoky, and sweet notes. Add black pepper to taste at the end to bring out the pungency of the turmeric.

2 tablespoons nutritional yeast

1 teaspoon ground turmeric

½ teaspoon smoked paprika

2 teaspoons Dijon mustard

1 teaspoon dried or fresh chives

¼ teaspoon ground cumin

¼ teaspoon cayenne pepper (optional)

½ teaspoon salt or black salt (see Pro Tip)

60 ml unsweetened soy milk

2 teaspoons olive oil or stock

50 g thinly sliced spring onions (green parts only)

175 g chopped courgette

60 g baby spinach

450 g extra-firm tofu, drained and pressed (see Pro Tip on page 84)

Freshly ground black pepper (optional)

4 to 8 slices sourdough bread, toasted

1. In a small bowl, mix together the yeast, turmeric, paprika, mustard, chives, cumin, cayenne, and salt. Add in the soy milk to create a thin sauce. Add 1 tablespoon water, as needed, to thin.

2. Heat the olive oil in a large frying pan over medium heat. Add the chopped spring onions and courgettes and cook until softened, about 5 minutes. Add the baby spinach, then cover with a tight-fitting lid to steam for 1 to 2 minutes.

3. Crumble the tofu with your hands or a fork into small pieces. Move the vegetables to one side of the pan and add the tofu. Cook the tofu for 2 minutes, then add the sauce to the tofu and the vegetables. Stir to combine and cook for about 5 minutes or until the tofu is slightly golden brown. Season to taste, adding in more salt/pepper as desired.

4. Serve immediately with the sourdough toast.

FF UNLEASHED:

If you are not following a low FODMAP approach, you can use 1 teaspoon of garlic powder instead of the chives.

PRO TIP:

Black salt, or kala namak, will give an eggy taste to the scramble. It can be found online or in speciality food shops.

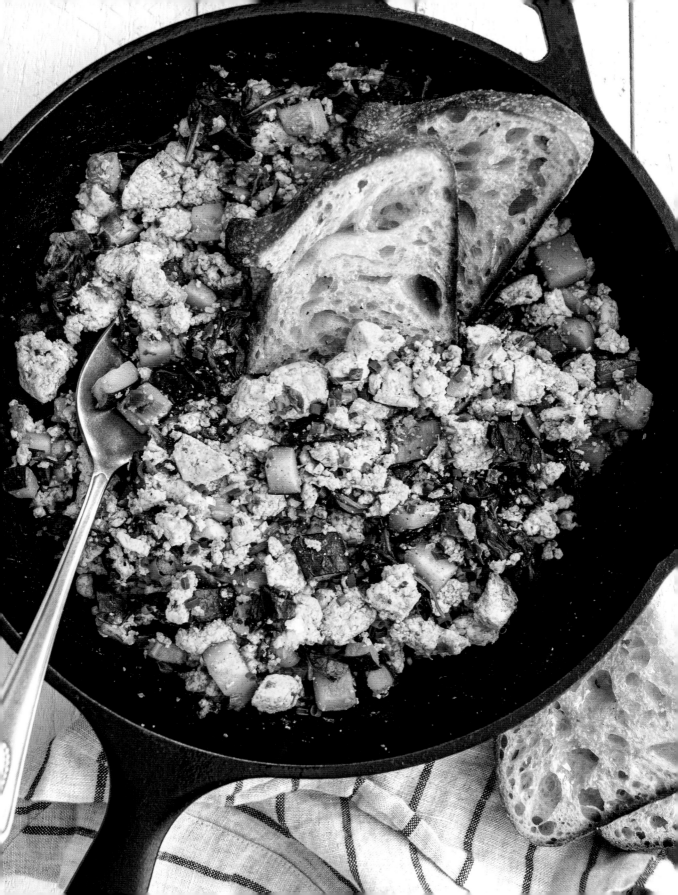

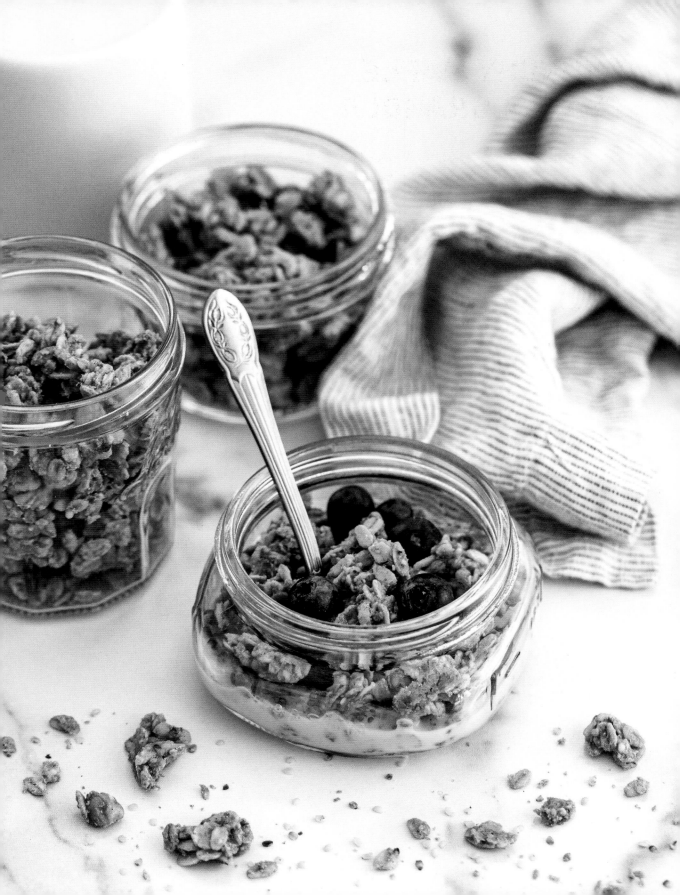

CRUNCHY MAPLE PEANUT GRANOLA

4 Plant Points

Makes 4 or more servings

Whether it's a smoothie bowl topping, breakfast on the go, or a little munch-and-crunch snack, it's always nice to have some delish granola around.

175 g jumbo oats

40 g walnuts, chopped

2 tablespoons hemp seeds

1 teaspoon ground cinnamon

¼ teaspoon salt

2 tablespoons avocado oil

60 g peanut butter

60 ml 100% maple syrup

1 teaspoon vanilla extract

1. Preheat the oven to 175°C. Line a rimmed baking tray with parchment paper or a silicone baking mat.

2. In a large bowl, mix together the oats, walnuts, hemp seeds, cinnamon, and salt.

3. In a small saucepan, melt the avocado oil and peanut butter until combined. Remove from the heat and add the maple syrup and vanilla.

4. Pour the wet mixture over the oats mixture and stir until completely combined.

5. Spread the granola mixture onto the prepared baking tray in a single even layer.

6. Bake for about 12 minutes, press the granola down, then bake for another 7 minutes, or until golden brown.

7. Allow the granola to cool on the baking tray completely (about 45 minutes) before breaking into clusters.

SIMPLE SOURDOUGH SAMMY AND CHIA JAM

CHIA JAM

2 Plant Points

Makes 240 ml

It's a smart move to sneak in chia seeds wherever possible, like this recipe. They're a great source of plant-based omega-3 healthy fats and fibre. They also have this mystical property of transforming from a seed into a gelatine when wet. Abracadabra!

300 g frozen strawberries	1 tablespoon freshly squeezed orange juice
2 tablespoons chia seeds	

1. Allow the frozen berries to thaw on the worktop for at least 2 hours.

2. Place the strawberries, chia seeds, and orange juice in the bowl of a food processor or blender and blend until combined.

3. Place the jam in a sealable storage container; it will be runny at this point. Allow it to set in the fridge for at least 30 minutes to thicken.

4. Store in the fridge for up to 2 weeks.

SIMPLE SOURDOUGH SAMMY

5 Plant Points

Makes 1 sandwich

This recipe is rich in omega-3 healthy fats, protein, and fibre. Not too shabby for quick and easy. For those wondering, edible hemp seeds and marijuana come from different varieties of *Cannabis sativa*, with the main difference being the THC content. Hemp seeds won't get you high, but they will get you healthy! They have the same amount of protein by weight as beef or lamb plus added fibre to satisfy your hunger, making them great for those with the munchies.

2 slices wholegrain sourdough	2 tablespoons peanut butter
2 tablespoons Chia Jam	1 teaspoon hemp seeds

1. Toast the slices of bread to your preference.

2. Spread one slice of bread with the chia jam and the other slice of bread with the peanut butter.

3. Sprinkle the toast with the hemp seeds.

4. Enjoy with the two slices of toast smashed together to make a sammy, or leave separate and enjoy as an open-faced sandwich.

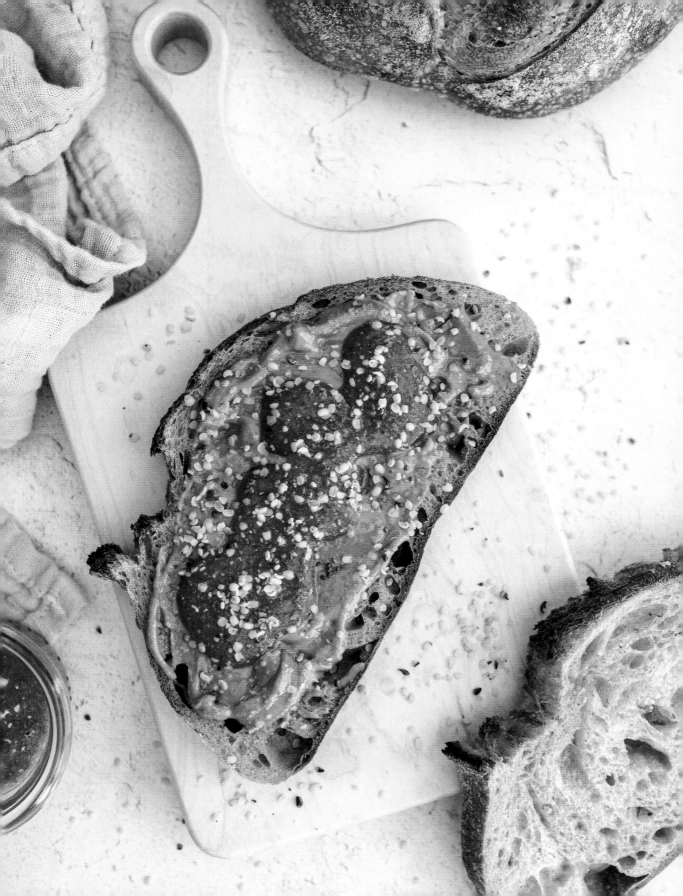

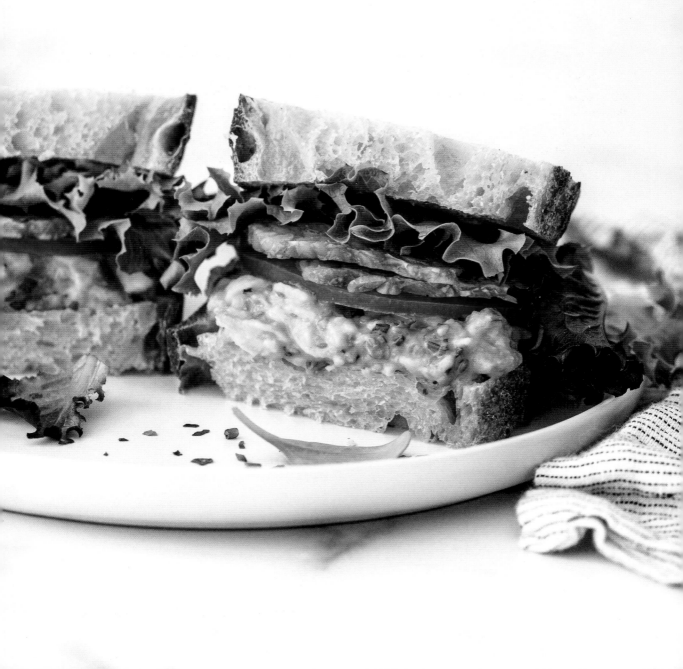

CREAMY AUBERGINE SANDWICH

8 Plant Points

Makes 1 sandwich

Just because you're eliminating sliced cold meats doesn't mean you have to skip out on delicious sandwiches. A ripe tomato is a little firm, a little soft, but not too much of either. Look for tomatoes that are ripe throughout and (given the choice) avoid the ones that look underripe near the stem end.

2 slices sourdough

2 teaspoons olive oil

60 g tempeh, cut into flat, thin strips

2 tablespoons Roasted Aubergine Dip (page 74)

2 slices fresh tomato

1 handful salad greens

Pinch salt

1. Toast the sourdough until lightly browned.

2. While the sourdough is toasting, heat a small frying pan over medium heat. Add the olive oil to the pan, then add the tempeh to the pan and cook for 2 minutes on each side, or until golden brown.

3. Build your sandwich by spreading the aubergine dip on each slice of bread. Then top one slice of bread with the tomatoes, salad greens, seared tempeh, a pinch of salt, and the second slice of bread.

ROASTED AUBERGINE DIP

4 Plant Points

Makes about
6 servings

An ideal aubergine is firm with tight, shiny skin. Fresher aubergines will feel heavier. When you press the aubergine with your finger, it should temporarily indent and then bounce back into shape. This dip will make more than you need; enjoy leftovers with raw vegetables for snacking, on sourdough toast, in the Creamy Aubergine Sandwich (page 73), or in the Aubergine Hummus Buddha Bowl (page 120).

1.1 kg aubergine

60 g tahini

1 to 2 tablespoons freshly squeezed lemon juice

¾ teaspoon salt

1 tablespoon garlic-infused olive oil (optional; see Pro Tip, page 87)

¼ teaspoon ground cumin

2 tablespoons chopped fresh flat-leaf parsley

Freshly ground black pepper

1. Preheat the oven to 230°C. Cut a slit into the aubergines and place on a baking tray lined with parchment paper or a silicone baking mat.

2. Roast the aubergines for about 60 minutes, turning halfway, until soft to the touch and noticeably very tender. Remove the aubergines from the oven and let cool to the touch.

3. Peel and discard the skin from the aubergines. Remove and discard the stems. Place the aubergine flesh in a large bowl. If the aubergine has a lot of moisture on it, gently shake it to remove as much liquid as possible so your dip isn't runny. Add the tahini and lemon juice and mash the flesh with a fork or potato masher. For a smoother dip, you can use a food processor. For a richer, creamier dip, drizzle in the garlic-infused olive oil as you finish mashing the aubergine.

4. Stir in the cumin and parsley, then place in a large bowl. Season to taste, adding more salt, pepper, or lemon juice as needed.

FF UNLEASHED:

If you are not following a low FODMAP approach, add 1 crushed garlic clove.

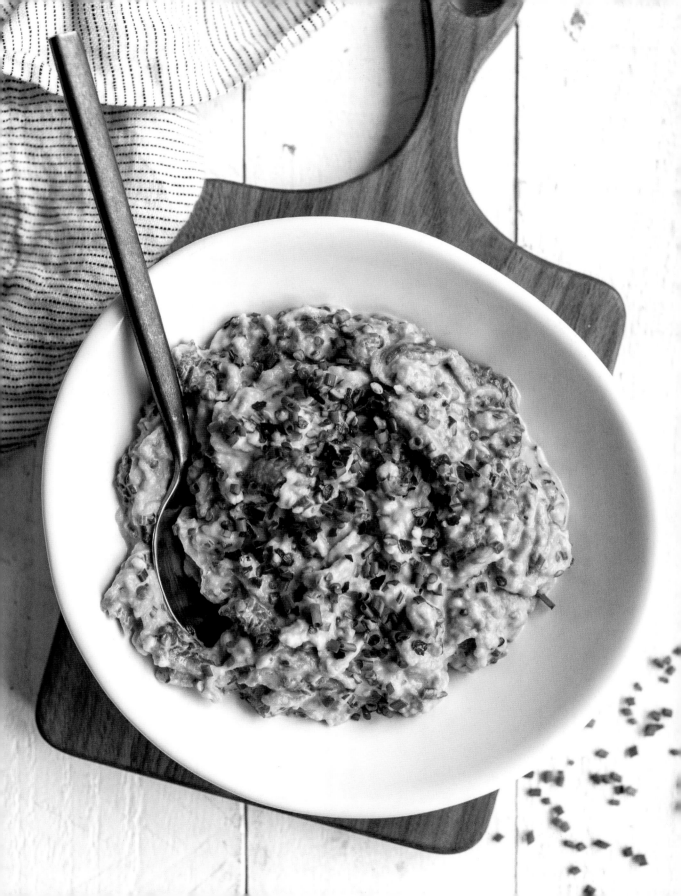

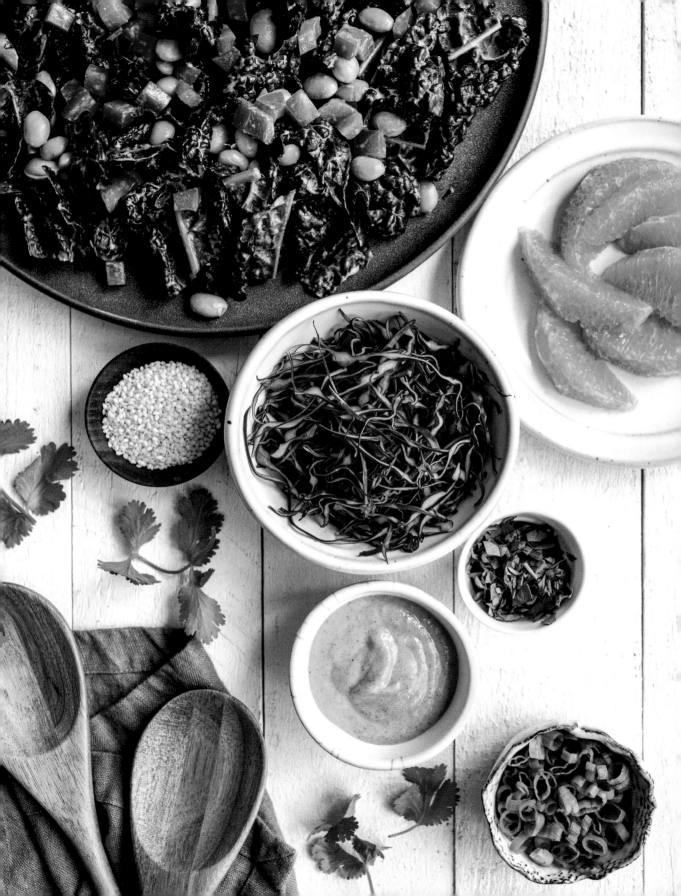

EDAMAME KALE SALAD

6+ Plant Points

Serves 2 as a main,
4 as a side

Call me weird if you must, but I think massaging your food makes you feel more connected to it and then you enjoy the flavours more. While you get your hands involved, consider that the word "edamame" means "beans on a branch." Edamame contains isoflavone phytochemicals associated with lower rates of breast cancer, prostate cancer, and osteoporosis and can improve perimenopausal symptoms. Best food massage ever!

3 tablespoons creamy almond butter

1 tablespoon low-sodium soy sauce or tamari

2 teaspoons finely grated fresh ginger

1 medium orange, peel removed

¼ teaspoon crushed red pepper flakes

420 g chopped kale leaves, stems removed

150 g shelled edamame

1 medium sweet red pepper, seeded and diced

Supercharge it! (optional toppings):

Orange segments, membranes removed

25 g thinly sliced spring onions, green parts only

2 tablespoons sesame seeds

70 g finely shredded red cabbage

10 g finely chopped fresh coriander leaves

Turmeric Tofu from Coconut Curry Bowl (page 93)

1. Place the almond butter, soy sauce, ginger, orange, red pepper flakes, and 1 to 2 tablespoons water in the base of a small food processor or blender and purée until creamy and smooth (see Pro Tip). Set aside.

2. Place the kale in a large bowl along with 2 tablespoons of the dressing. Using your hands, massage the dressing into the kale for 1 to 2 minutes, until the kale is slightly wilted and the dressing is well incorporated.

3. Add in the edamame and sweet red pepper, then toss together again. Divide among bowls and top with the remaining dressing and toppings of your choice.

PRO TIP:

You can substitute 3 to 4 tablespoons freshly squeezed orange juice in place of the orange and whisk together until very smooth and creamy.

LEMON LENTIL SALAD

8 Plant Points

Serves 4

I can't decide if this is a summer salad or an autumn/winter salad. The sweet potatoes and carrots feel like cooler-weather foods, but then the courgette, yellow squash, and lemon are such classic summertime favourites. I guess it's just versatile for all seasons. What do you think?

FODMAP note: 175 g diced courgette is a low FODMAP–friendly serving.

260 g diced sweet potatoes

2 medium carrots, diced

1 small courgette, diced

1 small yellow squash, diced

¼ teaspoon smoked paprika

½ teaspoon ground cumin

¼ teaspoon salt

¼ teaspoon freshly ground black pepper

Olive oil (optional)

1 teaspoon Dijon mustard

2 tablespoons freshly squeezed lemon juice

2 tablespoons tahini

10 g finely chopped fresh flat-leaf parsley

300 g canned lentils, drained and rinsed

1. Preheat the oven to 200°C. Place the sweet potatoes, carrots, courgette, and squash in a large bowl and add the paprika, cumin, salt, and pepper. Drizzle in olive oil, if using, then toss well to cover the mixture with the spices. Place in a single layer on a large baking tray and bake for 25 to 30 minutes, until golden brown and tender.

2. While the vegetables are cooking, whisk together the mustard, lemon juice, tahini, and 2 tablespoons water until creamy and smooth. Add in the parsley along with salt and pepper to taste.

3. Mix together the canned lentils and cooked vegetables with the dressing and serve.

PRO TIP:

Want to roast your veggies oil-free? Let's do it! Simply steam the starchy vegetables (that is, the sweet potatoes and carrots) until just tender. Combine them with your raw non-starchy veggies (that is, the courgette and squash) in a large bowl and add enough moisture to help the spices adhere. Now add the spices (Step 1 above), mix, and set aside for 10 to 20 minutes before roasting to allow the spices to absorb moisture. Boom! Delish.

FF UNLEASHED:

If you are not following a low FODMAP approach, add more courgette and add 1 crushed garlic clove to the dressing.

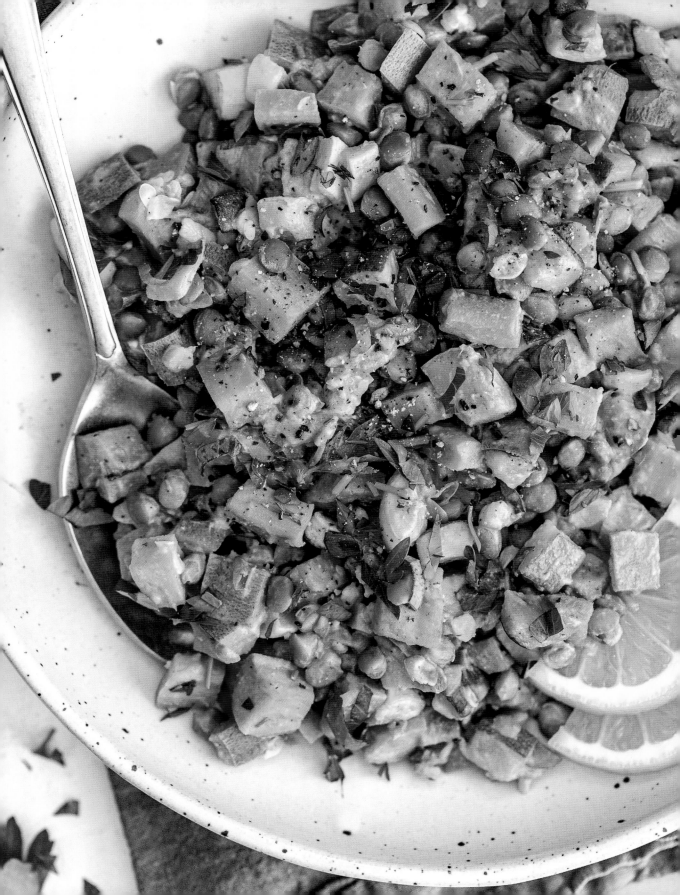

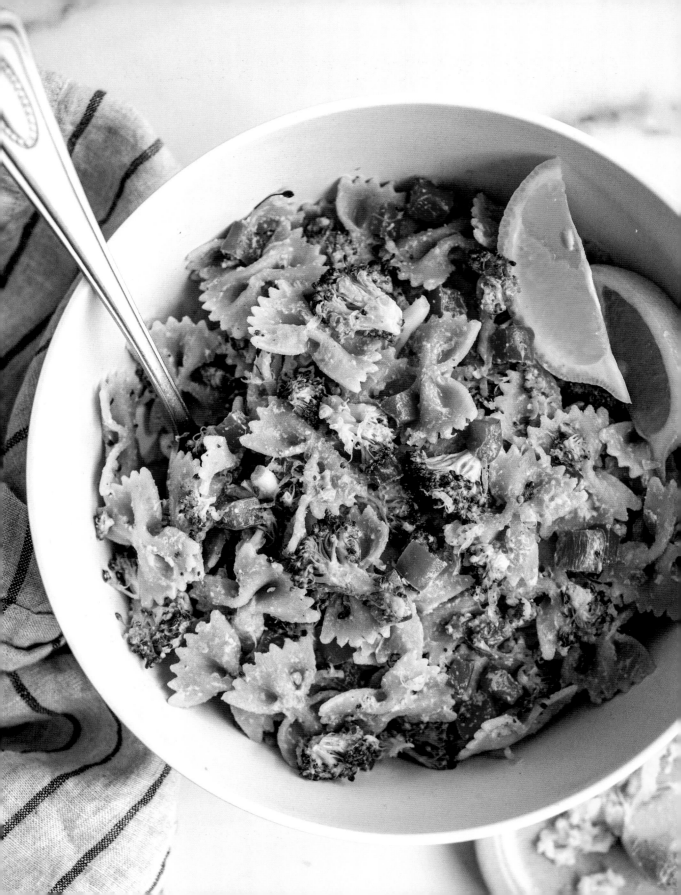

GINGER BROCCOLI PASTA SALAD

5 Plant Points

Serves 2 to 3

The green from the broccoli and the red from the sweet red peppers are easy on the eyes, aren't they? But it's more than just good looks. The vitamin C from the peppers actually increases absorption of the iron in the broccoli. They're complementary in every way.

175 g roughly chopped broccoli florets (see Pro Tip)

1 medium sweet red pepper, seeded and diced

Salt and freshly ground black pepper

2 teaspoons olive oil (optional)

225 g uncooked pasta of choice (gluten-free or quinoa farfalle (butterfly)

2 tablespoons freshly squeezed lemon juice

½ teaspoon lemon zest

2 tablespoons tahini

1 teaspoon Dijon mustard

1 teaspoon apple juice or ½ teaspoon 100% maple syrup

1 teaspoon low-sodium tamari or soy sauce

1 teaspoon grated fresh ginger

1. Preheat the oven to 200°C. Toss the broccoli and diced pepper with the olive oil and a pinch of salt and pepper until well coated. Place in a single layer on a large baking tray and roast for 15 to 20 minutes, until the broccoli is lightly browned but still has a slightly crunchy texture. (If you want to roast the broccoli and pepper without oil, see the Pro Tip on page 78.)

2. While the broccoli is cooking, bring a large pot of water to a boil. Cook the pasta according to the packet directions, then drain and set aside.

3. While the pasta is cooking, make the dressing. Whisk together the lemon juice, lemon zest, tahini, mustard, maple syrup, tamari, and ginger. Taste and adjust to preference, adding in more lemon juice for a brighter dressing, more ginger or more tahini for a creamy dressing. Add salt and pepper, if desired.

4. Toss together the crispy roasted broccoli, red pepper, and pasta with the dressing.

PRO TIP:

Cruciferous veggies produce cancer-fighting phytochemicals called isothiocyanates (like sulforaphane) when they are chopped or crushed. To maximize the cancer-fighting phytochemicals, we want to CHOP our broccoli, then STOP for 10 minutes to let the chemical reaction take place. CHOP then STOP with cruciferous veggies!

GREAT GREEK GRAIN SALAD

9+ Plant Points

Serves 4

Say that five times fast! It's hard to beat the combination of flavours in a Greek salad—olives, cucumbers, basil, parsley, a fresh squeeze of lemon. I love to eat this with plant-based Homemade Tofu Feta. Note that the feta needs to be made at least an hour ahead, but it's amazing and worth it. I like to close my eyes when I eat this and imagine the sun radiating down on my skin while the Mediterranean laps against my toes in the sand. Never mind the children jumping on the couch with permanent markers—reality can wait.

FODMAP note: 40 g of chickpeas per serving is low FODMAP.

370 g cooked quinoa

40 g hulled hemp seeds

60 g diced cucumber

70 g sliced pitted black or Kalamata olives

50 g thinly sliced spring onions, green parts only

1 medium sweet red pepper, seeded and chopped

10 g finely chopped fresh basil

10 g finely chopped fresh flat-leaf parsley

2 tablespoons freshly squeezed lemon juice

Salt and freshly ground black pepper

Extra-virgin olive oil (optional)

40 g canned chickpeas (optional)

Homemade Tofu Feta (page 84; optional)

1. In a large bowl, toss together the quinoa, hemp seeds, cucumber, olives, spring onions, sweet pepper, basil, and parsley. Add the lemon juice and toss again, then season to taste as needed with salt and pepper. If desired, drizzle on olive oil and toss once more.

2. Enjoy as is, or with canned chickpeas or Homemade Tofu Feta.

FF UNLEASHED:

If you are not following a low FODMAP approach, you can add more chickpeas and also add chopped tomato.

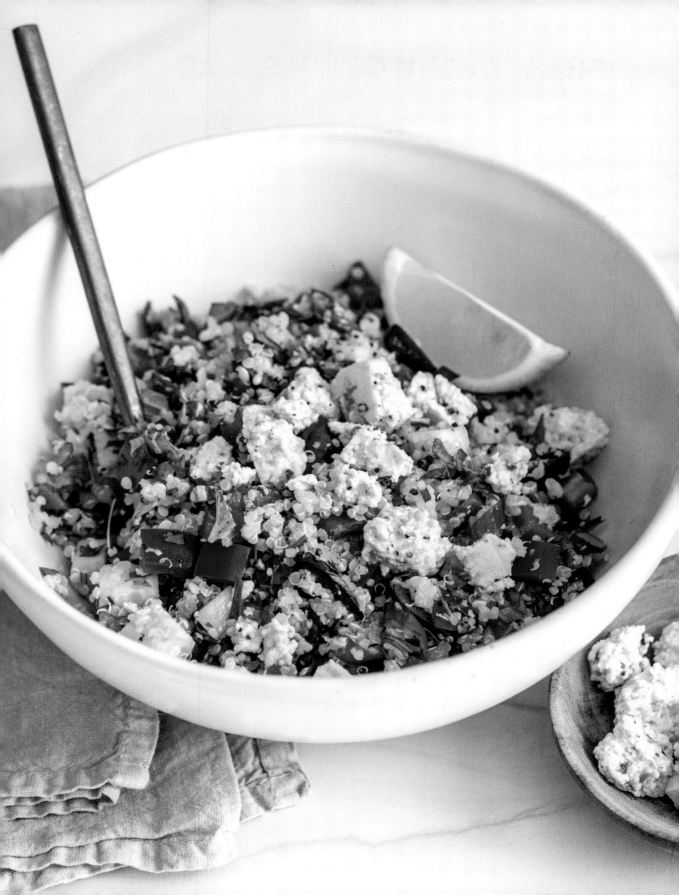

HOMEMADE TOFU FETA

3 Plant Points

Makes 4 servings

Before you make this recipe, you should figure out who you're going to call first to tell them that you just had the most amazing, completely plant-based feta. Let them know that this is an act of love, to share the *Fibre Fuelled* tofu feta recipe.

1 tablespoon white miso

2 tablespoons freshly squeezed lemon juice

1 tablespoon apple cider vinegar

½ tablespoon nutritional yeast

½ teaspoon dried oregano

¼ teaspoon salt

¼ teaspoon freshly ground black pepper

225 g extra-firm tofu, drained and pressed (see Pro Tip)

1. In a bowl, whisk the miso, 2 tablespoons water, the lemon juice, vinegar, nutritional yeast, oregano, salt, and pepper until the miso is dissolved. Crumble in the tofu, then gently fold together until the tofu is well covered with the wet ingredients.

2. Cover and place in the fridge for at least 1 hour. The feta becomes more flavourful as it sits!

PRO TIP:

Pressing tofu removes the excess moisture to increase firmness and hold its shape. You can use a tofu press, or simply place the tofu on a layer of paper towels, then cover with another layer of paper towels. Put something heavy on top, like a big, thick book and some cans from the store cupboard. Let it sit for at least 30 minutes, until the paper towels stop absorbing moisture. Then cut the tofu into whatever your desired shape is and store in the fridge or freezer.

LOW FODMAP BIOME STOCK

Makes about 2 litres

While on a low FODMAP diet, you want a stock recipe that packs the flavour without leaning on garlic and onions. This recipe establishes your foundation as you build to the future and are able to add those flavour foods in by training your gut. Before you know it, you'll be graduating to the Biome Stock Unleashed recipe (page 239).

1 large piece dried kombu

130 g chopped carrots

100 g chopped celery

15 g dried shiitake mushrooms or
1 teaspoon mushroom powder

2.5 cm piece fresh ginger, sliced

2 tablespoons nutritional yeast

2 tablespoons olive oil

3 tablespoons low-sodium tamari

¼ teaspoon ground turmeric

1. Place the kombu, carrots, celery, mushrooms, ginger, nutritional yeast, olive oil, tamari, turmeric, and 2 litres water in a slow cooker and simmer on low for at least 6 hours. Alternatively, place in a large stockpot and simmer on low for at least 2 hours, stirring occasionally.

2. Let cool, then strain through a fine-mesh strainer. Divide into glass containers, placing some in the freezer for use later in the week and the following week and some in the fridge for immediate use.

PRO TIP:

Save your scraps! Biome Stock can help reduce food waste. Simply create a storage container in your freezer that you can throw your plant scraps—peelings, rinds, cores, tips, leaves, shoots, bulbs and heads—for later use in your Biome Stock. Feel free to experiment with variations on the formula and post them to social media for all to enjoy! To keep it low FODMAP, make a special container that only low FODMAP ingredients go into.

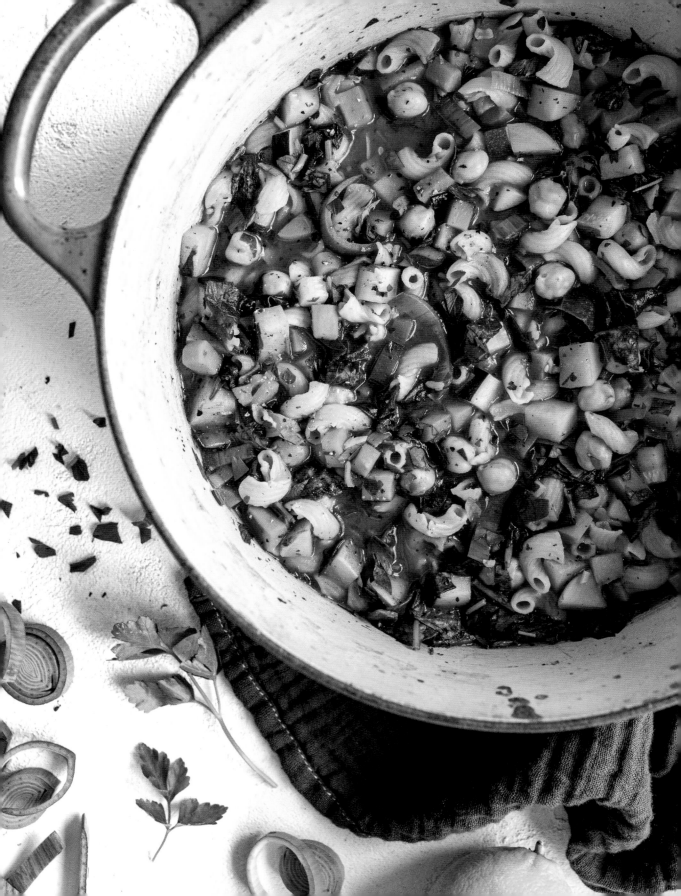

WEEKNIGHT MINESTRONE SOUP

9+ Plant Points

Serves 4

Minestrone was my favourite soup as a child. I loved the spice pattern and how hearty and filling it was on a cold day in Syracuse, New York.

1 tablespoon garlic-infused olive oil or stock (see Pro Tip)

45 g leeks (green tips only), thinly sliced

2 medium carrots, diced

1 small Desiree or Maris Piper potato, diced

2½ teaspoons Italian seasoning (garlic-free for low FODMAP)

¼ teaspoon smoked paprika

¼ teaspoon salt

¼ teaspoon freshly ground black pepper

175 g diced courgette

120 ml bottled or canned tomato sauce

1 litre Low FODMAP Biome Stock (page 85) or other vegetable stock

170 g canned chickpeas, drained and rinsed

125 g gluten-free pasta (elbows or shells)

60 g roughly chopped baby spinach

1 tablespoon freshly squeezed lemon juice

10 g chopped fresh flat-leaf parsley

1. In a large pan, heat the olive oil over medium heat and add the leeks and carrots. Sauté for 5 minutes, stirring occasionally. Add in the potato, Italian seasoning, paprika, salt, and pepper and cook another 10 minutes, stirring often to prevent sticking. If the vegetables are sticking, add in a splash of water or stock.

2. Add in the courgettes, tomato sauce, stock, 240 ml water, chickpeas, and pasta and bring to the boil. Reduce the heat to low and simmer for 5 minutes, then turn off the heat and let sit another 5 minutes, until the pasta is tender. (If you are using gluten-free pasta, it will likely become mushy as this soup sits. If planning leftovers, cook the pasta separately and add to the soup right before serving.)

3. Just before serving, add the spinach and stir until wilted. Stir in the lemon juice and parsley.

PRO TIP:

Garlic-infused olive oil gives low FODMAP recipes a great flavour boost. FODMAPs are not lipid soluble, so you can add the flavour of garlic to oil without the FODMAPs coming along. To make garlic-infused olive oil, warm 120 ml olive oil and 4 slightly crushed garlic cloves in a small saucepan over low heat for 5 minutes. Remove from heat and allow to cool completely, then remove the garlic cloves and place the oil in an airtight container. Store in the refrigerator for up to 1 month.

FF UNLEASHED:

If you are not following a low FODMAP approach, you can substitute 1 large white or yellow onion and 2 garlic cloves for the leek.

HEALING MISO SOUP

5+ Plant Points

Serves 4

Miso is brought to life from soybeans by a fungus named *Aspergillus oryzae*, also known as koji mould. *A. oryzae* is also responsible for creating soy sauce, sake, and rice vinegar. Recent research has discovered that koji contains abundant amounts of glycosylceramide, which has been found to have prebiotic benefits on the gut microbiota. Scientists speculate that this may in part explain the longevity of populations who consume these foods.

2 litres Low FODMAP Biome Stock (page 85)

1 to 2 teaspoons finely chopped fresh ginger

1 teaspoon low-sodium soy sauce or tamari

3 medium carrots, thinly sliced

225 g extra-firm tofu, drained, pressed, and cubed

75 g thinly sliced pak choi leaves

3 to 4 tablespoons white miso

Supercharge It! (optional toppings):

Green spring onion

Coriander

Sesame seeds

Nori strips

1. Bring the stock to the boil in a large stockpot. Add in the ginger, soy sauce, and carrots and cook for 4 minutes, until the carrots are just softened.

2. Add in the tofu and pak choi and cook for another 5 minutes, stirring occasionally.

3. Remove from the heat and whisk in the miso. Start with 3 tablespoons, then add more depending on your preference.

4. Divide into bowls and top with your preferred toppings: green spring onion tops, coriander, sesame seeds, and/or nori strips.

FF UNLEASHED:

If you are not following a low FODMAP approach, you can add 2 crushed garlic cloves with the ginger.

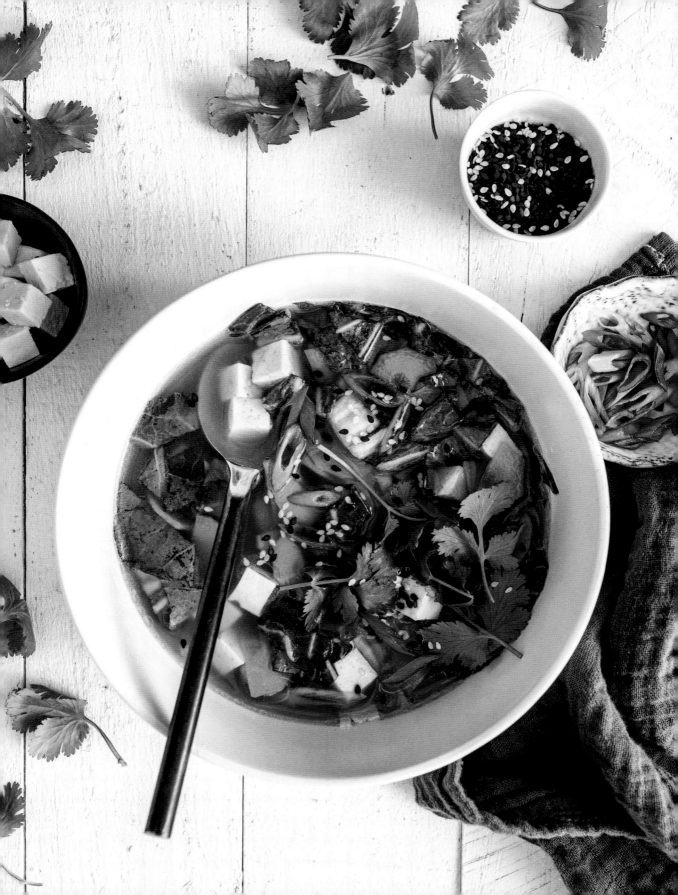

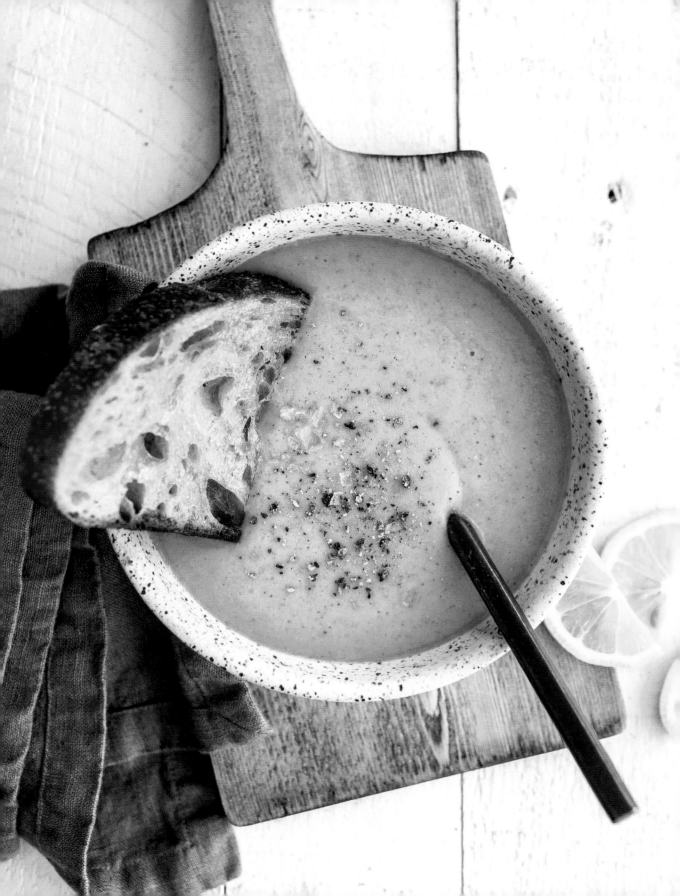

CHEESY BROCCOLI AND POTATO SOUP

7 Plant Points

Serves 4

Who says you can't have creamy, cheesy broccoli soup on a low FODMAP diet? Nutritional yeast is a species of yeast known as *Saccharomyces cerevisiae* that imparts the cheesy flavour. It has protein, B vitamins, trace minerals, and prebiotic fibre. It's also deactivated and not alive. That said, the only people that I recommend not to consume nutritional yeast are those with Crohn's disease, as there is concern that it could worsen the disease.

1 medium carrot, diced

450 g peeled and diced Desiree or Maris Piper potatoes

4 to 5 tablespoons nutritional yeast

3 to 4 teaspoons freshly squeezed lemon juice

2 tablespoons water (or olive oil, for a richer flavour)

¼ to ½ teaspoon smoked paprika

½ to 1 teaspoon salt

2 teaspoons garlic-infused olive oil (see Pro Tip, page 87)

90 g green leek tips, roughly diced

1 small courgette (ends trimmed), diced

210 g chopped broccoli florets

1 litre Low FODMAP Biome Stock (page 85) or low FODMAP stock

25 g raw walnuts

Freshly ground black pepper

1. Place the carrot and 225 g of the potatoes in a medium saucepan and cover with water. Bring to the boil, then reduce the heat to medium-low and cook for 10 to 15 minutes, until tender. Drain and place in the base of a blender along with 2 tablespoons of the nutritional yeast, 2 teaspoons of the lemon juice, the water, paprika, and salt. Purée until very creamy and smooth, scraping down the sides as needed. The cheesy sauce should be very thick, but if it's too thick to blend, add in a tablespoon or two of water or broth. Season to taste and place in a large saucepan.

2. Wipe out the medium saucepan used for the carrots and potatoes. Heat the garlic-infused olive oil in the saucepan over medium heat. Add the leek and cook for 4 minutes, stirring occasionally, then add in the remaining 225 g potatoes, the courgette, and the broccoli. Cook for an additional 5 minutes, stirring often to prevent sticking.

RECIPE CONTINUES

3. Add the stock, walnuts, 2 tablespoons of the remaining nutritional yeast, and 1 teaspoon of the remaining lemon juice. Cover with a tight-fitting lid and simmer over medium heat for 15 minutes, until the vegetables are tender.

4. Transfer the courgette-potato stock to the base of a blender and purée until creamy and smooth (you can also enjoy it chunky—just pulse a few times in the blender/food processor for the desired consistency), then add to the saucepan with the cheesy sauce. Stir together and season to taste, adding more freshly ground pepper, salt, lemon juice, nutritional yeast, and/or smoked paprika as desired.

5. Enjoy it as is or with sourdough bread. Leftovers freeze great for a quick meal.

PRO TIP:

To make cheesy croutons for the soup, toss cubed bread with nutritional yeast and a little olive oil (and garlic powder if you are not restricting FODMAPs) and bake at 200°C for about 5 minutes, or until crispy.

FF UNLEASHED:

If you are not restricting FODMAPs, you can substitute cashews instead of walnuts and add 2 crushed garlic cloves to the soup.

COCONUT CURRY BOWL

4+ Plant Points

4 servings

In a study of more than two thousand recipes, scientists discovered that the secret behind curry's popularity is the diverse mix of spices that have very different flavour profiles. Effectively, this creates an explosion of flavour that tickles the taste buds. Diversity of spices for the win!

FODMAP note: Many prepared veggie stocks contain garlic and onion, as well as other high FODMAPs like celery. Since it's hard to know the serving size of each vegetable included, we recommend a vegetable stock that's garlic-free and onion-free, or specifically low FODMAP. The Low FODMAP Biome Stock (page 85) is designed to serve this purpose.

400 g extra-firm tofu, drained, and pressed (see Pro Tip, page 84)

3 teaspoons olive oil

1 teaspoon ground turmeric

¼ to ½ teaspoon freshly ground black pepper

¼ teaspoon chilli powder (garlic-free for low FODMAP)

1 tablespoon plus 1 teaspoon low-sodium tamari or soy sauce

2 teaspoons curry powder

½ teaspoon arrowroot powder (optional)

225 g rice noodles

25 g thinly sliced green spring onion tops

1 teaspoon grated fresh ginger

140 g torn kale leaves, stems removed

240 ml canned coconut milk

480 ml Low FODMAP Biome Stock (page 85) or other low FODMAP vegetable stock

2 tablespoons freshly squeezed lime juice

Supercharge It! (optional toppings):

Jalapeño pepper, seeded and diced

Chopped fresh coriander leaves

Sesame seeds

1. Preheat the oven to 200°C.

2. Dice the tofu and toss with 1 teaspoon of the olive oil, ½ teaspoon of the turmeric, the black pepper, chilli powder, 1 tablespoon of the tamari, 1 teaspoon of the curry powder, and the arrowroot powder, if using. Place in a single layer on a rimmed baking tray and roast for 15 minutes, turning halfway through the cooking.

3. Soften the noodles according to the packet directions while the tofu cooks, then set aside.

4. In a medium saucepan, heat the remaining 2 teaspoons olive oil over medium heat and add the spring onion and ginger. Stir, cooking, for 30 seconds, until just fragrant. Add in the torn kale leaves and cook another 30 seconds, then add in the remaining teaspoon of tamari,

RECIPE CONTINUES

½ teaspoon turmeric, and 1 teaspoon of curry powder along with the coconut milk and stock.

5. Bring to a simmer and let cook for 10 minutes. Remove from the heat and stir in the lime juice.

6. Divide the tofu and noodles among four bowls. Top with coconut curry stock and optional toppings.

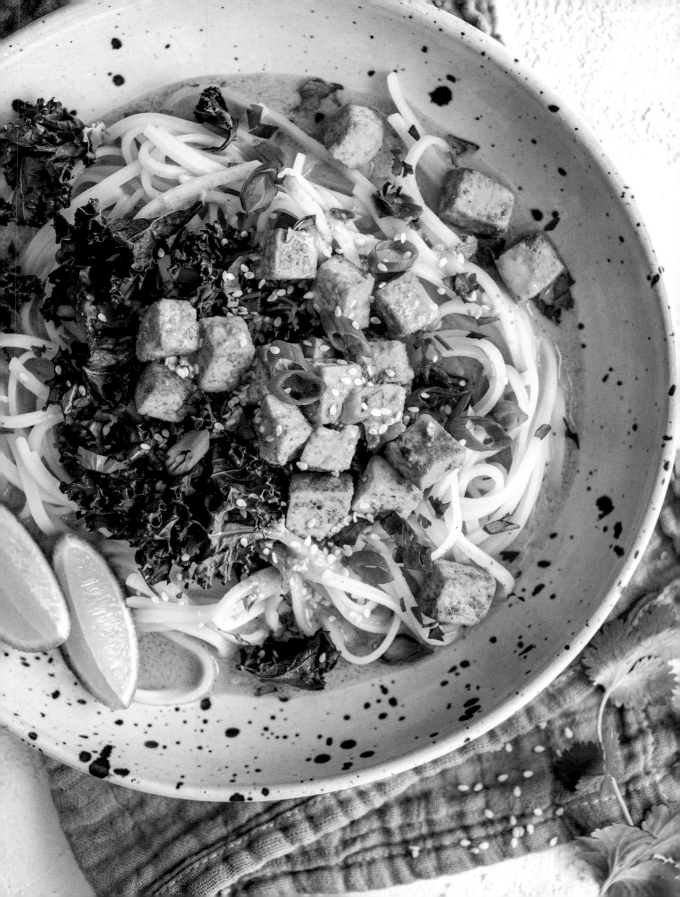

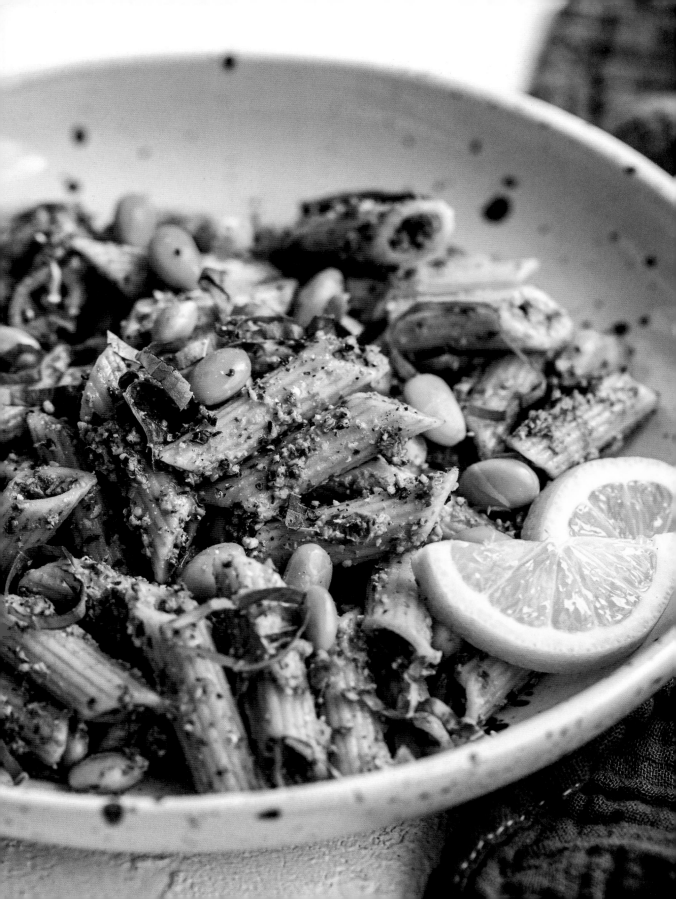

EDAMAME PESTO PASTA
(with quinoa pasta/gluten-free pasta)

4 Plant Points

Serves 4

Pesto originates from Genoa, a port city in the northwest corner of Italy. Its name is derived from the Italian word *pestare*, which means "to pound." According to tradition, the ingredients are "pounded" in a marble mortar using the circular motion of a wooden pestle. Embrace the tradition! Let me know if you pull out the mortar and pestle.

340 g gluten-free or quinoa rotini or penne

225 g cooked edamame

50 g fresh basil, plus 10 g torn basil for garnish

60 g spinach leaves

1 tablespoon nutritional yeast

1 to 2 tablespoons freshly squeezed lemon juice

2 tablespoons garlic-infused olive oil (see Pro Tip, page 87) or Low FODMAP Biome Stock (page 85)

½ teaspoon salt

Supercharge It! (optional toppings):

Halved cherry tomatoes (5 cherry tomatoes are low FODMAP friendly)

Pine nuts

1. Bring a large pan of water to the boil. Add the pasta and cook until al dente according to the packet directions. Drain, reserving 120 ml of the pasta water. Set aside in a large bowl.

2. Add 170 g of the edamame to the base of a food processor and pulse 10 to 15 times until roughly chopped. Add in the 50 g basil, the spinach leaves, and nutritional yeast and pulse another 10 times, until well combined.

3. With the motor running, add in the lemon juice and olive oil until well combined. Add in the salt and season to taste. With the motor running, slowly add in the pasta water, 1 tablespoon at a time, until the desired consistency is reached (I usually end up using 80 ml).

4. Toss the edamame pesto and remaining edamame with the cooked pasta, adding in 1 tablespoon or so of reserved pasta water as needed to thin. Add the torn basil leaves and toss with the pasta. Stir in the additional supercharged toppings of choice.

PRO TIP:

If you buy a hydroponic basil plant, store it on the worktop in a vase of water and change the water once a day. Similarly, you can store cut basil in the same way. Basil is a warm-weather herb, so the refrigerator is a bit too cold for it.

FF UNLEASHED:

If you are not following a low FODMAP approach, you can use wholewheat or legume-based pasta. Add 2 garlic cloves before blending the pesto and top with cherry tomatoes.

ZIPPY CORIANDER BOWL

11+ Plant Points

4 servings

I'm a huge fan of sauces. I think it's the chance to pour flavour at your will onto dishes. Anyone else feel that way? Well, putting fresh coriander with lime juice in a sauce is a little slice of heaven for me. Ever notice how some people hate coriander, though? Scientists discovered that there is actually a gene that determines those strong feelings. The haters can't help it; they're wired that way.

FODMAP note: Kabocha squash is low FODMAP. A 40 g of canned chickpeas is a low FODMAP–friendly serving.

95 g brown rice
or 90 g quinoa

230 g peeled, seeded, and diced Kabocha squash

2 large carrots, diced

2 teaspoons olive oil

¼ teaspoon salt

¼ teaspoon freshly ground black pepper

140 g finely shredded red cabbage

40 g rocket leaves

50 g thinly sliced spring onions (green parts only)

125 g canned chickpeas, drained and rinsed

20 g fresh coriander leaves

20 g fresh flat-leaf parsley

80 ml freshly squeezed lime juice

3 tablespoons tahini

2 tablespoons olive oil, stock, or water

Supercharge It!:

4 tablespoons pumpkin seeds

2 tablespoons sunflower seeds

Sprouts, alfalfa

1. Combine the brown rice and 240 ml water in a medium saucepan and bring to the boil. Reduce the heat to low, cover with a tight-fitting lid, and cook for 40 to 45 minutes, until the rice is tender and the water is absorbed. Fluff with a fork, then set aside to cool. You can do this ahead of time for easy meal assembly.

2. Preheat the oven to 200°C. Place the pumpkin and carrots in a large bowl along with the olive oil, salt, and pepper. Toss together until well coated, then place in a single layer on a rimmed baking or roasting tin. Cover with foil and roast for 25 to 30 minutes, until the vegetables are tender. Remove the foil for the last 5 minutes of cooking to allow for browning. (If you want to roast the pumpkin and carrots without oil, see the Pro Tip on page 78.)

3. While the pumpkin and carrots are roasting, place the cabbage, rocket, spring onions, chickpeas, and brown rice in a large bowl. Set aside.

RECIPE CONTINUES

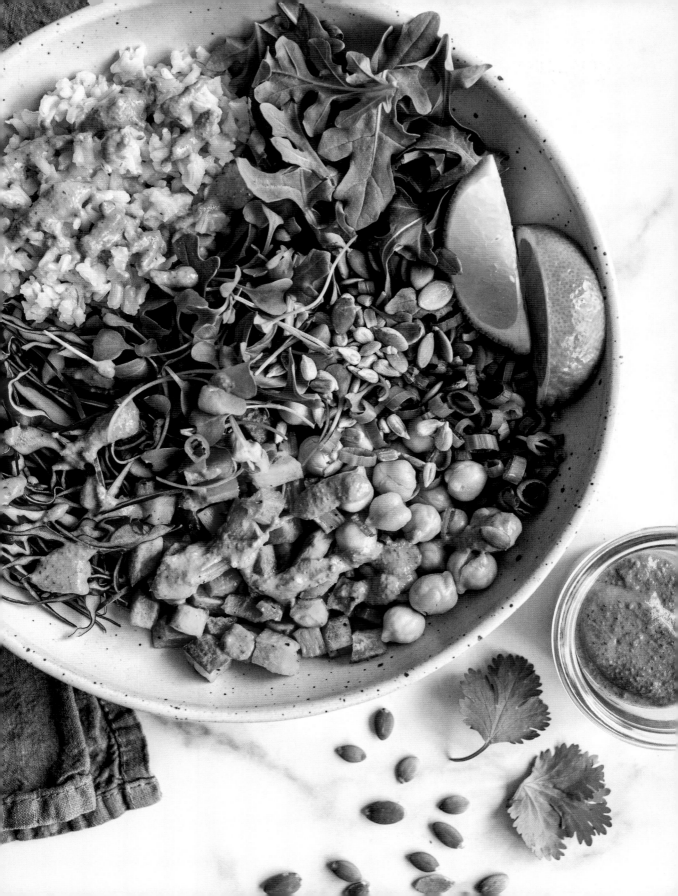

4. Make the dressing. Place the coriander, parsley, lime juice, and tahini in the base of a blender or food processor. Pulse together 10 to 15 times, until the herbs are very finely chopped. With the motor running, add in the olive oil until a creamy dressing forms. Taste, adding salt and pepper as desired or more lime juice and/or tahini as needed.

5. When the pumpkin and carrots are done, remove and let cool slightly. Toss with the rice and other veggies and dressing and serve with the supercharged toppings, as desired.

FF UNLEASHED:

If you are not following a low FODMAP approach, you can make this dish with all squash instead of carrots, or sub in butternut squash or sweet potato.

SP&L BURGER PATTIES

10+ Plant Points

Makes 15 patties—
freeze for later

Does SP&L stand for So Perfect and Lovely or Sweet Potato and Lentils? I'm not answering. These burgers take a while to prepare, but they are amazing and totally worth it. Enjoy them as a burger, or crumbled onto your favourite salad. They can be frozen for quick meals throughout the week. The ideal time to cook them is when you have extra cooked grains in the fridge because the brown rice and quinoa need to be cooked and cooled ahead of time.

FODMAP note: Dried lentils and chickpeas are high FODMAP, but servings of 40 g canned chickpeas or 100 g canned lentils are low FODMAP. Canning actually reduces the FODMAP content. The reason is that the FODMAPs are water soluble, so they will migrate into the water that you then pour off. You can further reduce the FODMAP content by thoroughly rinsing them.

450 g peeled and cubed sweet potatoes

2 tablespoons chia seeds

265 g canned lentils or black beans (not low FODMAP)

100 g thinly sliced spring onions (green parts only)

15 g chopped fresh coriander

195 g grated carrots

100 g sweet red pepper, seeded and diced

60 ml freshly squeezed lime juice

1 teaspoon lime zest

1 teaspoon smoked paprika

1 teaspoon ground cumin

1 teaspoon dried oregano

½ to 1 teaspoon salt

1 teaspoon chipotle powder

½ teaspoon freshly ground black pepper

¼ teaspoon cayenne pepper (optional)

250 g cooked brown rice

230 g cooked quinoa

6 tablespoons gluten-free bread crumbs

Olive oil, for greasing the parchment paper and brushing the tops of the patties

RECIPE CONTINUES

1. Place the sweet potatoes in a microwave-safe bowl with a splash of water and cover with a tight-fitting lid. Cook on high in the microwave for 4 minutes or until soft. Alternatively, steam until soft and set aside.

2. Whisk together the chia seeds and 5 tablespoons boiling water in a small bowl and set aside.

3. Drain and rinse the canned lentils, reserving 85 g. (If you are not restricting FODMAPs, you can substitute canned black beans for lentils.)

4. Place the spring onion, coriander, carrots, red pepper, lime juice, lime zest, paprika, cumin, oregano, salt, chipotle powder, black pepper, cayenne, cooked sweet potato, and lentils into the base of a food processor and pulse until just combined, scraping down the sides as needed. Taste, adding more seasoning/salt/lime juice as preferred.

5. Transfer the mixture to a large bowl and add in the brown rice, quinoa, reserved lentils, bread crumbs, and chia mixture. Mix until well combined, adding in more salt/pepper/seasonings as desired.

6. Preheat the oven to 200°C.

7. Line a baking tray with parchment paper and brush with olive oil. Using an ice cream scoop as a measure, scoop the mixture and form into a patty with your hands. Place on the tray to flatten slightly, then repeat until the remaining mixture is used. You will likely need two baking trays, depending on their size. Brush the tops of the finished patties with olive oil and bake for 25 to 30 minutes, until lightly browned, flipping halfway through.

8. These patties will last in the fridge for 4 days, or in the freezer for 4 months. When freezing, place on a lined baking tray in a single layer until frozen, then transfer to an airtight container. To reheat, microwave for 1 minute or panfry for 2 to 3 minutes per side until warmed through and crispy.

FF UNLEASHED:

If you are not following a low FODMAP approach, you can substitute black beans instead of lentils and 150 g cooked onions instead of spring onions. Add 2 crushed garlic cloves, and use chilli powder instead of chipotle powder.

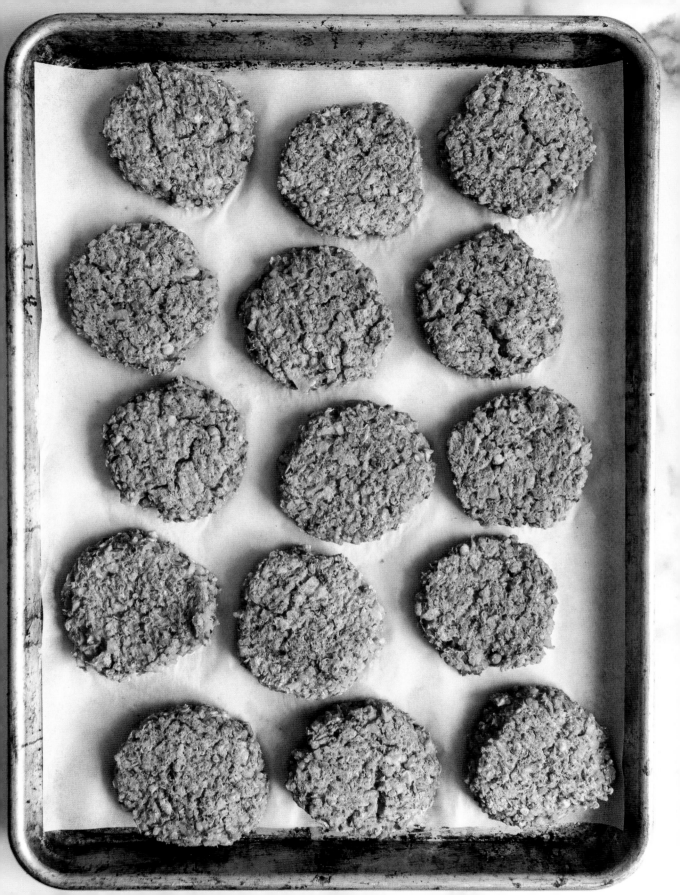

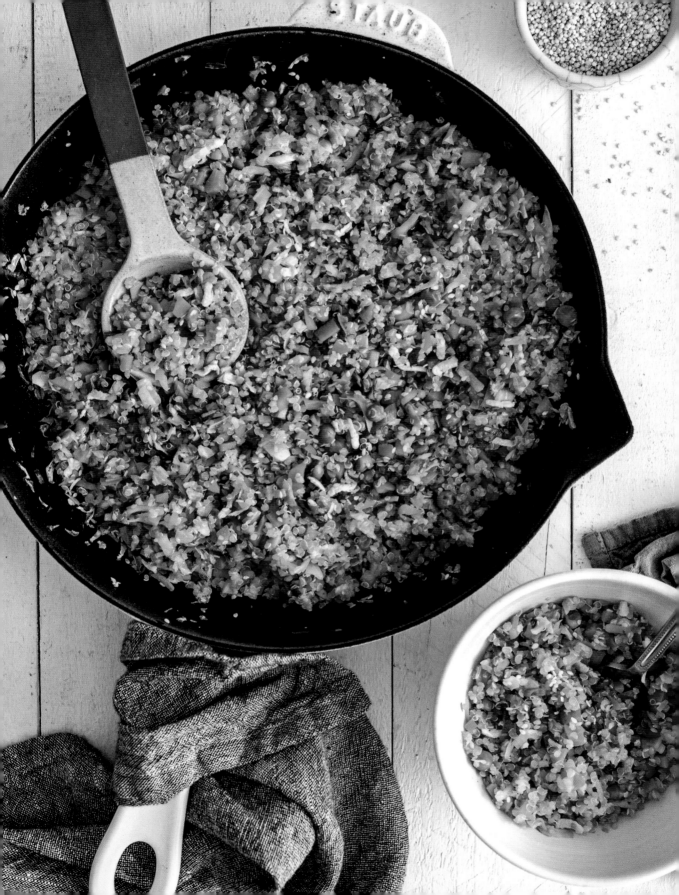

QUINOA FRIED RICE

8 Plant Points

Serves 4

Quinoa is high in protein, B vitamins, minerals, and plant-based omega fats. Some call it a "superfood," but the Incas, who originally cultivated it, called it "mother grain." Funnily enough, it's more closely related to beetroot and spinach than wholegrains, making it a pseudo grain. Yeah, that was a curveball for me, too.

2 tablespoons low-sodium soy sauce or tamari

2 tablespoons 100% pineapple juice or ½ teaspoon 100% maple syrup

2 tablespoons rice wine vinegar

1 teaspoon finely chopped fresh ginger

1 teaspoon sriracha (optional)

1 to 2 tablespoons toasted sesame oil, garlic-infused olive oil (see Pro Tip, page 87), or stock

250 g diced extra-firm tofu

3 medium carrots, finely diced

40 g green peas

140 g finely chopped cabbage

50 g thinly sliced spring onions (green parts only)

550 g cooked and cooled quinoa

3 tablespoons sesame seeds

1. In a small bowl, whisk together the tamari, 2 tablespoons water, the pineapple juice, vinegar, ginger, and sriracha, if using. Set aside.

2. Heat the oil in a large frying pan or wok. Add in the tofu and cook 2 to 3 minutes, stirring often, until the tofu is just golden brown.

3. Add in the carrots, peas, and cabbage and cook another 10 minutes, stirring often, until the vegetables are just tender. If the vegetables begin to stick, add in an extra splash or two of stock.

4. Add in the spring onions, quinoa, sauce mixture, and sesame seeds. Toss together another minute or two, until the quinoa is heated through. Season to taste and serve.

FF UNLEASHED:

If you are not following a low FODMAP approach, you can add 2 crushed garlic cloves when you add the quinoa to the frying pan.

SWEET AND SPICY PEANUT TEMPEH WRAPS

8 Plant Points

Makes 8 lettuce wraps

Originating in Indonesia, tempeh starts as boiled soybeans and is transformed by a fungus, *Rhizopus oligosporus*. The end result contains twenty-five different microbes. A small study of humans found that tempeh consumption increased the growth of *Akkermansia muciniphila*, a friendly bacteria that protects against obesity, type 2 diabetes, and inflammatory bowel disease.

5 tablespoons smooth peanut butter

3 tablespoons freshly squeezed lime juice

3 tablespoons low-sodium tamari

¼ to ½ teaspoon crushed red pepper flakes

1 teaspoon grated fresh ginger

250 g chopped fresh pineapple

1 tablespoon toasted sesame oil (see Pro Tip)

225 g tempeh, coarsely chopped

8 large butter lettuce leaves

130 g shredded carrot

70 g finely shredded red cabbage

1. Place the peanut butter, lime juice, tamari, red pepper flakes, ginger, and 80 g of the pineapple in the base of a small food processor or blender and purée until creamy and smooth. If needed, add in a tablespoon of water to thin. Reserve 60 ml of the sauce and set aside.

2. Heat the sesame oil in a large, non-stick frying pan over medium heat. Add the tempeh and cook for 5 to 6 minutes, stirring often, until crispy and golden brown. Add in the peanut sauce and cook for an additional 3 to 4 minutes, stirring often, until the tempeh is coated and the sauce is warmed through.

3. Fill the lettuce leaves with the shredded carrot, remaining pineapple, cooked tempeh, and shredded cabbage. Drizzle with the remaining peanut sauce.

FF UNLEASHED:

If you are not following a low FODMAP approach, you can add 2 teaspoons chilli garlic sauce, such as sambal oelek, to the peanut sauce.

PRO TIP:

The toasted sesame oil provides a traditional taste and allows the tempeh to become crunchy. You can use an alternative oil, if desired, or omit.

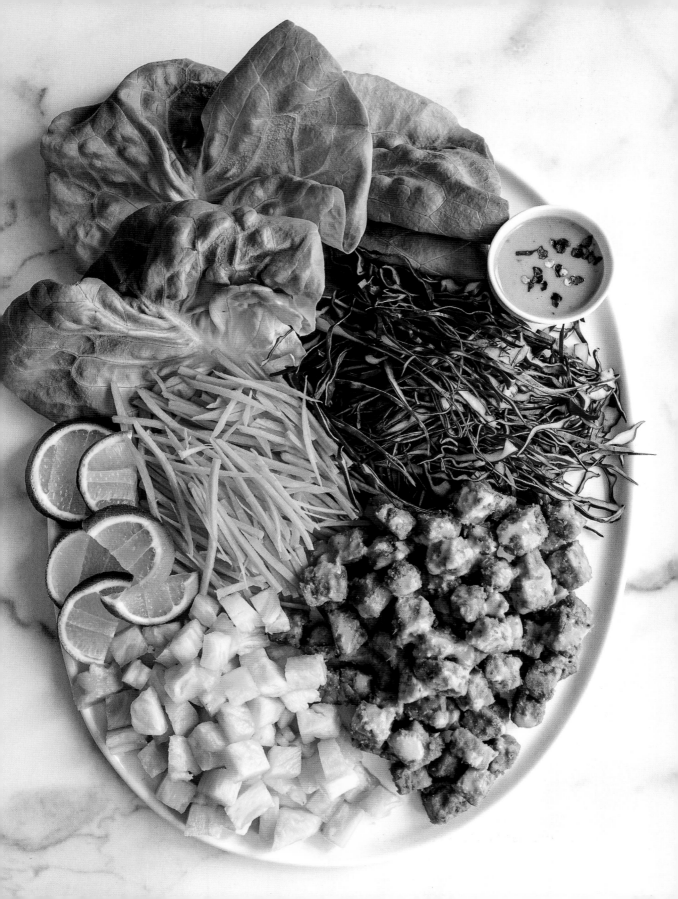

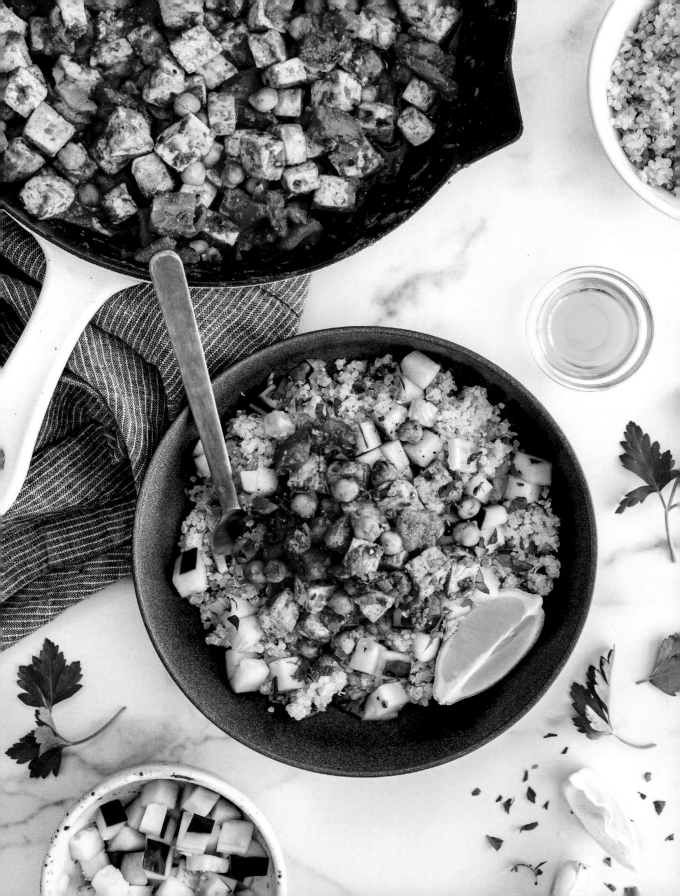

CHICKPEA GLOW BOWL

8 Plant Points

Serves 4

During the era of Indian maharajas and maharanis, royal chefs created exuberant spice blends for a complex, aromatic culinary experience. The composition of garam masala differs regionally across India, and may include up to thirty different ingredients. According to Ayurvedic tradition, garam masala is properly named for its ability to enhance digestive fire, or agni, which supports strong immunity and a long, healthy life.

FODMAP note: This recipe uses 170 g of chickpeas to make 4 servings. Note that 40 g of canned chickpeas is considered low FODMAP, while 80 g is considered moderate FODMAP.

2 teaspoons garlic-infused olive oil (see Pro Tip, page 87) or stock, plus more as garnish (optional)

2 tablespoons chives (fresh or freeze-dried)

2 teaspoons smoked paprika

2 teaspoons ground cumin

½ teaspoon garam masala

½ teaspoon ground turmeric

½ teaspoon salt

¼ teaspoon freshly ground black pepper

¼ teaspoon cayenne pepper

170 g canned chickpeas, drained and rinsed

400 g tofu, drained and cut into cubes

One 400 g can dhopped tomatoes

370 g cooked quinoa

Juice of 1 lemon

180 g diced cucumber, to garnish

Fresh flat-leaf parsley, to garnish

1. Heat the garlic-infused olive oil in a large frying pan over medium heat. Add the chives, paprika, cumin, garam masala, turmeric, salt, black pepper, cayenne, chickpeas, and tofu. Stir occasionally and cook for about 5 minutes, until the tofu starts to get a little crisp on the outside.

2. Add the chopped tomatoes and allow the mixture to simmer for about 20 minutes while you prep the rest of the ingredients.

3. To assemble the bowls, fill with a base of cooked quinoa, then top with the chickpea-tofu mixture. Drizzle with lemon juice and more olive oil, if desired. Garnish with the diced cucumber and fresh parsley.

"I CAN'T BELIEVE THIS IS FODMAP FRIENDLY" PASTA SAUCE

5 Plant Points

Serves 4

Everyone needs a delicious pasta sauce in their life. Unfortunately, onions, garlic, and tomato paste make most pasta sauces high FODMAP. No worries, though. You'll be happy to usher in a new era of pasta sauce with this "I Can't Believe This Is FODMAP Friendly" recipe.

1 tablespoon garlic-infused olive oil (see Pro Tip, page 87)

3 carrots, finely chopped

45 g finely chopped fennel bulb

2 tablespoons balsamic vinegar

1 tablespoon low-sodium soy sauce or tamari

2 tablespoons tomato paste

1 teaspoon dried sage

½ teaspoon dried rosemary

½ teaspoon dried oregano

Pinch ground cinnamon

½ teaspoon freshly ground black pepper

1 teaspoon 100% maple syrup or apple juice (optional)

225 g extra-firm tofu, pressed

One 400 g can crushed tomatoes

240 ml Low FODMAP Biome Stock (page 85)

Salt

Crushed red pepper flakes (optional)

10 g chopped fresh basil

340 g cooked gluten-free pasta of choice, for serving

1. Heat the olive oil in a large saucepan over medium heat. Add in the carrots and fennel and sauté until very well browned, 10 to 15 minutes.

2. While the carrots are cooking, in a small bowl, whisk together the vinegar, soy sauce, tomato paste, sage, rosemary, oregano, cinnamon, and pepper. If you prefer your red sauce on the sweeter side, add in the maple syrup. Otherwise, leave it out.

3. Add the tomato mixture to the carrots and deglaze, scraping up any browned bits at the bottom of the pan. Reduce the heat to low and crumble in the tofu along with the tomatoes and stock. Simmer for at least 20 minutes, allowing the mixture to thicken and come together. Season, adding in salt and pepper to taste. If tolerated, add in red pepper flakes to taste.

4. Right before serving, stir in the basil and serve over cooked pasta.

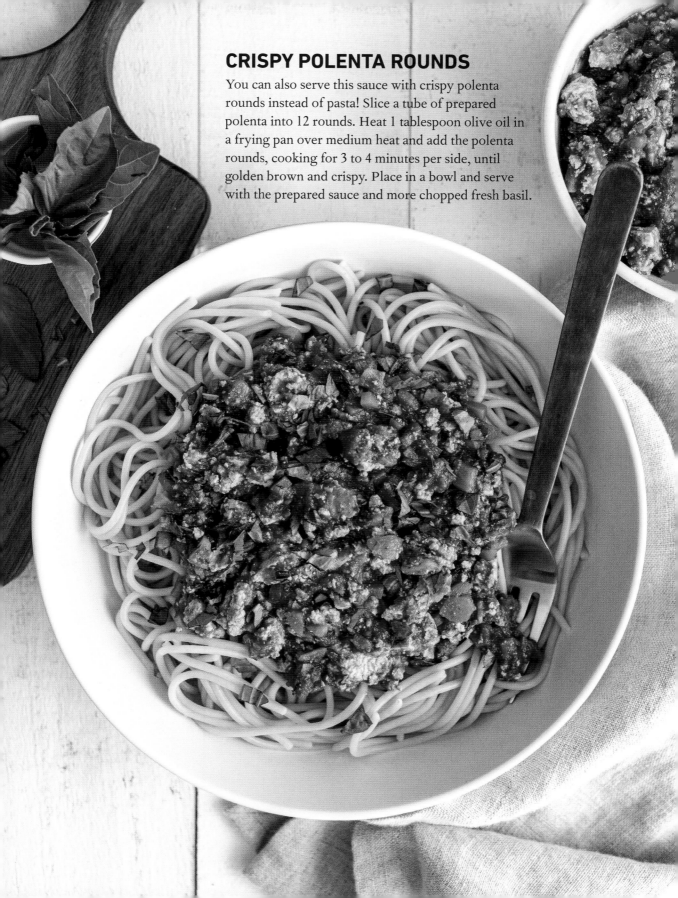

CRISPY POLENTA ROUNDS

You can also serve this sauce with crispy polenta rounds instead of pasta! Slice a tube of prepared polenta into 12 rounds. Heat 1 tablespoon olive oil in a frying pan over medium heat and add the polenta rounds, cooking for 3 to 4 minutes per side, until golden brown and crispy. Place in a bowl and serve with the prepared sauce and more chopped fresh basil.

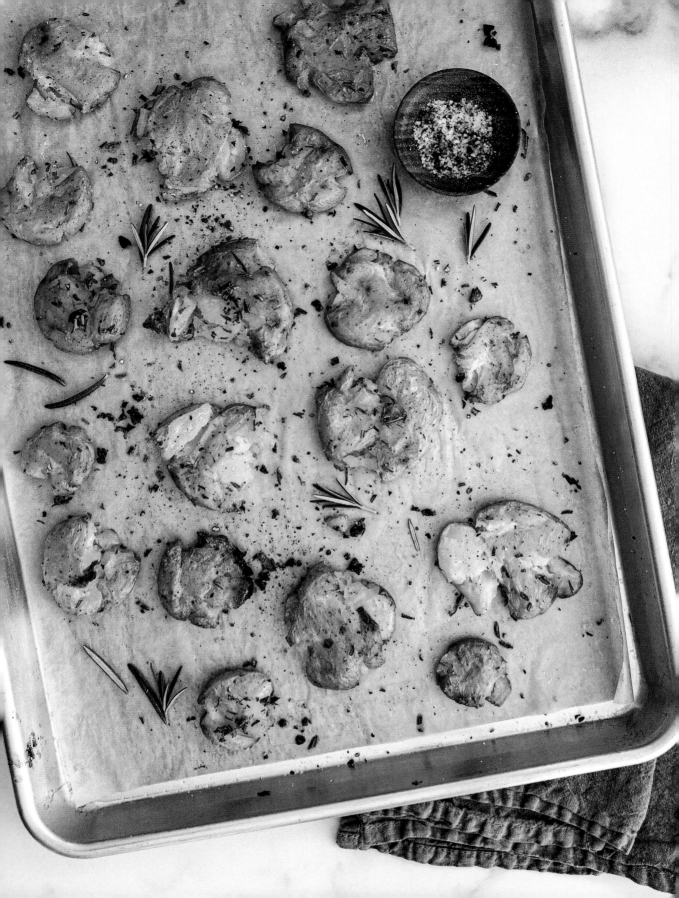

ROSEMARY SMASHED POTATOES

1 Plant Point

Serves 4

"Smashed" is such a great culinary word. This is the perfect side dish for the SP&L Burger Patties (page 101). Potatoes are low FODMAP, so you can enjoy a heaped serving of these.

450 g golden or russet potatoes, scrubbed and chopped

1 tablespoon olive oil

½ teaspoon dried rosemary or 1½ teaspoons chopped fresh rosemary

Salt and freshly ground black pepper

1. Preheat the oven to 220°C. Line a baking tray with parchment paper or a non-stick mat and set aside.

2. Place the potatoes in a large saucepan and cover with water. Bring to the boil and cook for 15 minutes, or until just tender, taking care not to overcook. Drain.

3. Place the potatoes on the prepared baking tray and gently smash them with a potato masher or the back of a wooden spoon. Drizzle with the olive oil, rosemary, salt, and pepper. Use your hands to gently cover all of the potatoes with the spices.

4. Bake for 30 to 40 minutes, until golden brown and crispy.

PRO TIP:

If you have leftovers, store them in the fridge and then panfry them for 2 to 3 minutes until hot and crispy.

TEMPEH STIR-FRY
with Saffron Rice

8+ Plant Points

Serves 4

Saffron is the most expensive spice in the world. China's Buddhist monks dyed their robes red with saffron, and Cleopatra soaked in a saffron-scented bath. Now you get to enjoy this timeless classic with dinner on a random Tuesday. Lucky you!

1½ tablespoons low-sodium soy sauce or tamari

1 tablespoon plus 1 teaspoon olive oil or water

1 teaspoon date paste or 100% maple syrup

2 teaspoons freshly squeezed lime juice

1 teaspoon chipotle powder (optional)

1 garlic clove, crushed (optional; not low FODMAP)

½ teaspoon freshly ground black pepper

½ teaspoon dried oregano

½ teaspoon freeze-dried or fresh chives

½ teaspoon smoked paprika

½ teaspoon ground cumin

225 g tempeh, crumbled

1 small courgette, sliced

1 sweet red pepper, seeded and chopped

3 tablespoons thinly sliced spring onions (green parts only)

5 g chopped fresh coriander

¼ teaspoon good-quality saffron threads

1 teaspoon extra-virgin olive oil

190 g brown basmati rice, rinsed

½ teaspoon salt

1. In a large mixing bowl, whisk together the soy sauce, ½ tablespoon of the olive oil, the date paste, lime juice, chipotle powder, if using, garlic, if using, black pepper, oregano, chives, paprika, and cumin. Add the tempeh, courgette, sweet red pepper, spring onions and coriander to the bowl and toss to coat. Cover, then place in the fridge for at least 1 hour or overnight to marinate.

2. When ready to eat, place the saffron threads in a small bowl and cover with hot water to bloom. Heat the extra-virgin olive oil in a medium saucepan over medium heat and add in the rinsed rice. Toast for 1 to 2 minutes, until the rice is fragrant and golden brown. Add in the reserved saffron mixture, salt, and 300 ml water, then bring to the boil. Reduce the heat to low, cover with a tight-fitting lid, and cook for 40 minutes, or until the rice has absorbed the water and is tender.

3. Heat the remaining ½ tablespoon olive oil in a large frying pan over medium heat.

RECIPE CONTINUES

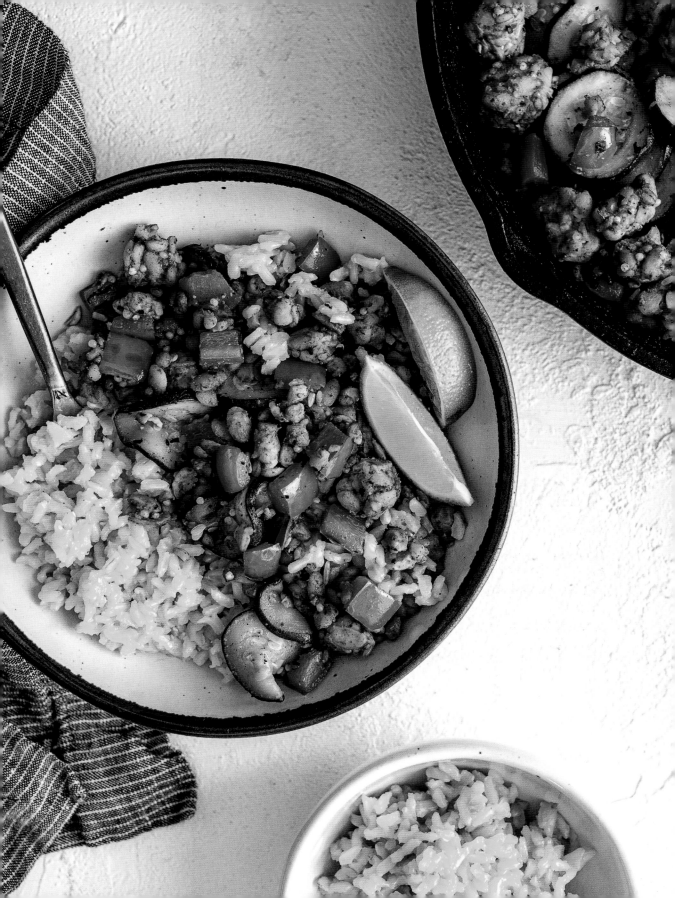

Add in the tempeh and vegetable mixture and cook, stirring often, for 10 minutes, until the tempeh is crispy and the vegetables are cooked through. If the tempeh starts to stick, add in a little water, vegetable stock, or oil. Taste, adding more salt as needed. I usually add ¼ teaspoon more with a little more black pepper.

4. Serve with the saffron rice.

PRO TIP:

The key compounds and pigments in saffron—picrocrocin, safranal, and crocin—dissolve better in water than oil but need time to steep and escape. Grind with a mortar and pestle and steep for at least 20 minutes (up to 24 hours) for optimal release.

FF UNLEASHED:

If you are not following a low FODMAP approach, you can add 1 crushed garlic clove and substitute 1 teaspoon chilli pepper instead of chipotle powder to the marinade and add whatever vegetables you desire to the recipe—more peppers, tomatoes, onion, etc.

CRISPY TEMPEH RICE BOWLS
with Steamed Greens

6+ Plant Points

Makes 2 bowls

My favourite parts of this dish are the different textures: crispy tempeh, chewy rice, soft greens. Textures aren't discussed enough. They add so much to our dietary experience and aren't to be underrated.

95 g uncooked brown rice

70 g broccoli florets, cut into small pieces

3 tablespoons low-sodium tamari or soy sauce

140 g kale, stems removed, chopped

Juice of 1 large lemon

1 tablespoon olive oil or stock

115 g tempeh, very finely chopped

1½ tablespoons tahini

1 teaspoon date paste or 100% maple syrup

¼ teaspoon crushed red pepper flakes (optional)

Supercharge It! (optional toppings):

½ cucumber, chopped

2 spring onions, chopped (green parts only)

1 tablespoon hemp seeds

2 teaspoons sesame seeds

1. Bring a large pan of water—at least 720 ml—to a boil. Add the brown rice and reduce the heat to low and allow to simmer, covered, for 30 minutes. Taste for doneness; the rice should be almost al dente. Next, add in the broccoli and cook for about 5 more minutes, until just tender.

2. Drain the rice and broccoli and return them to the pot. Season with 1 tablespoon of the tamari and set aside.

3. While the rice is cooking, set up a steamer basket in a large pan with water on the bottom. Bring to the boil, then add the kale to the steamer basket and reduce the heat to low. Steam for 7 minutes, or until the kale is tender.

4. Remove the cooked kale from the pan, drain the water, and remove the steamer basket. Return the kale to the pan and toss with half the lemon juice.

5. While the greens are steaming, heat the olive oil in a frying pan over medium heat. Sauté the tempeh until slightly brown and crisp, 5 to 8 minutes. Remove from the heat and set aside.

RECIPE CONTINUES

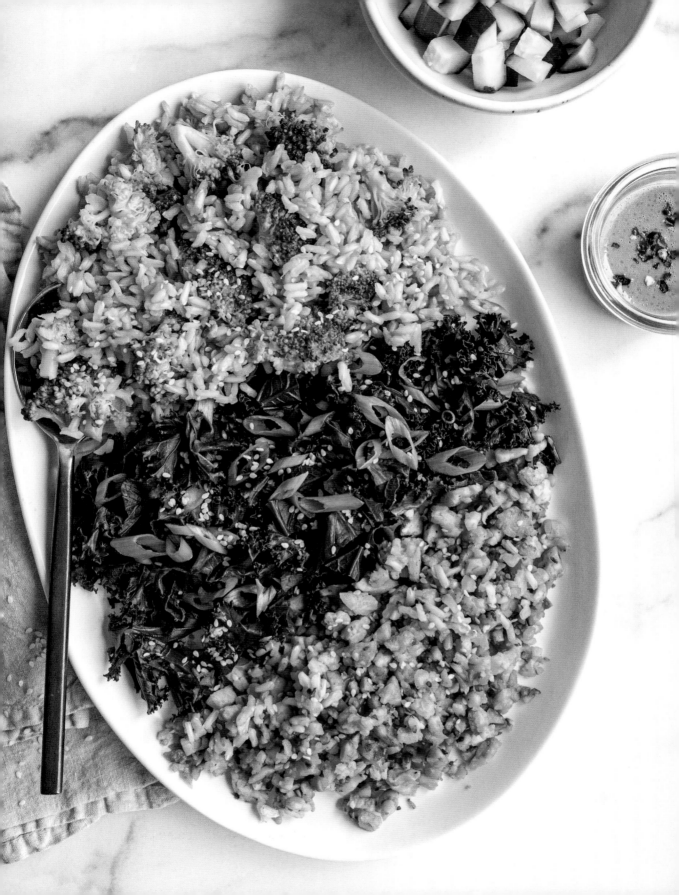

6. While the tempeh is cooking, whisk together the remaining 2 tablespoons tamari, the remaining lemon juice, the tahini, date paste, and red pepper flakes, if using. Slowly drizzle in 2 tablespoons water until the dressing is creamy and thick. Season to taste, adding in more lemon/salt/pepper/tahini as desired.

7. To serve, divide the rice and broccoli mixture between two bowls. Add half of the kale to each bowl and sprinkle the cooked tempeh on top. Garnish with the supercharged toppings of your choice, then drizzle with the dressing.

PRO TIP:

Steaming your greens reduces the oxalic acid content by up to 53 per cent, which increases the bioavailability of minerals like calcium, iron, and magnesium.

AUBERGINE HUMMUS BUDDHA BOWL

11 Plant Points

Makes 2 bowls

Buddha bowls are always a winner for colour, beauty, plant diversity, and flavour. I highly recommend adding some tofu feta on this one (for Homemade Tofu Feta, go to page 84)!

FODMAP note: 40 g canned chickpeas per serving and 5 cherry tomatoes per serving is low FODMAP.

85 g canned chickpeas, drained and rinsed

1 teaspoon garlic-infused olive oil (see Pro Tip, page 87), stock, or water

¼ teaspoon ground cumin

¼ teaspoon smoked paprika

Salt and freshly ground black pepper

300 g cooked brown rice

120 g Roasted Aubergine Dip (page 74)

10 g chopped fresh flat-leaf parsley

80 g Kalamata olives, roughly chopped

100 g cherry tomatoes, halved

1 medium cucumber, thinly sliced into half moons

1 medium carrot, grated

1. Preheat the oven to 200°C. Line a rimmed baking tray with parchment paper or a silicone baking mat and set aside.

2. Toss the chickpeas with the garlic-infused olive oil, cumin, smoked paprika, salt, and pepper on the prepared baking tray. Bake for about 15 minutes, or until slightly crisp.

3. To assemble the bowls, divide the brown rice between two bowls, then top each with the aubergine dip, parsley, olives, tomatoes, cucumber, carrots, and crispy chickpeas.

FF UNLEASHED:

If you are not following a low FODMAP approach, you can add more canned chickpeas or substitute dried, cooked chickpeas if you are not restricting FODMAPs. You can also add more than 5 cherry tomatoes per serving.

>> *To view the 69 scientific references cited in this chapter, please visit www.theplantfedgut.com/cookbook.*

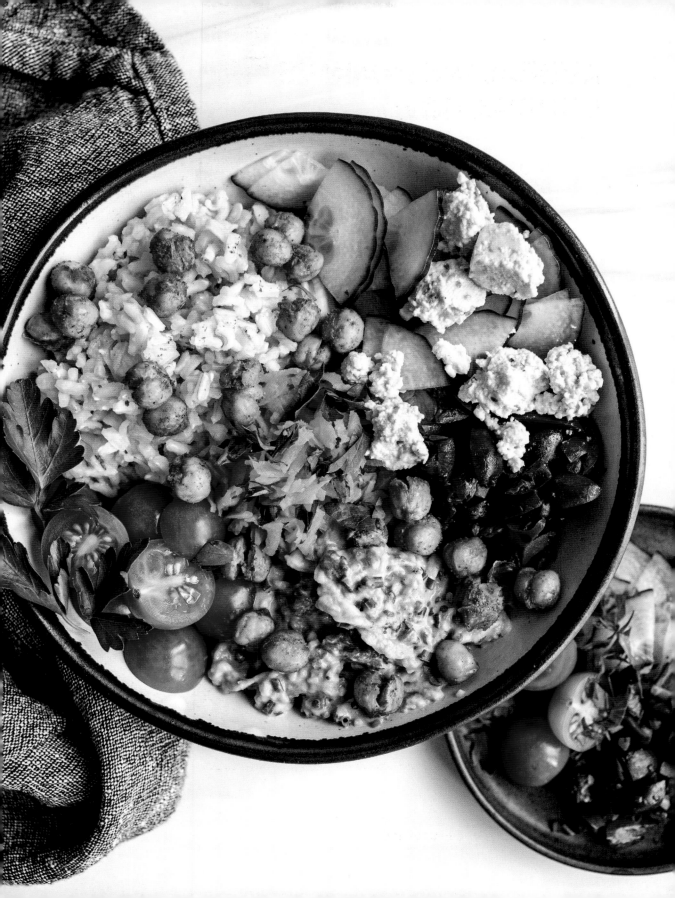

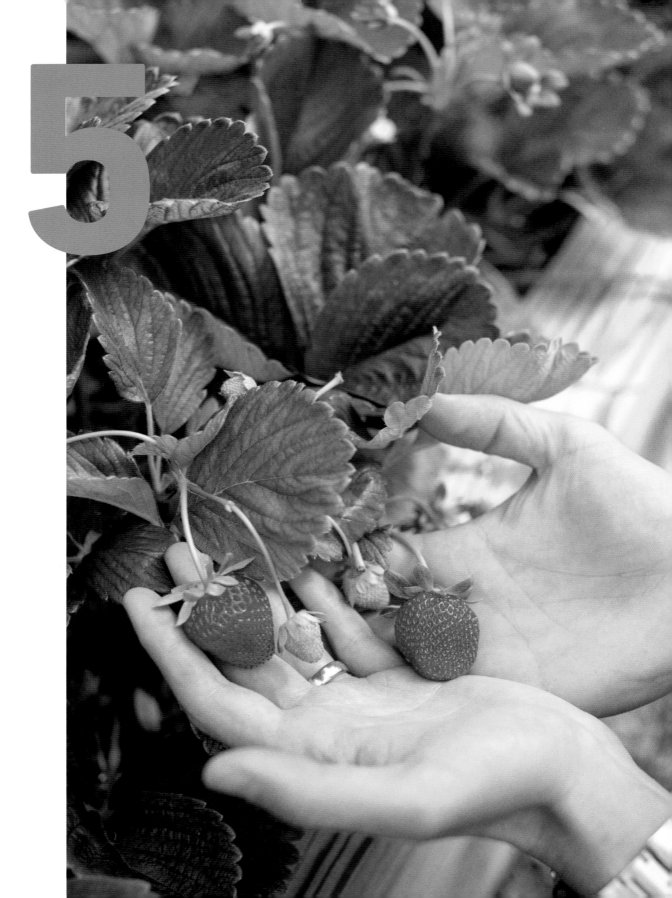

Hope for Histamine Intolerance

Histamine may be the cause of your symptoms. Here are the knowledge and recipes you need to figure it out.

Do you remember where you were in May 2020? Most of the world was in lockdown due to the rapidly evolving global pandemic, and I was launching my first book, *Fibre Fuelled*. But Sweden chose a contrarian approach and kept restaurants and most businesses open. It's during this time that there was an outbreak of people with swelling, hives, irregular heartbeat, headaches, nausea, diarrhoea, and vomiting across the country. Thirty people in the first outbreak, nine more in early June, and then another twenty in July—all in different locations. The authorities got involved, and the epidemiologists traced everything back to three restaurants. Were these superspreader events the result of the novel coronavirus punishing Sweden for its open table policy? No. It was a case of bad tuna.

Scombroid poisoning is what happens when you ingest fish that has extremely high histamine levels due to improper processing or storage. Believe it or not, it's not an infection at all. It's purely the effect of excessive histamine. Histamine is a chemical produced in the body that is involved in a number of normal, healthy bodily functions. We actually need histamine to function properly. But when we ingest an overwhelming amount all at once, we can get the reaction you see on the right, which is known as histamine intoxication. It also can occur with bad cheese (although most cases are due to fish). In this outbreak, they were able to trace the tuna back to one common source overseas.

Behold the power of histamine! Histamine and FODMAP intolerance are the two most important food intolerances based upon my clinical experience. FODMAP intolerance is much more mainstream, while histamine intolerance doesn't usually get much attention. I'm excited to introduce you to it because I sincerely believe this is life-changing information that's going to connect some dots and be an aha moment for a few of you.

Histamine intolerance can present with digestive problems; it can also be the root cause of lots of other issues: migraine headaches, dizziness or light-headedness, rapid or irregular heartbeat, flushing, eczema, hives, itchy skin, shortness of breath, wheezing, or allergy symptoms like runny nose, congestion, and sneezing. I'll help you apply the GROWTH strategy to properly identify whether or not you have histamine intolerance and what you can do about it.

One of my goals is to shine a light on the broad effects of histamine in the body. Whether it's you or someone you know, histamine intolerance could potentially be both the source of the problem *and* the solution. So don't be shy about sharing what you learn in this chapter—you can help me get this book into the hands of those who need it! Post your favourite facts to social media. Help me get the word out! There are far too many people out there suffering with these symptoms who have no clue that *this* may be their problem.

Histamine Explained

Let's take it from the top: Histidine is one of the twenty amino acids that are the building blocks of protein, and it also happens to be the precursor to histamine. When histidine comes into contact with an enzyme—L-histidine decarboxylase for my fellow nerds out there—it gets converted into histamine. Many species of bacteria have this enzyme and do this as a normal part of fermentation or in the life cycle of food (ripening before decaying). You'll also find these same bacteria as a part of the normal gut flora. But the main source of histamine inside the body is produced by immune cells called basophils and mast cells. There are also nerves, blood platelets, and cells lining the intestine that store histamine and are prepared to release it when stimulated.

Histamine is a normal and important part of human physiology. There are four different histamine receptors spread throughout the body in the digestive tract, skin, heart and peripheral blood vessels, the brain, lungs, bone marrow, and uterus. Yeah, that's almost everything. Histamine is a signalling molecule with broad and far-reaching effects: stimulating smooth muscle constriction in the lungs or gut, increasing acid production in the stomach, relaxing blood vessels. In women, histamine increases oestrogen production. In men, histamine plays a role in penile erection. When the body is in balance, histamine is an important part of that balance and poses absolutely no threat to us. We have those receptors for good reasons, not because it's bad.

Histamine intolerance is caused by the loss of balance within the body, leading to excessive histamine stimulation of those receptors. The end result can be the manifestation of the aforementioned symptoms. In a recent review of patients with confirmed histamine intolerance, they found the number one symptom was bloating. Almost everyone had bloating. After that, the symptoms scatter in literally thousands of directions. There were more than twenty-four different symptoms registered. A total of 97 per cent had three or more different symptoms. The average number of symptoms experienced by an individual patient was eleven! This is the first of several challenges when it comes to histamine intolerance. The presentation can be wildly varied, making it extremely difficult to assign a pattern of symptoms to the condition.

Respiratory system
Runny nose
Nasal congestion
Sneezing
Shortness of breath

Cardiovascular system
Heart palpitations
Rapid heart rate
Irregular heart rhythm
Light-headedness
Low blood pressure
High blood pressure

GI tract
Bloating
Fullness after meals
Diarrhoea
Abdominal pain
Constipation
Cramping
Belching
Nausea
Vomiting
Heartburn

Skin itching
Flushing
Rash/eczema
Hives
Swollen, reddened eyelids

Other symptoms
Painful menses
Dizziness
Insomnia
Headache
Migraine
Fatigue
Ringing in ears

Histamine and Hormones

Histamine is a normal part of women's health. For better or for worse, histamine and oestrogen are tied together like Bonnie and Clyde. Oestrogen promotes more histamine. Histamine promotes more oestrogen. When they surge, they surge together. Things are great when they are in balance. Histamine plays a role in women's libido, ovulation, and even the implantation of a fertilized egg into the uterus—all important things. But when histamine and oestrogen go "ride or die," things get a little bit scary. Oestrogen levels surge during ovulation, immediately before menstruation. Histamine levels surge in parallel. This may explain why some women experience headaches or worsening of digestive symptoms at this point during their cycle. But here's an interesting thing: During pregnancy, when oestrogen levels are through the absolute roof, histamine intolerance symptoms often improve. It's paradoxical, until you realize that the placenta produces five hundred to a thousand times more of the enzyme that breaks down histamine (diamine oxidase, or DAO) than is typical before pregnancy. Seriously, the intelligence of the human body and nature is just amazing, isn't it? The takeaway point here is that hormones and histamine are interconnected and this may explain differences in food sensitivity or the manifestation of symptoms at specific points during the menstrual cycle.

Despite the complexity of it all, understanding histamine intolerance doesn't need to be difficult. In fact, it's quite simple: If you suffer from two or more of these symptoms, then you should consider whether the cause is histamine intolerance. Take a look at the list on page 125. Do you have two of those symptoms? If you were sitting across from me in the clinic, I would look you in the eyes and say, "Histamine intolerance is one of the things that we need to consider here. If you're not getting better, then we need to take the steps necessary to determine whether or not this is the source of your problem." In the GROWTH strategy, we start by identifying the genesis of our symptoms. Could histamine intolerance be the genesis for you? In this chapter, I will be showing you how to Restrict, Observe, and Work It Back In to determine if it is.

Histamine Balance and How We Get Tipped Over

The body thrives on balance and rhythm. When the body is in balance, histamine that is in our diet gets broken down in the small intestine and colon by an enzyme called DAO. The gateway for histamine into the body is the single layer of cells lining the intestine called the epithelium. DAO serves as our defence system to neutralize the histamine before it crosses that barrier.

Histamine intolerance is a condition of histamine excess relative to the body's neutralizing systems. Picture DAO as the soldiers lined up in front of your castle wall (the epithelium), making sure it doesn't get overrun with histamine. When DAO levels are adequate and the castle wall is intact, histamine is entirely neutralized. But if the histamine levels overwhelm the defences, then it enters into the citadel. That is when we manifest symptoms.

It is a threshold event. If you stay below the threshold, then you will remain symptom-free. But if you cross the threshold, you'll start to run into trouble. The problem is that the threshold can be a moving target, different for every single one of us and even fluctuating from day to day. If we want to understand histamine intolerance, then we need to dig deeper into the three main factors that determine whether we have histamine harmony:

1. Excessive histamine: We know that histamine is formed by bacteria as a part of fermentation as well as the ripening and deterioration of perishable food. What this means is that the histamine content of a food varies based upon what stage in its maturation process it is. For example, we talked about the case of the bad tuna in Sweden. If you had consumed that same tuna immediately at the time of catch, this would never have happened. But it was the time between catch and the poor preservation of the fish that allowed the microbes to work on the histidine in the fish and produce the histamine.

General Pointers to Avoid Higher Histamine Levels

In a moment, we will review the specific foods that you need to be cautious with on a low-histamine diet. But before we discuss specifics, let's discuss themes:

- Eat fresh food whenever possible. Most fresh fruits and vegetables are totally in play!
- Perishable food has the least histamine at harvest, and histamine levels will then continue to rise.
- Cooling slows down histamine production. Freezing slows it even more. If a product is frozen immediately after harvest, this protects against histamine release.
- All fermented foods are high in histamine.
- Alcohol is a fermented food. So is chocolate. And vinegar. Sorry!
- Try to avoid canned foods, ready meals, and processed perishable foods.
- Frying and grilling foods increases histamine levels.

» Histamine in your diet isn't the only potential way for you to have excessive histamine levels. The other route is by stimulating your own immune cells to release their histamine. There are some foods—citrus, for example—that are not inherently high in histamine but are thought to trigger histamine release. Don't worry, I'm going to make it super simple for you. The master list of foods that produce excessive histamine will include all of this, so you don't need to sweat the details. I just want you to have a complete understanding of how this works before I provide the simple solutions.

» There are also microbes living inside our gut that have the enzymes to produce histamine. We don't have evidence yet that production of histamine by our own gut microbes is a driver of histamine intolerance, but it's worth noting that our gut microbes do have this functionality and therefore may play a role in histamine balance.

2. Inadequate DAO activity: DAO is our soldier standing at the gates, defending us from histamine overload. But there are a number of ways that DAO levels can be impaired and ultimately become inadequate to control histamine breakdown.

» DAO is produced by the cells lining our intestine. If you damage those cells, you may impair their ability to produce DAO. Coeliac disease, Crohn's disease, ulcerative colitis, small intestine bacterial overgrowth, irritable bowel syndrome, short bowel syndrome, and gastrointestinal surgeries are some of the conditions that have been linked to reduced DAO production. Treat the root cause, and DAO levels will rise.

» It's possible to have a gene that alters the function of DAO, reducing the rate of histamine degradation. It's also possible to have very minor substitutions in the code for the amine oxidase copper-containing 1 gene, known as AOC1. These small alterations, which can affect 27 per cent or more of individuals, have been associated with reduced production of DAO. It's common enough that personal genetic reporting companies like SelfDecode can predict if a person has a higher likelihood of developing histamine intolerance.

» DAO activity can be inhibited by drugs, alcohol, and other foods. For example, there are food components called biogenic amines that are structurally similar to histamine and can alter DAO activity. In this case, DAO insufficiency is temporary and reversible by simply removing the offending agent. Don't worry, I will make it super simple with a list of the foods and medications to look out for on pages 132 and 133.

3. Gut microbiome disturbance: There's a strong association between food intolerance and irritable bowel syndrome (IBS). A full 80 per cent of IBS patients identify food as triggering their GI symptoms and more than half report worsening of their symptoms when consuming high-histamine foods. Perhaps we can understand histamine intolerance better by looking more closely at the condition it is most strongly associated with—irritable bowel syndrome. The old-school docs, like my mentor Dr. Doug Drossman, taught us that irritable bowel syndrome involves altered visceral hypersensitivity, where the five hundred million nerves lining

your gut become jumpy and overactive. The new-school docs like me emphasize the role of dysbiosis in irritable bowel syndrome, which includes deranged gut microbes, increased intestinal permeability, and leakage of intestinal contents into the bloodstream. But we're actually saying the same thing because increased intestinal permeability has been found to coexist with visceral hypersensitivity. The concern is that damage to the gut microbiota (dysbiosis) may make it easier to have food intolerances through these mechanisms. Could this be underlying histamine intolerance? Yes! Detailed microbiome analysis of patients with histamine intolerance revealed bacterial patterns and loss of diversity indicative of dysbiosis. In simple terms, I'm saying that a damaged gut lowers the threshold and makes it easier to have histamine intolerance. But the opposite is also true: If we heal the gut, then we can restore competence to the epithelial barrier like resurrecting a castle wall to its most powerful might and glory. Raising the wall will raise your threshold for histamine tolerance. Your gut can be healed, and when it is, you will be more equipped to handle histamines.

So Should We Take Probiotics to Treat Histamine Intolerance?

We have to be careful here. Some of the common probiotic strains—*Lactobacillus casei, Lactobacillus bulgaricus, Streptococcus thermophilus, Lactobacillus delbrueckii, Lactobacillus helveticus*—are known histamine producers. We also don't yet have a high-quality, randomized, placebo-controlled trial of probiotics for histamine intolerance. Given the complexity of histamine intolerance, we don't want to take chances with a multistrain probiotic. Instead, we want to keep it simple and lean on what we know. *Saccharomyces boulardii* is the most studied probiotic that exists. Its safety and efficacy have been studied in more than ninety clinical trials. It strengthens the intestinal barrier by repairing tight junctions, leading to reduced intestinal permeability. It improves the production of SCFAs, specifically butyrate. But perhaps most important for our discussion on histamine, *Saccharomyces boulardii* has been shown to increase DAO levels. Until we have randomized controlled trials of probiotics in histamine intolerance, the best available data suggest to me that *Saccharomyces boulardii* at a dose of 500 to 1,000 mg daily may be beneficial and a good choice for people with histamine intolerance. This is always with the caveat that if you feel like it is actually making your symptoms worse, then you should stop it.

Diagnosing Histamine Intolerance Using the GROWTH Strategy

"Is it possible that histamine intolerance is the cause of my symptoms?"

That's the first question for you to ponder. If you have two or more of the symptoms of histamine intolerance, then it would make sense for you to take the steps necessary to determine whether you in fact have the condition. If you don't have the symptoms, I have good news for you. In the pages that follow are some seriously delicious recipes developed for all to enjoy, whether you have histamine intolerance or not.

But for those of you looking to determine if you have histamine intolerance, getting a blood test for DAO unfortunately isn't a reliable way to diagnose histamine intolerance. The threshold for histamine intolerance is a moving target that isn't simply proportional to the amount of DAO circulating in the blood. It is the balance among histamine, DAO, and the competence of the intestinal barrier. This balance and whether it elicits symptoms (and which ones) is specific to you, and it will vary from day to day and from meal to meal.

Sounds complicated, right? This complexity, and the absence of a gold standard test, has contributed to our difficulties in identifying patients with histamine intolerance and also in conducting high-quality research.

But it doesn't need to be so complicated. We will simply apply the GROWTH strategy, which once again takes a complex process and makes it simple while simultaneously being reliable and guiding us toward healing.

G: Genesis

First, we need to make sure that the genesis of your symptoms isn't something else. Earlier I mentioned that coeliac disease, Crohn's disease, and ulcerative colitis are all associated with histamine intolerance because they disrupt the intestinal lining. There are also the diagnoses that we discussed in Chapter 3, such as constipation and gallbladder issues, that need to be considered. But going beyond these players, I want to introduce you to two new factors that need to be considered—food allergy and mast cell activation syndrome.

Food allergies can present with many of the same symptoms often attributed to histamine. We need to make the distinction because histamine intolerance is not an immune-mediated allergic condition, so if you have a food allergy, the treatment and approach will be different. In order to know whether you have histamine intolerance or a food allergy, keep a record of the food you eat and your symptoms. Histamine intolerance symptoms should occur with a broad mix of foods (the ones described on page 133), whereas a food allergy should be specific to specific foods. If needed, skin-prick and IgE antibody testing for food allergies could be considered with an allergist to help bring clarity to this question.

Mast cell activation syndrome is another condition sometimes confused with histamine intolerance. It is characterized by episodes with sudden onset of severe symptoms—hives, swelling, low blood pressure, difficulty breathing, and severe diarrhoea—all similar symptoms to histamine intolerance, albeit generally more intense. Mast cells are actually the body's innate carriers of histamine, and during mast cell activation they essentially pour their histamine into your blood. If your symptoms are intense and episodic, you may want to be checked for mast cell activation syndrome, which involves getting your blood checked for tryptase within two hours of an episode (I will generally give the laboratory order to my patient to have on hand) and a twenty-four-hour urine collection to look for specific markers of mast cell activation. Similar to food allergy, if you think mast cell activation syndrome is a possibility, then you should consult with an allergist.

It's also very common for people with histamine intolerance to simultaneously have *other* food intolerances, specifically lactose and fructose intolerance. Annoying? Absolutely. Surprising? Definitely not. The common thread is that food intolerances occur in people who have a damaged gut. You don't see intolerances in people with a healthy gut unless they have a genetic reason. As described above, there are a number of ways that dysbiosis can predispose us to struggle in processing our food. But if damage to the gut is the root of the problem, then we also know where we'll find our solution.

You may also be concerned you may have intolerance of both FODMAPs and histamine. If this is the case, I'd encourage you to start by first following the low FODMAP approach. In a randomized, controlled trial of high versus low FODMAP, researchers found that the low FODMAP diet actually reduced histamine levels eightfold. After you get control of the FODMAPs, you can always move forwards with evaluating histamine intolerance. Given the complexity, a registered dietitian would certainly come in handy.

Let's Talk about the Connection between Histamine and Gluten

There is a strong overlap between histamine intolerance and coeliac disease. In fact, a recent study discovered that among people with coeliac disease who are not improving on a gluten-free diet, more than 50 per cent of the time it is due to histamine intolerance. As we discussed in Chapter 3, you're going to want to make sure that coeliac disease is not present, as most of the symptoms that you find in histamine intolerance can also be coeliac disease. Definitive testing with genetic or small intestine biopsies is needed, and if coeliac disease is present, then gluten needs to be removed entirely from the diet.

But should everyone who is histamine intolerant be gluten-free? I haven't seen enough evidence to convince me that there's a great benefit to it, although generally reduction of gluten-containing food inadvertently leads to a reduction in histamine intake, which may improve symptoms. The problem is that it's a step towards further dietary restriction, which can lead to nutritional deficiencies and cause damage to the gut microbiota. If you choose to go gluten-free, I encourage you to make an effort to still get your wholegrains from the gluten-free wholegrains—quinoa, sorghum, teff, millet, amaranth, buckwheat, brown rice. Low-gluten diets have been associated with increased risk of type 2 diabetes and coronary artery disease, driven by the reduction in wholegrains by eliminating the gluten-containing foods. If you include gluten-containing foods, make them high-quality sources like organic whole wheat, Ezekiel, or rye bread. Either way, make sure to get your wholegrains, people! They have prebiotic fibre, oligosaccharides, and resistant starches. Your gut microbes love them.

Before we Restrict, Observe, and Work It Back In, let's pause and review your medication list. Remember what Dr. Lesesne taught us: "Step 1: Make sure it's not the meds." There are medications associated with histamine intolerance, and if you are using one of them, it may be worthwhile to have a conversation with your GP to discuss whether there would be a safe and appropriate substitution that could be made.

Medications Associated with Histamine Intolerance

Adapted from Comas-Baste et al., Biomolecules. 2020 Aug; 10(8): 1181.; Maintz et al., Am J Clin Nutr. 2007 May;85(5): 1185–96.

Acetylcysteine	Chloroquine	Ibuprofen	Pentamidine
Acetylsalicyclic acid	Cimetidine	Isoniazid	Pethidine
Alcuronium	Clavulanic acid	Metamizole	Prilocaine
Alprenolol	Clonidine	Metoclopramide	Prometazina
Ambroxol	Colistimethate	Morphine	Propafenone
Amiloride	Cyclophosphamide	Naproxen	Suxamethonium
Aminophylline	D-tubocurarine	Nonsteroidal anti-inflammatory drugs	Thiopental
Amitriptyline	Diclofenac		Verapamil
Cefotiam	Dihydralazine	Pancuronium	
Cefuroxime	Dobutamine		

R: Restrict

Every food has histamine. That histamine content varies based upon the context—specifically, whether a food is fresh, fermented, fried, smoked, canned, or cooled. Histamine cannot be fully avoided; there's no such thing as "histamine-free." It's also not to be vilified, because histamine is an important and necessary part of human physiology. But like breathing oxygen and drinking water, we want your histamine intake to be in balance with your body. Identifying that balance requires us to temporarily reduce the amount of histamine in your diet.

So our goal during this phase is not to avoid all histamine, because that's impossible, but to get you to a place where your symptoms improve. Then we'll figure out which histamines you're sensitive to and what your threshold is. Our plan is to enter into an initial, temporary restrictive phase for two weeks. In some cases, this may need to be extended beyond two weeks. There is no master list of histamine-containing foods—it boils down to your individual response. To keep it simple, I'm going to give you a list of foods that most frequently cause histamine intolerance and walk you through some key points about restriction. I'll also include space for you to write in foods you discover your unique gut has sensitivity to.

Foods to Avoid During a Histamine Restriction Phase

Adapted from Comas-Baste et al., Biomolecules. 2020 Aug; 10(8): 1181.; Maintz et al., Am J Clin Nutr. 2007 May;85(5): 1185-96.

Plants			Animal products
Alcohol	Lentils (canned)	Teas: black, green, maté	Cheese
Aubergine	Liquorice	Tomatoes	Eggs
Avocado	Mushrooms	Vinegar and vinegar-containing foods (pickles, olives)	Fish, canned or preserved fish, fish derivatives like sauces
Banana	Nuts and nut milks, walnuts, cashews		
Chickpeas (canned)			Ham
Chocolate, cocoa, cacao	Papaya		Milk, fermented milk
Citrus foods	Peanuts		Pork
Coffee (caffeinated)	Pineapple		Sausages, sliced deli meats, hot dogs, and other processed meats
Dried fruits: apricots, prunes, dates, figs, raisins	Plum		
	Spices		
	Spinach		Shellfish
Energy drinks	Soybeans (canned), soy milk, fermented and unfermented soy derivatives		
Fermented plant foods like sauerkraut, kimchi, tempeh, miso, etc.			
Fruit juices	Strawberries		
Kiwi			

It may seem like the list is long, so let's break this down a little bit.

- Spinach, aubergine, tomato, and avocado are the classic high-histamine plants. They are to be avoided during the restriction phase. But it's worth mentioning that their histamine content varies and depends on time relative to harvest. If you have a garden and harvest these plants for immediate consumption, their histamine content is relatively low.

- Soy milk and nut milks are on this list, but oat milk is fair game. It's actually super easy to make oat milk at home. I learned this recipe from my friend Dana Shultz of Minimalist Baker. Simply buzz 1 cup of water with ¼ cup of organic rolled oats in a blender for 30 to 45 seconds. Whoomp, there it is.

- Citrus fruits, papaya, pineapple, and strawberries are not inherently high in histamine, but they are thought to trigger the release of histamine within the body. Plan to eliminate them during histamine restriction, but then consider them for reintroduction during the maintenance phase.

- Apple cider vinegar is generally well tolerated in histamine intolerance, while most other vinegar is not. Makes it tough when you don't have citrus, either! Opt for apple cider vinegar that is pasteurized without "the mother" in this case.

- Spices are a bit tricky! There are also some simple substitutions to reduce histamine content. For example, if you use pink peppercorns instead of black peppercorns or sweet paprika instead of spicy paprika, you reduce histamine content. We also made the spices optional so that you can avoid them during the restriction phase, but then start working them back in once you're in the maintenance phase. And obviously, if you're not here to test histamine but want delicious recipes, keep the spices in there!

- Our traditional Biome Stock should be modified to make it lower in histamine. You'll find a low-histamine version on page 159.

- Legumes like beans, lentils, and peas contain biogenic amines that reduce DAO activity and are therefore likely to worsen histamine intolerance when consumed from a can. Therefore, I recommend using dried legumes. If you boil the legumes, you will transfer the biogenic amines into the boiling water, which you can then discard. But the ideal way to reduce the biogenic amine content is through pressure-cooking your legumes.

How to Pressure-Cook Your Legumes

1. Rinse and sort your dried legumes. Make sure no pebbles have snuck in.

2. Place 450 g dried beans and 2 litres water in the pressure cooker. You can add a bay leaf and half an onion if desired for added flavour.

3. Cook your legumes for the specified time:

Dried beans, lentils, and peas	Dry cooking time (minutes)
Black beans	20-25
Black-eyed peas	14-18
Broad beans	12-14
Chickpeas	35-40
Lentils	8-10
Peas	16–20
Pinto beans	25-30
Red kidney beans	15-20

4. Let the pressure release naturally for at least 20 minutes prior to opening the pressure cooker.

5. Add salt if desired after pressure-cooking.

6. Makes about 1 kilo of beans. The legumes can be stored with a little cooking liquid (to keep moist) in the fridge, or freeze for up to 3 months. With histamine intolerance, you'd prefer to consume them as close to preparation as possible unless frozen.

Dr. B's Advice

Many legumes are capable of actually producing the DAO enzyme when sprouted, creating a plant-based source of DAO enzyme to boost your defences against histamine intolerance. In fact, in many cases the DAO activity is substantially higher than that found in animal sources like pig kidneys. Properly sprouted peas have the highest activity, 77 per cent more than you'll find in pig kidneys! Does it get any cooler? Yeah, it does. On page 348, I will teach you how to create pea sprouts for maximum DAO activity from the friendly confines of your home. But bear in mind, all pea, lentil, soybean, and chickpea sprouts are DAO boosters, regardless of how many days and what condition they were sprouted in. It's part of the magic of sprouting that we will be covering in Chapter 11! If you have histamine intolerance and aren't sprouting yet, you have been served!

Boosting Your Nutrients

It's important to be mindful of potential nutritional deficiencies on a low-histamine diet. Vitamin B_6, magnesium, calcium, and iron are particular points of vulnerability. The answer? GREENS AND BEANS, baby.

Leafy greens (minus spinach) are the most nutrient-dense foods on the planet, so it's no surprise that they're also a great source of magnesium, calcium, and iron (not to mention fibre!). Lean into leafy greens while on a low-histamine diet to access all those sweet nutrients.

Beans are perhaps my favourite microbiome food. Like wholegrains, they have fibre, oligosaccharides, and resistant starches—all of which are prebiotic and feed your gut microbiota. They also happen to be a great source of magnesium, calcium, and iron and do often contain vitamin B_6, particularly chickpeas.

GREENS AND BEANS should be on the same level as some of the great pairs in history—Kermit and Miss Piggy, Snoop Dogg and Dr. Dre, Netflix and Chill. My heart flutters just considering the nutrient density of these two together.

GREENS AND BEANS can take you a long way, but we need to keep it real on vitamin B_6. By restricting bananas, tomato sauce, spinach, and avocado, we are also restricting access to many of our B_6 sources. This is problematic because B_6 is a cofactor in DAO activity, meaning that you need adequate stores of B_6 in order for DAO to function properly. You'll find B_6 in multivitamins, B-complex vitamins, and as a stand-alone supplement. Pyridoxal 5′-phosphate (P5P) is the most absorbable source of B_6, if absorption is a concern. The recommended dietary allowance for adults is between 1.3 and 1.7 mg per day, depending on age and gender. Deficiency is more common than you would expect, affecting about 1 in 4 Americans and even 11 per cent who are actually taking a B_6 supplement! The good news is that we have the ability to test levels, to make sure that while taking a B_6 supplement you are not only nutritionally adequate but also not overshooting.

Histamine-Friendly Flavour Substitutions

Higher Histamine	Lower Histamine
Aubergine	Courgette
Cinnamon/cloves/nutmeg	Ginger
Jelly/jam	Mash fresh blueberry, mango, or peach with a fork
Banana	Cantaloupe
Tomato sauce	1. Cook and purée a blend of root vegetables and squashes with a lot of basil and Italian spices to make a sauce and freeze it. 2. Sauté greens with onions and garlic to cover pasta.
Pumpkin	Sweet potato
Spinach	Baby kale or spring greens
Citrus/pineapple/kiwi	Mango, peach
Plum	Apricot, peach
Strawberries	Blackberries, blueberries
Peanut or cashew butter	Almond or sunflower butter
Whole/chopped cashews, walnuts, and peanuts	Pumpkin or sunflower seeds
Black peppercorns	Pink peppercorns (they don't grind easily, so the common practice is to grind them in a coffee or spice grinder or to use a mortar and pestle)
Spicy paprika	Sweet paprika
Sweeteners	Fresh fruit purée or fresh apple juice

O: Observe and W: Work It Back In

Throughout this process, maintaining a food sensitivity diary is crucial. Go back to page 31 to see how I set mine up. You want to keep track of how you feel while consuming a low-histamine diet, bearing in mind that the goal is significant improvement in symptoms and to identify what foods trigger your symptoms.

You can view this process as a restrictive phase and a maintenance phase. During the restrictive phase, you're actively lowering histamine to improve symptoms and give your body a break from the histamine war. This takes at least two weeks but may require more time for some.

It's worth mentioning that new research suggests there are perks to being strict during this initial phase. All study participants who strictly followed the low-histamine diet experienced improvement in symptoms, with more than half becoming totally symptom-free. Not only did their symptoms improve, but so did their DAO levels, from a median of 2.5 U/mL up to 7.9 U/mL. By comparison, those with rare or no compliance with the diet did not see any improvement in their DAO levels.

To put these gains into perspective, however, it's worth noting that a DAO level less than 10 U/mL is consistent with histamine intolerance. Strict dietary compliance did not normalize the DAO levels; it raised them. I point this out because we don't want to subject ourselves to a prolonged restrictive diet. Dietary restriction reduces access to the nutrients for the gut microbiota, which limits your ability to heal your gut, and in some cases may actually make your gut health worse. One of our principle strategies for recovery from histamine intolerance is to get your gut health back. It is with this in mind that once your symptoms improve on the low-histamine diet, it's time to move towards reintroduction.

The maintenance phase is where we work things back in and start to assess where our points of vulnerability exist. Throughout this process, we want to be recording about it and creating a log of our experience that we can refer back to in the future. If you have symptoms after consuming a food that you're introducing, make sure to document how much of that food you consumed so that we can establish thresholds.

Reintroducing foods is a stepwise process that should be done systematically and with patience. With dietary changes, low and slow is the way to go! Here's a suggested order to consider:

1. Citrus fruits, strawberries, papaya, kiwi, pineapple
2. Bananas, plums, mushrooms, spices
3. Nuts, teas, coffee
4. Vinegar, avocado
5. Spinach, tomatoes, aubergine

Keep your eyes on the prize. We want to restore balance and harmony to your body. That means putting an end to the histamine war that's been raging. That also means healing your gut.

Low-Histamine Breakfasts

5-Minute Blueberry Pear Oats

Mango Blueberry Smoothie

Sweet Potato Waffles

Blueberry Buckwheat Pancakes

Warm Apple Pie Porridge

Low-Histamine Salads, Soups and Sandwiches

Sunburst Summer Salad

Autumn Kale Salad

Rainbow Farro Salad with Tahini Dressing

Hearty Chopped Salad

Pesto Pasta Salad

Low-Histamine Biome Stock

Roasted Cauliflower Soup

Sweetcorn and Pepper Gazpacho

Very Vegetable Soup

Sweet Potato Hummus Wraps

White Bean Hummus Toast

Low-Histamine Hearty Mains

Sweet Potato and Black Bean Tacos

Sweet Potato Burritos

Quinoa, Corn and Black Bean-Stuffed Peppers

Beetroot Risotto

Sesame Broccoli Noodles

Gado-Gado Quinoa Bowl

Sweet Potato Shawarma Bowl

Mango Burrito Bowl

Stuffed Sweet Potatoes

Simple Spaghetti with Garlicky Kale

5-MINUTE BLUEBERRY PEAR OATS

4+ Plant Points

Serves 2

The soft, ripe pear adds plenty of sweetness to this dish without the use of added sweeteners, which is a beautiful thing.

100 g jumbo oats

Pinch salt

1 teaspoon hemp seeds, chia seeds, or milled flaxseed

½ teaspoon vanilla powder

60 g finely chopped soft, ripe pear

90 g frozen wild or regular blueberries

Supercharge It! (optional toppings):

Chopped mango

Blueberries

Blackberries

Hemp seeds

Chia seeds

Coconut flakes

Chopped pitted dates

Carob Topping (see Pro Tip)

1. Place the oats, 480 ml water, and salt in a medium saucepan over medium-high heat and bring to the boil. Reduce the heat to low and simmer for 5 minutes, stirring often, until thickened.

2. Stir in the hemp seeds, vanilla powder, pear, and blueberries and cook an additional minute to soften.

3. Divide between two bowls, top with supercharged toppings, as desired, and serve.

PRO TIP:

Carob powder is a histamine-friendly cocoa powder alternative. It's easy to make a healthy, vegan hot chocolate sauce called carob topping. Simply blend together 2 tablespoons maple syrup, 2 tablespoons carob powder, and 7 tablespoons warm water until smooth. If you are not restricting histamine, you can substitute cocoa powder if preferred.

FF UNLEASHED:

If you are not restricting histamine, we recommend adding a few chopped dates and stirring in a tablespoon of peanut butter or almond butter for added creaminess.

MANGO BLUEBERRY SMOOTHIE

5+ Plant Points

Serves 2

This smoothie checks all the boxes with healthy plant-based omega-3 fats, prebiotic-rich wholegrains, and polyphenol-laden fruits for a combination that will liven up the party for your gut microbes.

3 tablespoons jumbo oats

2 teaspoons chia seeds

2 tablespoons roughly chopped almonds

½ teaspoon vanilla powder (optional)

Small pinch salt

90 g frozen blueberries, plus more if needed

120 g frozen mango

Supercharge It! (optional toppings):

Chopped mango

Blueberries

Blackberries

Hemp seeds

Chia seeds

Coconut flakes

Carob Topping (see page 139)

1. Combine 360 ml water with the oats, chia seeds, almonds, vanilla powder, if using, and salt in the base of a blender. Blend on high until the chia seeds and almonds are fully broken down and the mixture begins to thicken.

2. Add the frozen blueberries and mango. Blend until creamy and smooth. Add more water/frozen blueberries to get the desired consistency. Top with supercharged toppings, if desired.

PRO TIP:

The classic way to make a smoothie bowl thick and creamy is to freeze the banana, but bananas are high-histamine foods. Therefore, we're using frozen mango, which give us the same nice-cream texture. You can still use a frozen banana, though, if you are not limiting histamine. If you'd like to turn this smoothie into a bowl, use 240 ml water instead of 360 ml water.

FF UNLEASHED:

If you are not restricting histamine, you can substitute vanilla extract for the vanilla powder.

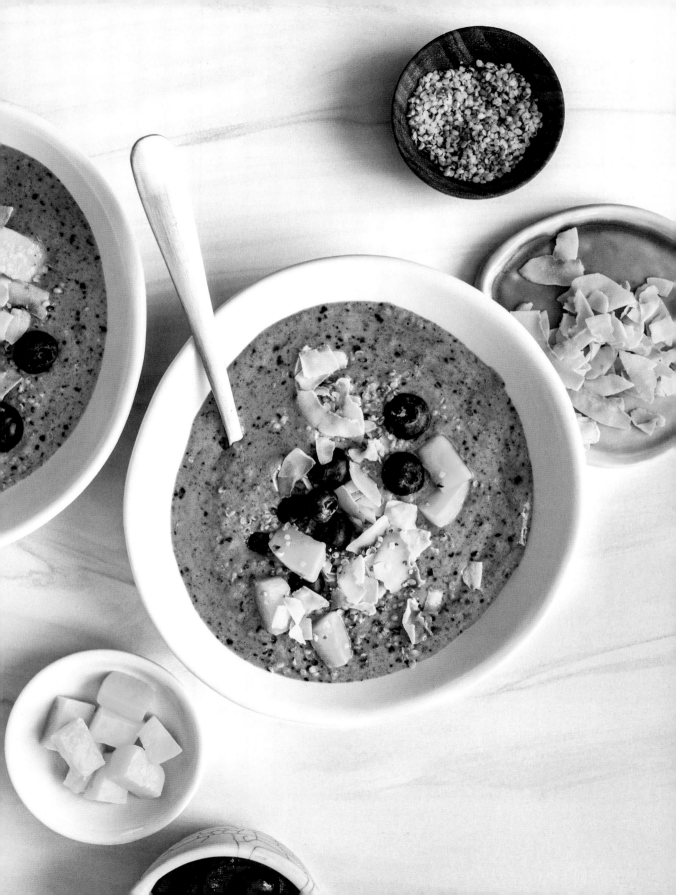

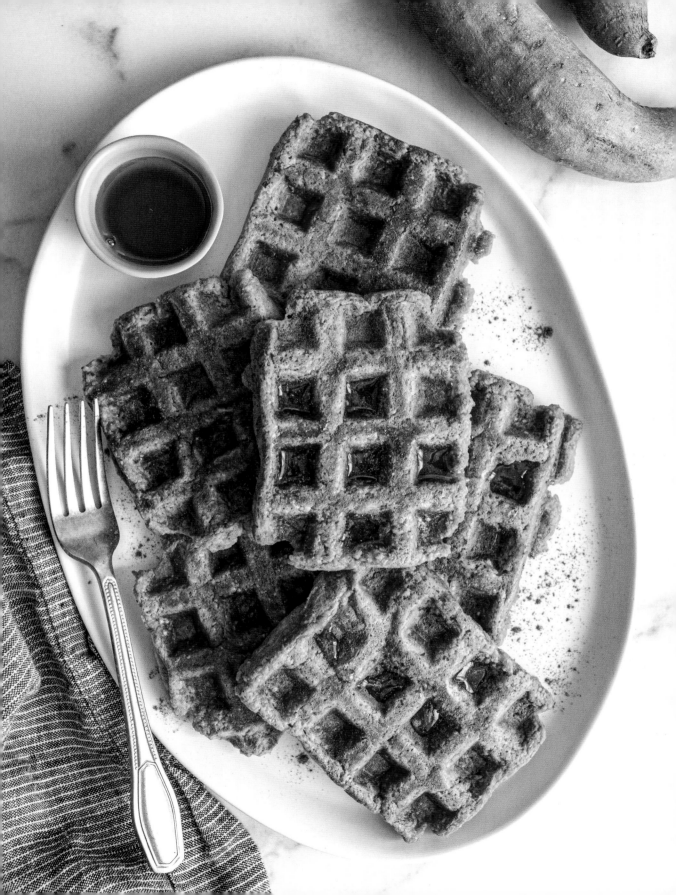

SWEET POTATO WAFFLES

3 Plant Points

Makes 6 waffles

It's a waffle, but made with sweet potatoes, which makes it fun. Orange waffles. Or purple if you're feeling crazy and substitute purple sweet potatoes. These work best on a traditional waffle maker.

1 medium sweet potato

Cooking spray, to grease the waffle maker

300 g jumbo oats

2 tablespoons milled flaxseed

1 tablespoon baking powder

½ teaspoon salt

1 tablespoon vanilla powder

¼ teaspoon ground ginger

⅛ teaspoon ground nutmeg

2 tablespoons avocado oil

1. Preheat the oven to 220°C. Cook the sweet potato in the oven until tender, 45 to 50 minutes. Or pierce the sweet potato with a fork, wrap it in a wet paper towel, and microwave on high for 5 to 6 minutes, until tender. Let cool, then scoop out the flesh and discard the peel.

2. Preheat the waffle maker according to the manufacturer's instructions. Lightly spray with cooking spray.

3. Place the oats in the base of a blender or food processor and process until a fine powder forms. Reserve 200 g of the oat flour for the waffles and reserve the rest to make the oat milk. Place the 200 g oat flour in a large bowl and whisk in the milled flaxseed, baking powder, salt, vanilla powder, ginger, and nutmeg until incorporated.

4. Place 240 ml water and the remaining oat flour in the base of the blender and purée to make oat milk. Add the avocado oil and sweet potato to the blender and purée until smooth. Add more water if too thick.

5. Add the sweet potato mixture to the flour and mix until just combined. It's okay if the batter is thick.

6. Scoop about 100 g of the batter onto the waffle maker, then cook according to the manufacturer's instructions.

FF UNLEASHED:

If you are not restricting histamine, add 1 teaspoon ground cinnamon to the batter.

BLUEBERRY BUCKWHEAT PANCAKES

4 Plant Points

Makes 8 pancakes

Blueberry Buckwheat Pancakes are an act of love for *someone* on a Saturday or Sunday morning. You can share them with others, but after a hard week you deserve a little self-care indulgence. For those wondering, buckwheat is not related to wheat and therefore these pancakes are gluten-free. Please don't let the word "wheat" trigger you.

100 g oat flour or buckwheat flour (or a mix of both)

1 teaspoon baking powder

½ teaspoon bicarbonate of soda

¼ teaspoon salt

⅛ teaspoon ground nutmeg

¼ teaspoon ground ginger

240 ml water or oat milk

1 tablespoon milled flaxseed mixed with 2½ tablespoons of water until gelled

½ teaspoon vanilla powder

90 g peeled, cored, and chopped fresh apple

1 to 2 tablespoons molasses, for sweetness (optional)

190 g frozen wild or regular blueberries

Olive oil or cooking spray, to grease the frying pan or griddle

1. In a large bowl, whisk together the flour, baking powder, bicarbonate of soda, salt, nutmeg, and ginger until well combined.

2. Place the water, milled flaxseed mixture, vanilla powder, apples, and molasses, if using, in the base of a blender and purée until smooth. Add the wet ingredients to the bowl with the dry ingredients and stir until just combined. Stir in the blueberries.

3. Heat a large non-stick frying pan or griddle over medium heat. Lightly coat with oil or cooking spray.

4. Pour the batter onto the pan in 60 ml servings (the batter will be thick) and shape into a circle. Let a few bubbles appear on the surface, then flip and cook the second side for 1 to 2 minutes, until easily lifted from the pan. The pancake colour will be darker than traditional pancakes if you use buckwheat flour. Repeat with the remaining pancakes, oiling the frying pan as needed to prevent sticking.

FF UNLEASHED:

If you are not restricting histamine, you can add ¼ teaspoon ground cinnamon; substitute ½ teaspoon vanilla extract for the vanilla powder.

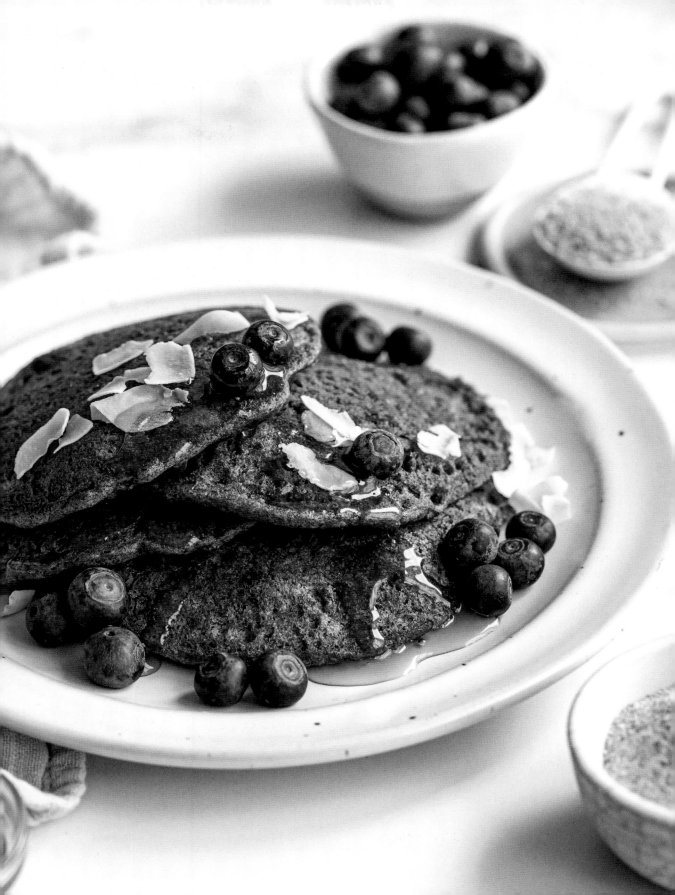

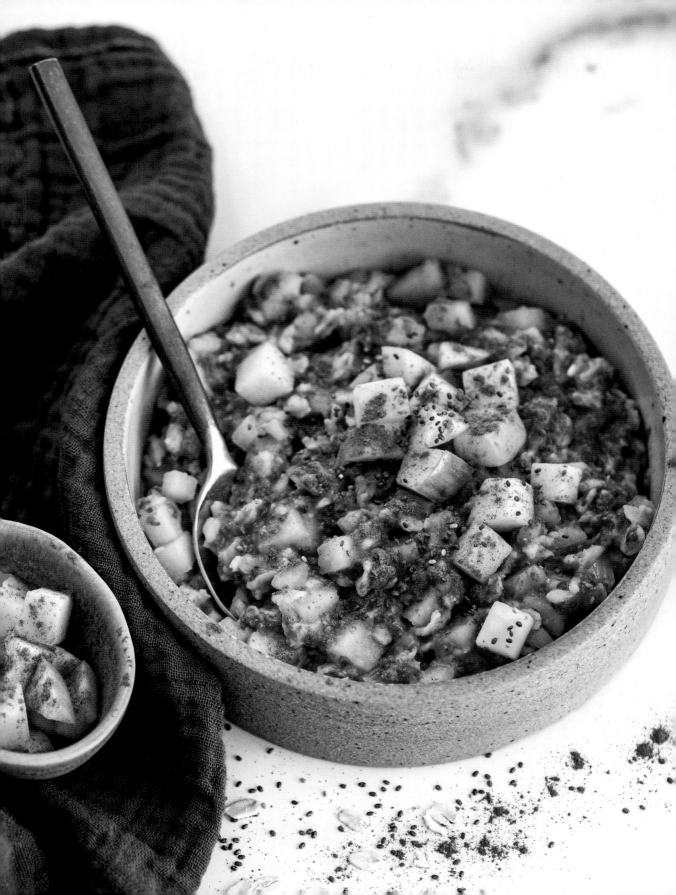

WARM APPLE PIE PORRIDGE

3+ Plant Points

Serves 2

Ginger has been shown to improve nausea and discomfort after meals. It's also been shown to accelerate stomach emptying. My suspicion is that the latter explains the former.

75 g jumbo oats

129 g peeled, cored, and finely chopped apple

1 teaspoon chia seeds

¼ teaspoon ground ginger

125 g unsweetened apple sauce

½ teaspoon vanilla powder

Supercharge It! (optional toppings):

Chopped mango

Blueberries

Blackberries

Hemp seeds

Chia seeds

Coconut flakes

Chopped pitted dates

Carob Topping (see Pro Tip, page 139)

1. In a medium saucepan over medium heat, whisk together the oats, chopped apple, chia seeds, ginger, apple sauce, and 240 ml water.

2. Cook for 10 minutes, stirring often, until the oats are soft and thick. If needed, add in an extra 2 to 3 tablespoons water for desired consistency. Stir in the vanilla powder and divide between two bowls.

3. Enjoy as is or with your favourite low-histamine toppings. If you prefer a sweeter porridge, drizzle 100% maple syrup on top, to taste.

FF UNLEASHED:

If you are not restricting histamine, you can add 1 teaspoon ground cinnamon and ⅛ teaspoon ground nutmeg; substitute ½ teaspoon vanilla extract for the vanilla powder.

SUNBURST SUMMER SALAD

9 Plant Points

Serves 4

Sweet peppers ripen on the vine, beginning with green (unripe) and transforming into different colours like autumn leaves. The yellow pepper gets its colour from lutein, a phytochemical that benefits eye health. Red peppers get their colour from capsanthin, another phytochemical that is thought to benefit our metabolism, including weight balance, blood sugar, and lipid control.

135 g quinoa, rinsed

360 ml water or Low-Histamine Biome Stock (page 159)

1 yellow sweet pepper, seeded and diced

1 red sweet pepper, seeded and diced

400 g cooked white beans or lentils

60 g rocket leaves

3 tablespoons thinly sliced spring onions (white and green parts)

35 g toasted sunflower seeds, pumpkin seeds, or other tolerated chopped nut/seed

10 g chopped fresh flat-leaf parsley

10 g torn fresh basil

3 tablespoons tahini

2 tablespoons apple cider vinegar

½ teaspoon dried dill

Pinch salt

Pinch ground pink peppercorn

Olive oil, water, or Low-Histamine Biome Stock (page 159), for drizzling

1. In a medium pan, place the quinoa and water and bring to the boil. Cover with a tight-fitting lid, reduce the heat to low, and cook for about 12 minutes, until the quinoa is tender and the water is absorbed. Remove from the heat and let cool for 5 minutes before removing the lid and fluffing with a fork. Set aside to cool, then place in a large bowl.

2. Add the sweet peppers, beans, rocket, spring onions, sunflower seeds, parsley, and basil. Mix together.

3. In a separate small bowl, whisk together the tahini, vinegar, dill, salt, and pink pepper. Drizzle with olive oil to make a thin dressing; I usually end up using 2 to 3 tablespoons. Add the dressing to the quinoa bowl and toss again to combine. Season to taste.

FF UNLEASHED:

If you are not restricting histamine, you can add 100 g halved cherry tomatoes; substitute 2 tablespoons lemon juice for the apple cider vinegar, and black peppercorns for the pink peppercorns. Garnish with 125 g Homemade Tofu Feta (page 84).

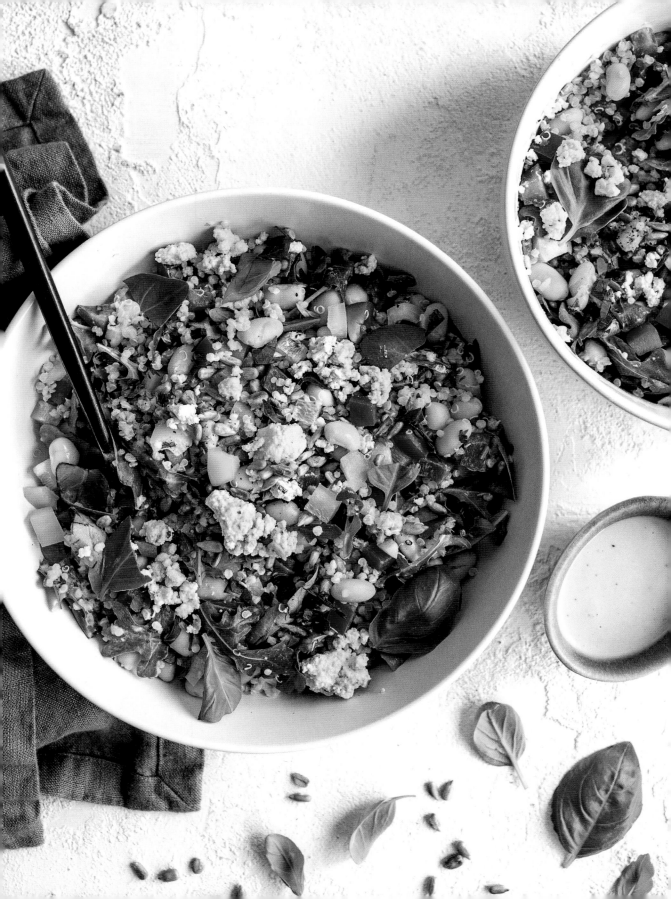

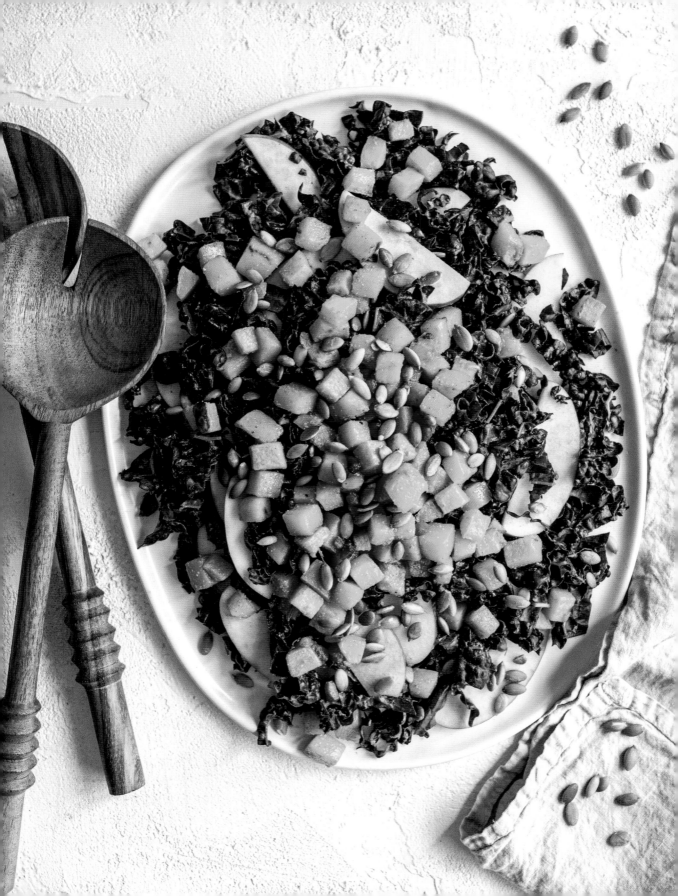

AUTUMN KALE SALAD

7 Plant Points

Serves 4

Butternut squash is not a sweet potato! Although the two share the orange pigment, which they get from beta-carotene, butternut squash is lower in calories and lower in sugar. Both are fantastic when the weather cools off.

820 g cubed butternut squash

2 teaspoons olive oil or Low-Histamine Biome Stock (page 159)

½ teaspoon salt

Pinch ground pink peppercorn

½ teaspoon ground cumin

½ teaspoon sweet paprika

½ teaspoon garlic powder

60 ml pomegranate juice

2 garlic cloves, crushed

¼ teaspoon mustard powder

60 g tahini

4 teaspoons apple cider vinegar

560 g cavolo nero or lacinato kale, stems removed and sliced into thin ribbons

30 g pumpkin seeds

2 sweet apples, diced

60 g pomegranate seeds

1. Preheat the oven to 220°C. Line a baking tray with parchment paper.

2. Place the squash on the baking tray and toss with the olive oil, salt, pink pepper, cumin, paprika, and garlic powder. Toss well. Cover with an upside-down baking tray or lightly tent with foil and roast for 20 to 25 minutes, until the squash is tender. Remove the cover for the last 5 minutes of cooking to lightly caramelize the squash.

3. While the squash is roasting, make the dressing. Whisk together the pomegranate juice, garlic, mustard powder, tahini, and vinegar. Season to taste, adding in salt and pink pepper as desired.

4. Place the kale in a large bowl and drizzle 1 to 2 teaspoons of the dressing, then use your hands to massage it into the kale for a few minutes. This helps to tenderize the kale.

5. Add in the cooked squash, pumpkin seeds, apple, and pomegranate seeds. Toss to combine, then divide onto serving plates. Drizzle with the remaining dressing.

FF UNLEASHED:

If you are not restricting histamine and you can tolerate them, add beans or lentils for a heartier meal. You can also substitute mustard for the mustard powder in the dressing, and black peppercorns for pink peppercorns.

RAINBOW FARRO SALAD
with Tahini Dressing

7 Plant Points

Serves 4

If it has farro, I'm there for it. I love the nutty taste and soft, chewy texture. Farro is an ancient wheat grain that originates from Mesopotamia and makes a great alternative to rice. A cup of farro has 20 grams of fibre. Gadzooks!

150 g cooked farro or other short grain

105 g finely chopped broccoli florets

½ red sweet pepper, seeded and thinly sliced

½ yellow or orange sweet pepper, seeded and thinly sliced

70 g finely shredded red cabbage

360 g cooked white beans

2 tablespoons tahini

2 tablespoons apple cider vinegar

2 tablespoons olive oil, stock, or water

2 garlic cloves, crushed

½ teaspoon salt

¼ teaspoon ground pink peppercorn

1. In a large bowl, combine the farro, broccoli, sweet peppers, cabbage, and white beans.

2. In a separate small bowl, whisk together the tahini, vinegar, olive oil, garlic, salt, and pink pepper. For a thinner dressing, whisk in an additional tablespoon or two of water. Season to taste, then add to the farro salad and toss well.

PRO TIP:

To pack for lunch, toss together the farro, vegetables, and beans. Add the dressing right before serving.

FF UNLEASHED:

If you are not restricting histamine, you can substitute black peppercorns for pink peppercorns.

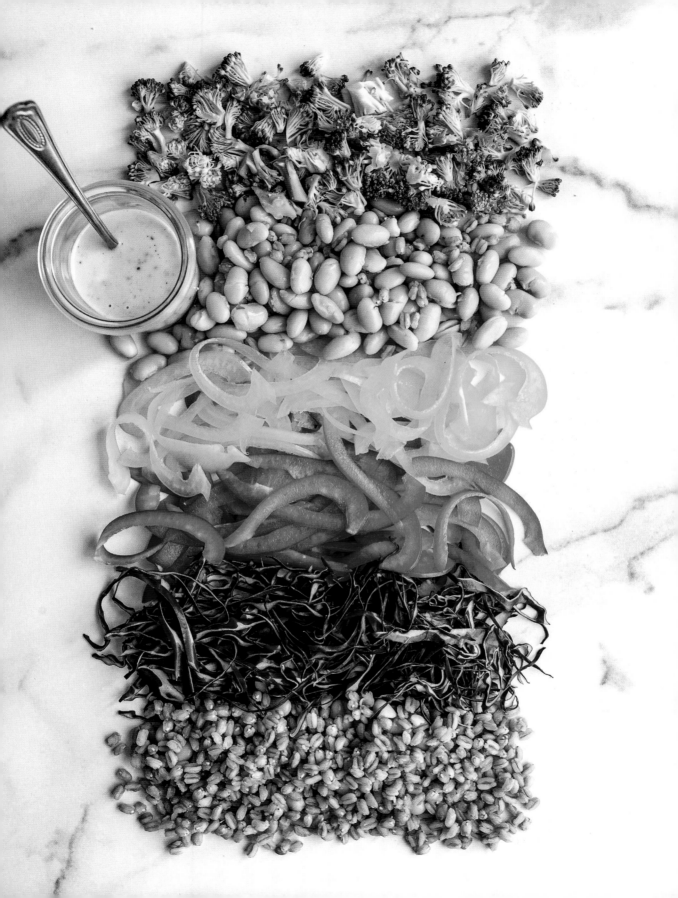

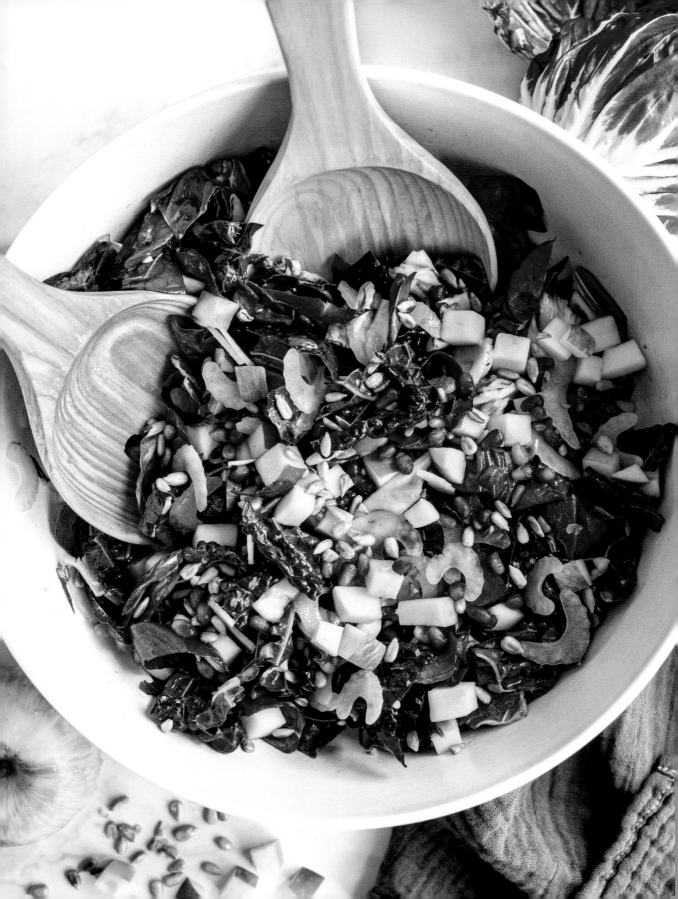

HEARTY CHOPPED SALAD

8+ Plant Points

Serves 4

Sweet pomegranate and apple pair perfectly with bitter radicchio and kale. The end result is balanced flavours within your mouth and balanced microbes devouring a diversity of plants in your gut. It's a win win win for you, your taste buds, and your microbes.

2 medium apples, cored and chopped into bite-size pieces

140 g chopped radicchio or thinly sliced red cabbage

420 g well-chopped kale leaves, stems removed

100 g very thinly sliced celery

85 g pomegranate seeds and/or blueberries

30 g toasted sunflower seeds

1 garlic clove, finely crushed

1 to 2 teaspoons apple cider vinegar

¼ teaspoon mustard powder

¼ teaspoon ground ginger

2 tablespoons tahini

3 tablespoons Low-Histamine Biome Stock (page 159), water, or olive oil

Salt and ground pink peppercorn

1. In a large bowl, combine the apples, radicchio, kale, celery, pomegranate seeds, and sunflower seeds.

2. In a separate small bowl, whisk the garlic into the vinegar until mostly dissolved. Add the mustard and ginger. Keep whisking, stirring in the tahini to make a creamy dressing, then add in the stock to create a pourable dressing. Season to taste with salt and pink pepper.

3. Add the dressing to the salad and toss very well.

PRO TIP:

To make ahead, add the dressing right before serving.

FF UNLEASHED:

If you are not restricting histamine, you can add 1 large chopped orange and 2 tablespoons orange or lemon juice to the dressing; substitute ½ teaspoon Dijon mustard for the mustard powder and black peppercorns for the pink peppercorns.

PESTO PASTA SALAD

4+ Plant Points

Serves 4

Diamine oxidase is produced by many legumes during germination to aid in development of the seedling. This is the same enzyme our body uses to reduce histamine levels. Sprouted green peas are particularly high in DAO and therefore make a nice addition to a low-histamine diet.

1 garlic clove, crushed

80 g fresh basil

80 g hemp seeds

15 g nutritional yeast

120 ml olive oil or Low-Histamine Biome Stock (page 159)

¼ to ½ teaspoon salt

340 g pasta, preferably organic wholewheat short pasta such as shells or macaroni

130 g frozen peas or sprouted green peas (see Pro Tip)

1. Place the garlic, basil, hemp seeds, and nutritional yeast in the base of a food processor. Pulse 10 to 12 times, until just combined. With the motor running, add the olive oil, stopping to scrape down the sides as needed. Add salt to taste.

2. Cook the pasta according to the packet directions. Two minutes before the pasta is done, add the frozen peas. Drain the pasta and peas and return to the cooking pot.

3. Add the pesto and toss to combine.

PRO TIP:

You can use sprouted green peas instead of the frozen peas in this recipe. When sprouted, they go from not producing DAO to producing tons of it. The highest DAO levels are achieved when the peas are sprouted in darkness. Sprouting peas is fun, inexpensive, quick, and insanely easy. See page 348 for more information on sprouting your own peas.

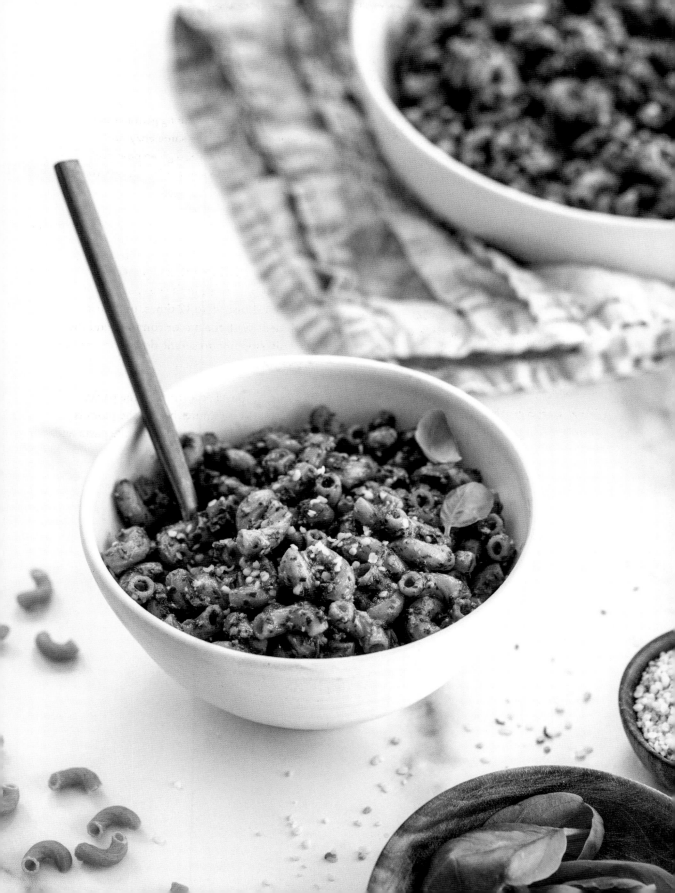

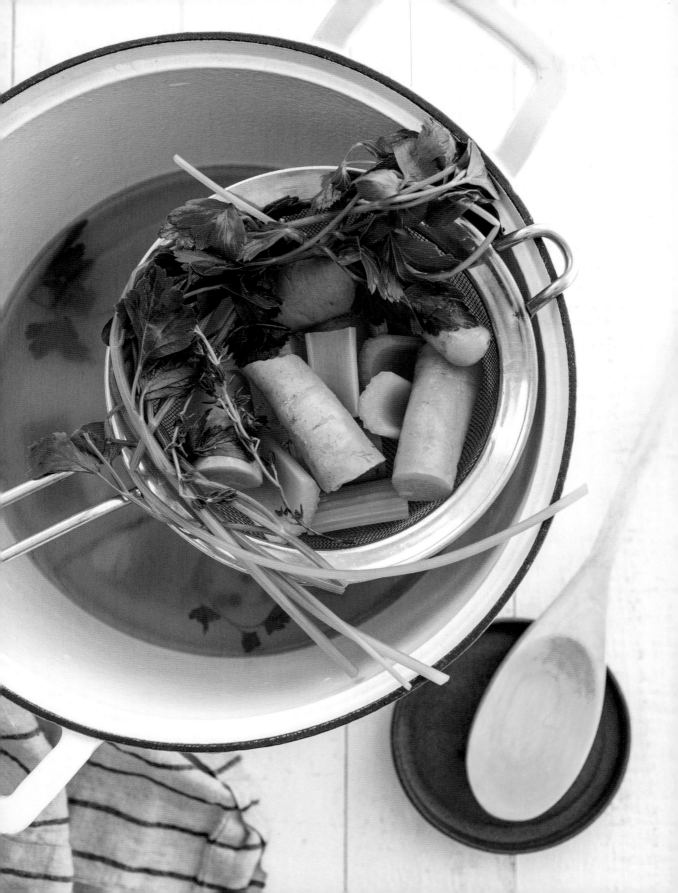

LOW-HISTAMINE BIOME STOCK

Makes 1.5 litres

Biome Stock is a foundational recipe for anyone who is following a Fibre Fuelled lifestyle. It's meant to be soothing to an upset gut and offers soluble fibre and polyphenols to nourish your little microbes. It was first introduced in *Fibre Fuelled*. In this version, we have reduced histamine content with maximum flavour.

1 medium white or yellow onion, quartered

1 to 2 large carrots, cut into chunks

3 celery sticks, cut into chunks

4 to 5 sprigs fresh flat-leaf parsley

2 to 3 sprigs fresh thyme

1 bay leaf

4 garlic cloves, crushed

6 whole pink peppercorns

2.5 cm piece fresh ginger, thinly sliced

½ teaspoon ground turmeric

Salt

1. Place the onion, carrots, celery, parsley, thyme, bay leaf, garlic, pink peppercorns, ginger, turmeric, and salt in the base of an Instant Pot or pressure cooker. Add 2 litres water. Cook on high pressure for 30 minutes, then naturally release for 10 minutes and quick release the remaining time.

2. Strain and enjoy.

PRO TIP:

The veggies can be saved, even frozen, for later use in other Biome Stock recipes. Or you can finely chop them and include them to make vegetable soup. If you do, this goes from stock to a low-waste, high-flavour 7 Plant Point Wild Biome Super Soup.

ROASTED CAULIFLOWER SOUP

3+ Plant Points

Serves 4

Cauliflower has been trending pretty hard in recent years—cauliflower pizza crust, cauliflower rice, cauliflower steaks. I'm happy to see it because cauliflower is a healthy food, high in fibre, cancer-fighting glucosinolates, and brain-healthy choline.

1 large head cauliflower, cut into bite-size florets

2 tablespoons extra-virgin olive oil

Salt and ground pink peppercorn

1 medium onion, chopped

2 garlic cloves, crushed

1 litre Low-Histamine Biome Stock (page 159), plus more as needed

⅛ teaspoon ground ginger

1 tablespoon apple cider vinegar, plus more as desired

Finely chopped fresh flat-leaf parsley, chives, and/or spring onions (green parts only), for garnish

Coconut cream, for drizzling (optional)

1. Preheat the oven to 220°C. Line a large baking tray with parchment paper.

2. Add the cauliflower and drizzle with 1 tablespoon of the olive oil and a generous pinch of salt and pepper, coat with your hands, then arrange in a single layer. Bake for 25 to 30 minutes, until tender and slightly caramelized.

3. In a soup pot set over medium heat, heat the remaining oil. Add the onion and cook for about 8 minutes, until softened, stirring often. Add the garlic and stir for 15 seconds, until just fragrant, then add the stock, scraping up any browned bits of the onion.

4. Add the cauliflower to the pot along with the ginger and bring to the boil. Reduce the heat to low and simmer 15 minutes more, until the cauliflower is very tender.

5. Transfer the soup to a blender (you may have to work in batches) or use an stick blender and purée until very creamy and smooth.

6. Add in the vinegar and blend again, then season to taste with salt, pepper, or vinegar as desired. For a thinner soup, add more stock.

7. Serve with garnish of choice.

PRO TIP:

When shopping for cauliflower, look for tight heads that are heavy for their size. If the heads are starting to separate, they are usually less fresh.

For a richer soup, drizzle over in a little coconut cream before serving.

FF UNLEASHED:

If you are not restricting histamine, you can substitute ⅛ teaspoon nutmeg for the ground ginger. Add 3 tablespoons raw cashews before you blend the soup.

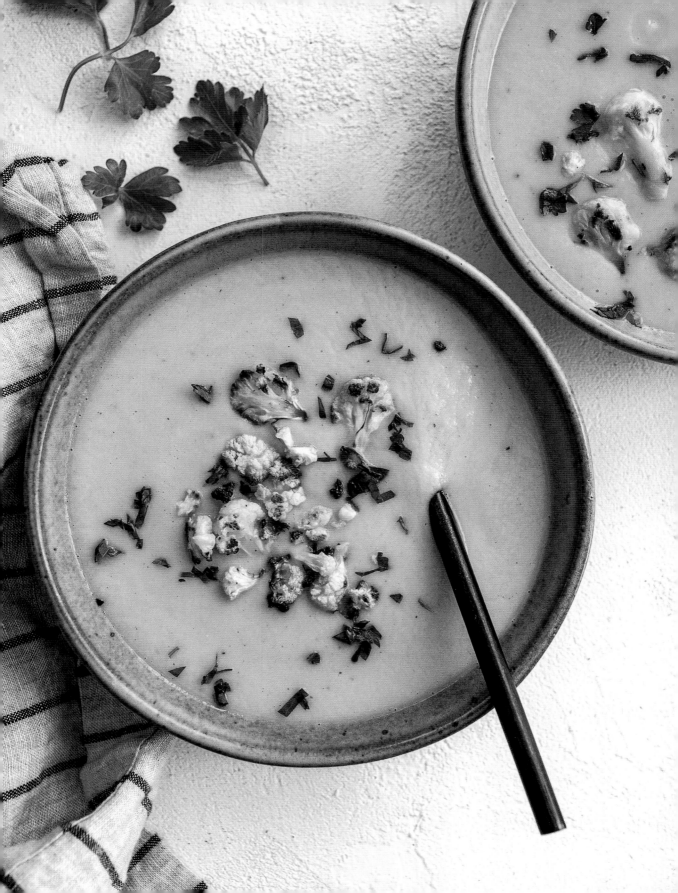

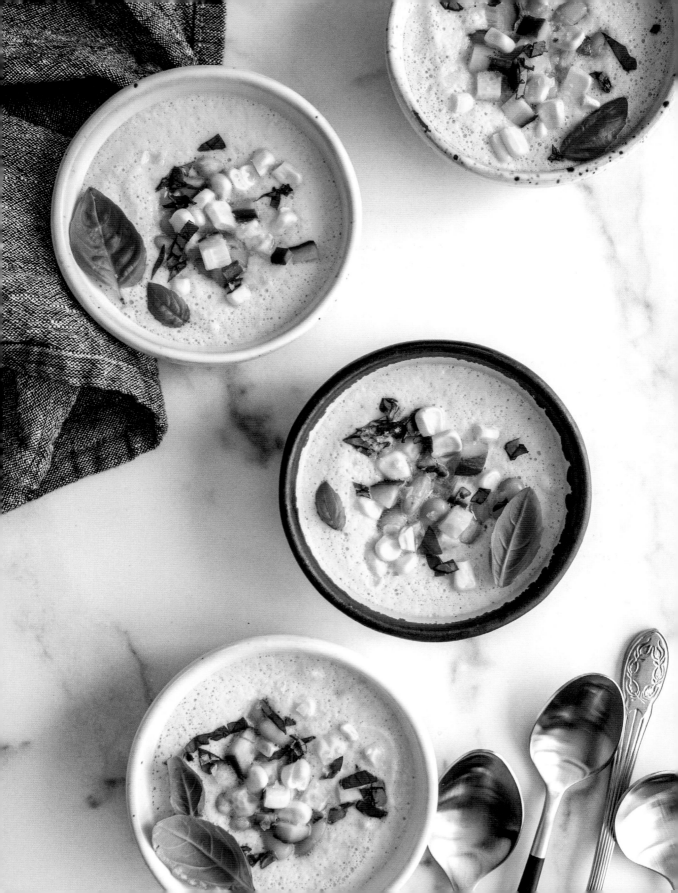

SWEETCORN AND PEPPER GAZPACHO

5+ Plant Points

Serves 4

Corn has developed a bad reputation due to field corn, which is a commodity crop used as livestock feed and to produce high-fructose corn syrup, ethanol, and a litany of ultra-processed foods. Sweetcorn, however, is distinctly different from field corn and is a classic summertime food to be enjoyed. Be sure to use fresh corn for this recipe—fresh corn is low histamine, while canned or frozen corn is not. My ideal sweetcorn is non-GMO and purchased less than twenty-four hours after harvest from a local farmer or other trusted source.

2 yellow sweet peppers, stemmed, seeded, and chopped

5 ears fresh corn, kernels and juices; reserve 75 g for garnish

2 garlic cloves

180 g cucumber, peeled and chopped, plus more for garnish

2 tablespoons extra-virgin olive oil or Low-Histamine Biome Stock (page 159), plus more olive oil for drizzling (optional)

2 tablespoons apple cider vinegar

½ to 1 teaspoon sea salt

Freshly ground pink peppercorn

180 g cooked white beans

Chopped fresh basil and/or chives, for garnish

1. Place the sweet peppers, corn kernels and juices, garlic, cucumber, olive oil, vinegar, salt, and pink pepper in the base of a blender or food processor and blend until smooth and creamy. Season to taste.

2. Divide into bowls and garnish with the white beans, fresh corn kernels, cucumber, basil, and chives as desired. Drizzle over extra olive oil, if desired.

FF UNLEASHED:

If you are not restricting histamine, you can add 1 to 2 yellow tomatoes; substitute 2 tablespoons traditional sherry vinegar for the apple cider vinegar, and substitute black peppercorns for pink peppercorns.

VERY VEGETABLE SOUP

8 Plant Points

Serves 4

Easy. Flexible. Inexpensive. Warming. Filling. Filled with fibre. Low in calories. A vehicle to deliver plants. Awesome as leftovers. Low on waste. Fun to share. There are TONS of good reasons to love this recipe.

1 tablespoon olive oil or 60 ml Low-Histamine Biome Stock (page 159)

1 white or yellow onion, diced

3 garlic cloves, finely chopped

2 carrots, halved and sliced

2 celery sticks, halved and sliced

½ teaspoon dried thyme

½ teaspoon dried oregano

½ teaspoon ground turmeric

¾ teaspoon sweet paprika

75 g frozen corn kernels

200 g chopped cauliflower florets

90 g quinoa, rinsed, or other gluten-free grains like buckwheat or sorghum

1 litre Low-Histamine Biome Stock (page 159)

360 ml coconut milk (optional)

2 teaspoons apple cider vinegar

10 g finely chopped fresh flat-leaf parsley

Salt and ground pink peppercorn

1. In a large saucepan set over medium heat, heat the olive oil. Add the onion, garlic, carrots, and celery and cook for about 10 minutes, until the vegetables are very soft.

2. Add the thyme, oregano, turmeric, and paprika and cook another minute or two, then add the corn, cauliflower, quinoa, and stock. Bring to the boil, then reduce to medium-low heat and simmer for 25 minutes, until the cauliflower is tender and the quinoa is cooked.

3. Add the coconut milk, if desired, the vinegar, and the parsley. Season to taste, adding salt and pepper as desired.

PRO TIP:

Coconut milk makes for a creamy soup, but you can omit it for a clearer version.

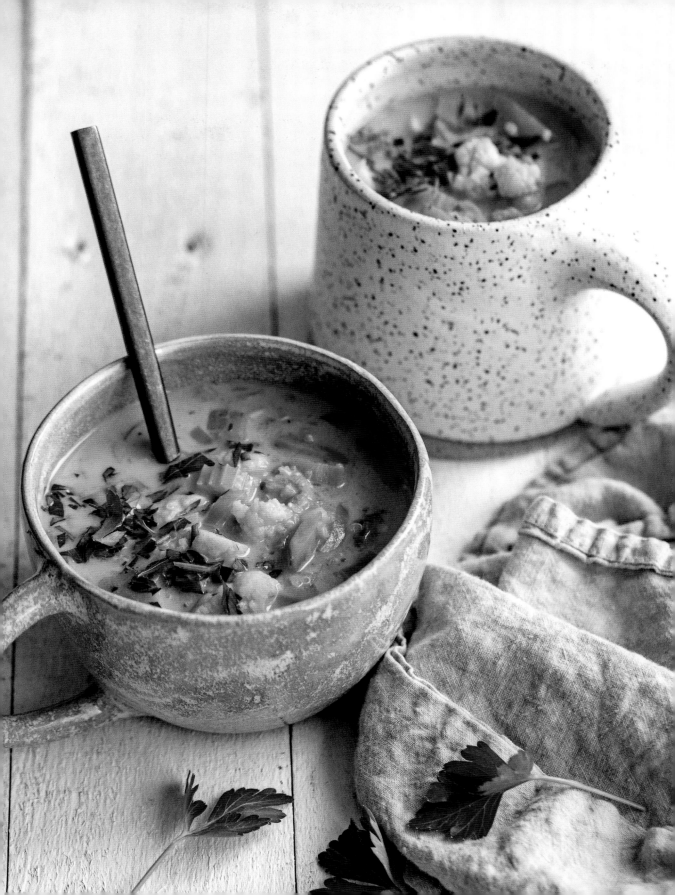

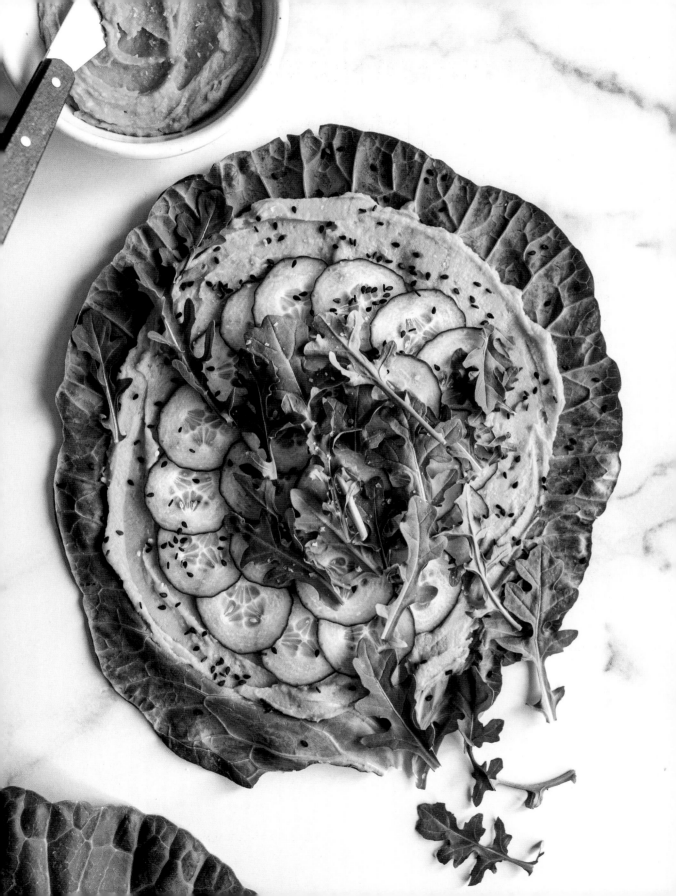

SWEET POTATO HUMMUS WRAPS

4+ Plant Points

Makes 4 wraps
(with some extra
hummus for snacking)

Sweet potatoes are relatively high in copper, which is important in the setting of histamine intolerance because copper is a cofactor for the DAO enzyme. In other words, we want to make sure we get enough copper in our diet if there is histamine intolerance.

400 g cooked sweet potato flesh

270 g cooked white beans

2 garlic cloves

180 ml Low-Histamine Biome Stock (page 159) or water

3 tablespoons tahini

½ teaspoon salt

¼ teaspoon sweet paprika

½ teaspoon ground cumin

2 teaspoons apple cider vinegar

4 wholewheat wraps of choice or spring green wraps

8 lettuce leaves

Supercharge It! (optional toppings):

60 g sliced cucumber

Handful fresh sprouts

Sliced spring onions (white and green parts)

Sliced radishes

1. Place the sweet potato, beans, garlic, and 120 ml of the stock in the base of a food processor or blender and purée until smooth and creamy. Add in the tahini, salt, paprika, cumin, and vinegar, then pulse to incorporate.

2. With the motor running, gradually drizzle in a tablespoon of the remaining stock. Stop the motor, scrape down the sides, and check for consistency. It should be creamy like hummus; if more liquid is needed, then turn on the motor again and slowly add in more stock. Depending on how thick and creamy you like your hummus, you may add up to 60 ml stock.

3. Season to taste, adding more salt, paprika, or cumin as desired.

4. Spread 2 to 3 tablespoons of hummus on the wrap and layer on the leaves, cucumber, sprouts, or other preferred toppings. Wrap, slice in half, and enjoy.

FF UNLEASHED:

If you are not restricting histamine, you can substitute 2 teaspoons lemon juice instead of the apple cider vinegar; add 180 g sliced cherry tomatoes and 1 large cubed avocado.

WHITE BEAN HUMMUS TOAST

3+ Plant Points

Makes 350 g
hummus

180 g cooked white beans contains 11 grams of fibre. The average Westerner gets just 15 grams of fibre per day. Just sayin'...

90 g dried white beans, rinsed

½ teaspoon salt

3 garlic cloves

2 tablespoons tahini or olive oil

1 teaspoon apple cider vinegar (optional)

Bread of choice, for serving

Supercharge It! (optional toppings):

Chopped fresh basil

Roasted artichoke hearts

Sliced radishes

Pea sprouts

Red onion

Sliced cucumber

1. Place the beans, salt, and garlic in the base of an Instant Pot. Cover with water by a few centimetres.

2. Set the valve to sealed, then cook at high pressure for 30 minutes. Natural release or quick release by moving the valve to vent.

3. Drain, reserving 120 ml of the cooking liquid. Place the beans, tahini, and vinegar, if using, in the base of a food processor and process until finely chopped. With the motor running, slowly drizzle in some of the reserved cooking liquid until the desired consistency is reached.

4. Serve on toasted bread with supercharged toppings of choice.

SWEET POTATO AND BLACK BEAN TACOS

3 Plant Points

Makes 8 tacos, with enough filling for the Sweet Potato Burritos (page 173)

Chimichurri is an uncooked sauce of Argentine origin that's classically served as a condiment with meat, but I think it's even better paired with complex flavours and spices in these tacos. Serve drizzled with Quick Coriander Chimichurri Sauce (see page 170).

2 large sweet potatoes, diced

75 g diced white or yellow onion

2 teaspoons ground cumin

½ teaspoon sweet paprika

½ teaspoon dried oregano

½ teaspoon garlic powder

½ teaspoon each salt and freshly ground pink pepper

Olive oil or Low-Histamine Biome Stock (page 159), enough to drizzle over diced sweet potatoes

720 g cooked black beans

8 tortillas of choice, warmed

Quick Coriander Chimichurri Sauce (page 170)

1. Preheat the oven to 200°C.

2. In a large bowl, place the sweet potatoes, onion, cumin, chilli powder (if not low histamine), paprika, oregano, garlic powder, salt, and pink pepper and drizzle with olive oil. Toss well, coating the sweet potato as much as possible with the seasonings.

3. Place in a single layer on a baking tray lined with parchment paper and roast for 30 to 35 minutes, until tender and cooked through. Remove and add in the black beans. Stir, then return to the oven for 5 minutes to warm through.

4. Divide the sweet potato filling between the warmed tortillas, and top with chimichurri sauce.

PRO TIP:

When fresh garlic and onions are CHOPPED, you activate an enzymatic reaction to create a chemical called allicin that has tremendous health benefits. Be sure to STOP after you CHOP for 10 minutes to let this reaction occur and maximize the production of allicin.

FF UNLEASHED:

If you are not restricting histamine, you can add 2 teaspoons chilli powder; substitute black peppercorns for pink peppercorns.

QUICK CORIANDER CHIMICHURRI SAUCE

2 Plant Points

Makes about 120 ml

25 g fresh coriander leaves, flat-leaf parsley leaves, or a combination of the two

2 garlic cloves, crushed

1 teaspoon apple cider vinegar

¼ teaspoon salt

Pinch ground pink peppercorn

60 ml extra-virgin olive oil

Place the coriander, garlic, vinegar, salt, 2 tablespoons water, and the pink pepper in the base of a food processor or blender and pulse 5 or 6 times, until coarsely chopped. Add in the olive oil and pulse again, 8 to 10 times, until the coriander is finely chopped but some texture remains. Season to taste, adding in more salt and pepper as desired.

FF UNLEASHED:

If you are not restricting histamine, you can swap in 2 tablespoons lime juice for the apple cider vinegar.

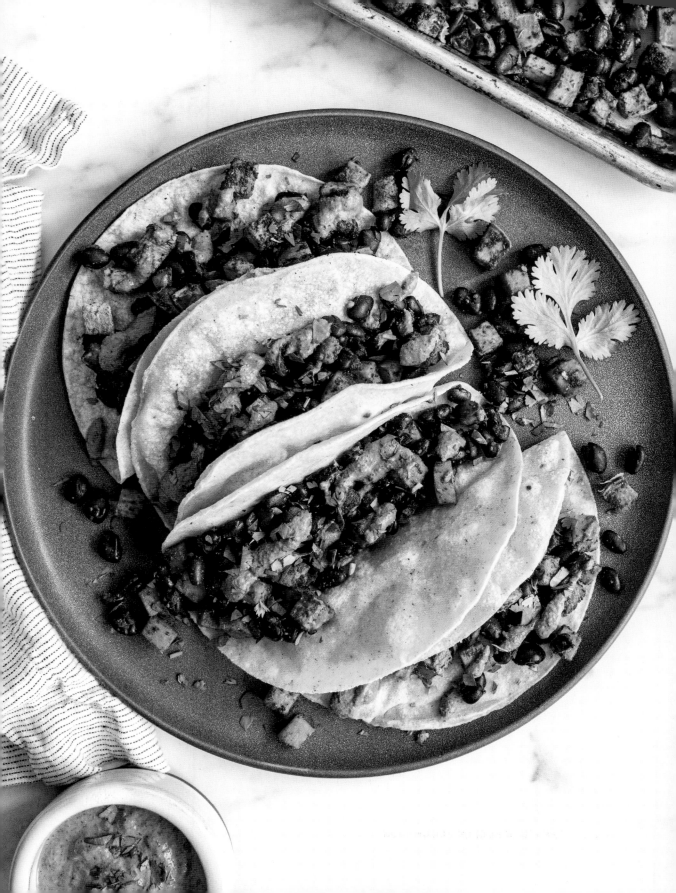

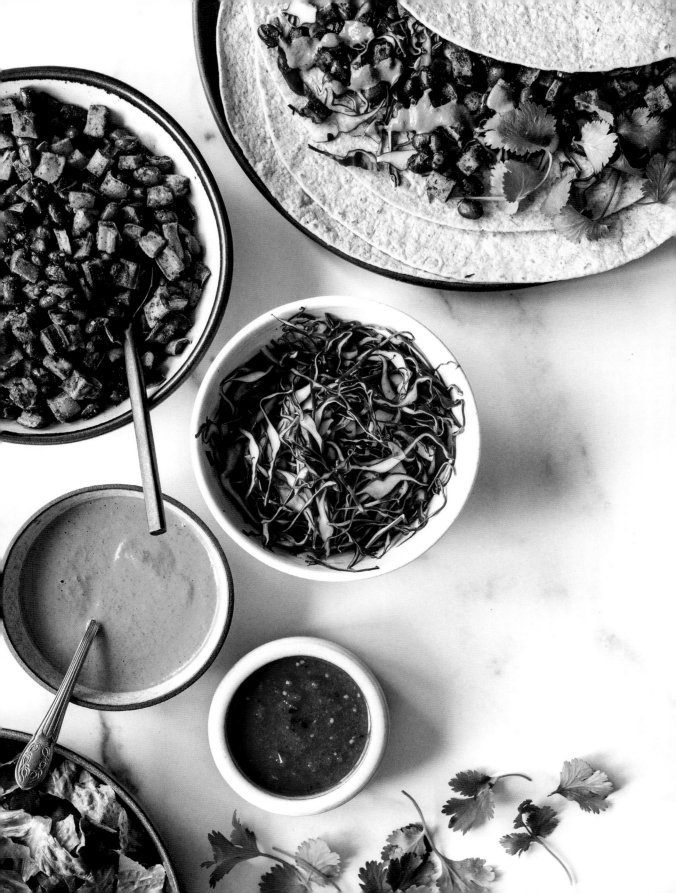

SWEET POTATO BURRITOS

5+ Plant Points

Makes 4 burritos

Cook once, eat twice. For a variation on the sweet potato & black bean Mexican dish, use the filling from the tacos for these simple burritos.

400 g Sweet Potato and Black Bean Tacos filling (page 169)

4 burrito-size tortillas of choice, warmed

90 g finely shredded red cabbage

10 g chopped coriander

Quick Coriander Chimichurri Sauce (optional) (see page 170)

1. Warm the sweet potato and black bean filling.

2. Warm the tortillas according to the packet directions. This will make it easier for rolling. Add 100 g of the filling on the tortilla along with the cabbage, coriander, and any other toppings as desired.

3. Roll, then slice in half. Serve with chimichurri sauce, if desired.

FF UNLEASHED:

If you are not restricting histamine, you can add in 1 large sliced avocado and salsa to taste.

QUINOA, CORN AND BLACK BEAN-STUFFED PEPPERS

7+ Plant Points

Makes 4 stuffed peppers

Sweet peppers contain a molecule called sweet pepper pyrazine, which is responsible for their distinctive scent. The human nose has an incredible capacity to detect this smell, even in exceedingly light concentrations. For example, you may notice a sweet pepper nuance to Cabernet Sauvignon wine due to the gentle presence of this molecule.

5 large fresh red sweet peppers, halved and seeded

2 tablespoons diced white onion

Fresh coriander, to taste

135 g quinoa, rinsed

360 ml Low-Histamine Biome Stock (page 159) or water

279 g cooked black beans

150 g sweetcorn kernels, frozen or thawed

2 teaspoons ground cumin

1½ teaspoons garlic powder

½ teaspoon salt

Pinch ground pink peppercorn

Avocado oil or olive oil, for brushing the exteriors of the sweet peppers

Supercharge It! (optional toppings):

Coriander

Red or white onion, diced

1. Preheat the oven to 230°C. Place two sweet pepper halves flat-side down on a lined baking tray. Roast on the middle or top rack for about 20 minutes, rotating halfway through, until slightly charred and soft.

2. Place the roasted red pepper, white onion, and coriander in the base of a food processor and pulse to create a chunky salsa. Season to taste with salt and pepper, then set aside.

3. Add the quinoa and vegetable stock to a saucepan and bring to the boil over high heat. Once boiling, reduce the heat, cover with a tight-fitting lid, and simmer for about 15 minutes, until all of the liquid is absorbed and the quinoa is fluffy.

4. Reduce the oven temperature to 190°C and lightly grease a 22 × 33 cm baking dish or rimmed baking tray.

RECIPE CONTINUES

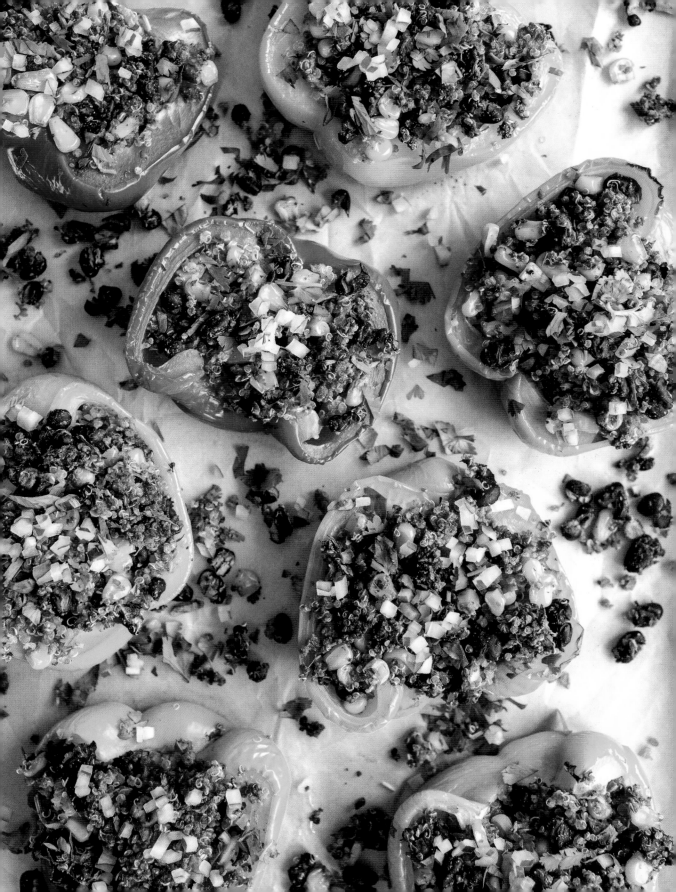

5. In a small bowl, combine the red pepper salsa, black beans, corn, cooked quinoa, cumin, garlic powder, ½ teaspoon salt, and a pinch of pink pepper.

6. Brush avocado or olive oil on the exterior of the peppers to prevent them from drying while baking. Scoop the filling into the peppers.

7. Cover the stuffed peppers with foil and bake for 30 minutes. Remove the covering, then bake for another 20 to 25 minutes, until the peppers are tender.

8. Garnish with supercharged toppings of your choice and serve.

FF UNLEASHED:

If you are not restricting histamine, you can substitute bottled roasted peppers instead of roasting your own peppers for the stuffing. Add 1½ teaspoons chilli powder to the stuffing and substitute black peppercorns for the pink peppercorns in steps 2 and 5.

BEETROOT RISOTTO

5 Plant Points

Serves 4

Think of the distinctive earthy smell that's recognizable after a summer rainfall or when you freshly dig up some soil. That smell is the result of geosmin, an organic compound produced by bacteria that live in the soil. Geosmin is also responsible for the earthy aroma of beetroot. Recent research indicates that the soil microbes actually produce geosmin to attract forest creatures that will help facilitate the spread of microbial spores. In other words, what you're smelling is a microbial pheromone. Fascinating, right? I like to use a "semi-stir method" when making this dish—it's more hands-off than traditional risotto but still yields the same creamy results.

2 large beetroot, peeled and cut into bite-size pieces

2 to 3 teaspoons olive oil or stock

¼ teaspoon salt

Pinch ground pink peppercorn

1 white or yellow onion, finely chopped

900 ml to 1 l vegetable stock or Low-Histamine Biome Stock (page 159)

3 garlic cloves, crushed

220 g Arborio rice or other short-grain rice

2 tablespoons tahini

1 tablespoon apple cider vinegar

60 ml coconut cream, water, or more stock (optional, to alter the consistency)

1. Preheat the oven to 200°C. Line a baking tray with parchment paper or a non-stick silicone baking mat. Place the chopped beetroot on the baking tray and drizzle with 1 to 2 teaspoons of the olive oil, the salt, and the pink pepper. Then use your hands to mix the seasonings and oil into the beetroot, taking care to coat each piece. Spread in a single layer and roast for 30 to 40 minutes, until tender.

2. While the beetroot is cooking, in a large saucepan set over medium heat, heat the remaining oil. Add the onion and cook for about 5 minutes, until softened.

3. While the onion is cooking, warm the stock over low heat in a separate saucepan.

4. Add the garlic and Arborio rice to the pan with the onion and cook for 30 seconds to 1 minute, stirring constantly, toasting the

RECIPE CONTINUES

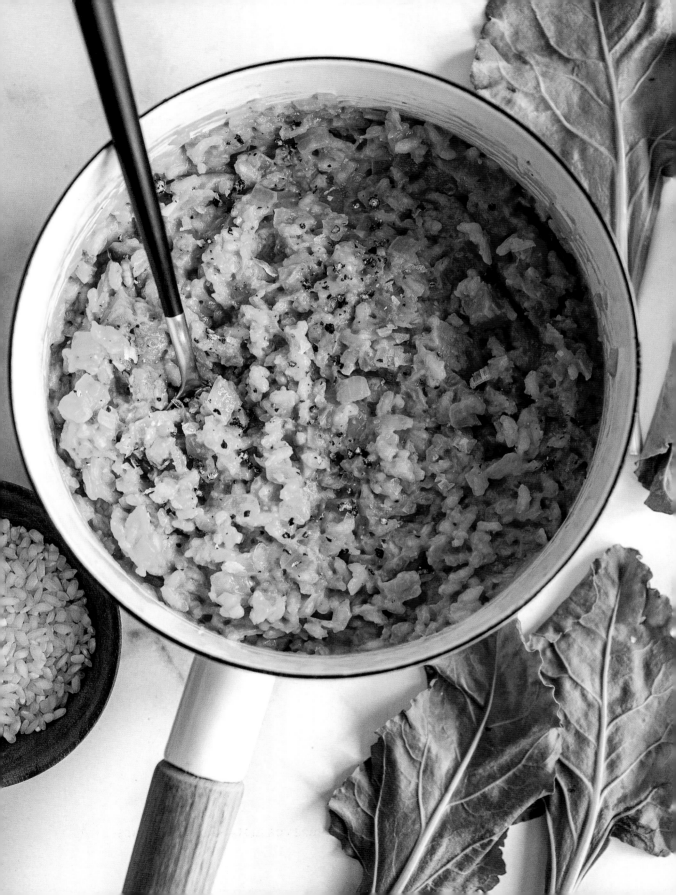

rice and garlic. Vigorously stir in 240 ml of the warmed stock, then cover with a tight-fitting lid and let simmer for 10 minutes to let the rice cook, then remove the lid, stir again, and repeat with more stock. Repeat for about 25 minutes, until the rice is cooked, adding more stock as needed.

5. Place half of the cooked beetroot in the base of a blender with the tahini, vinegar, and coconut cream. Pulse, scraping down the sides as needed, to form a thick paste.

6. Once the rice is al dente, add in the beetroot paste and cook for another few minutes, stirring often. Add a splash of water, oat milk, or stock as needed to achieve a creamy consistency. Then, add the remaining cooked beetroot and season to taste as needed.

FF UNLEASHED:

If you are not restricting histamine, you can substitute black peppercorns for pink peppercorns.

SESAME BROCCOLI NOODLES

5 Plant Points

Serves 4

In this recipe, black sesame seeds are best for their stronger, slightly bitter flavour. Pale sesame seeds serve best in gentle, sweet recipes.

225 g uncooked noodles, such as linguine or rice noodles

1 teaspoon olive oil, stock, or water

140 g chopped fresh or frozen broccoli

½ teaspoon salt, plus more for the broccoli

Pinch ground pink peppercorn

4 garlic cloves, crushed

2 tablespoons tahini

2 tablespoons apple cider vinegar

1 tablespoon sesame oil or Low-Histamine Biome Stock (page 159)

2 teaspoons apple juice or 1 teaspoon 100% maple syrup

1 tablespoon grated fresh ginger

½ teaspoon crushed red pepper flakes

30 g roughly chopped sunflower seeds

2 tablespoons sesame seeds

1. Bring a large pan of water to a boil. Cook the noodles according to the packet directions. Drain and set aside.

2. While the pasta is cooking, heat the olive oil in a large non-stick frying pan over medium-high heat. Add the chopped broccoli and season with a pinch of salt and a pinch of pink pepper. Cook for 4 to 5 minutes, stirring occasionally. If needed, add in a splash or two of water or stock if the broccoli is sticking to the pan.

3. Add 2 of the crushed garlic cloves and continue cooking for another minute. Once the garlic is fragrant, remove the pan from the heat and set aside.

4. To make the sauce, place the remaining 2 garlic cloves, the tahini, 60 ml water, vinegar, sesame oil, apple juice, ½ teaspoon salt, a pinch of pink pepper, ginger, and the red pepper flakes into the bowl of a small food processor or blender and combine until creamy.

5. Return the pasta to the pan and mix in the cooked broccoli and garlic, sunflower seeds, sesame seeds, and the sauce. Stir to thoroughly combine.

6. Serve immediately, or store in a sealed container in the fridge for up to 3 days.

FF UNLEASHED:

If you are not restricting histamine, you can substitute black peppercorns for pink peppercorns.

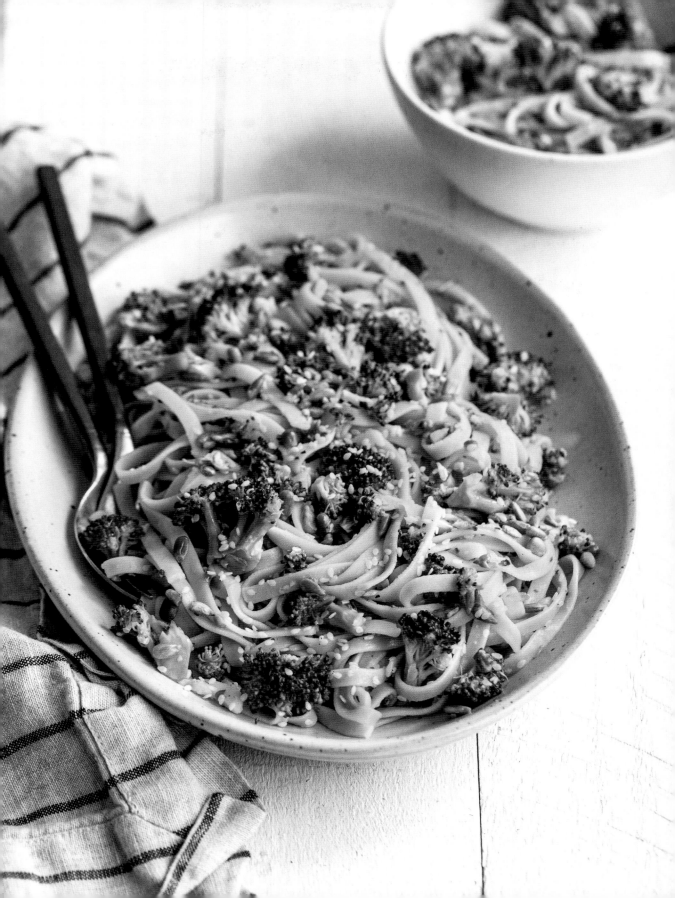

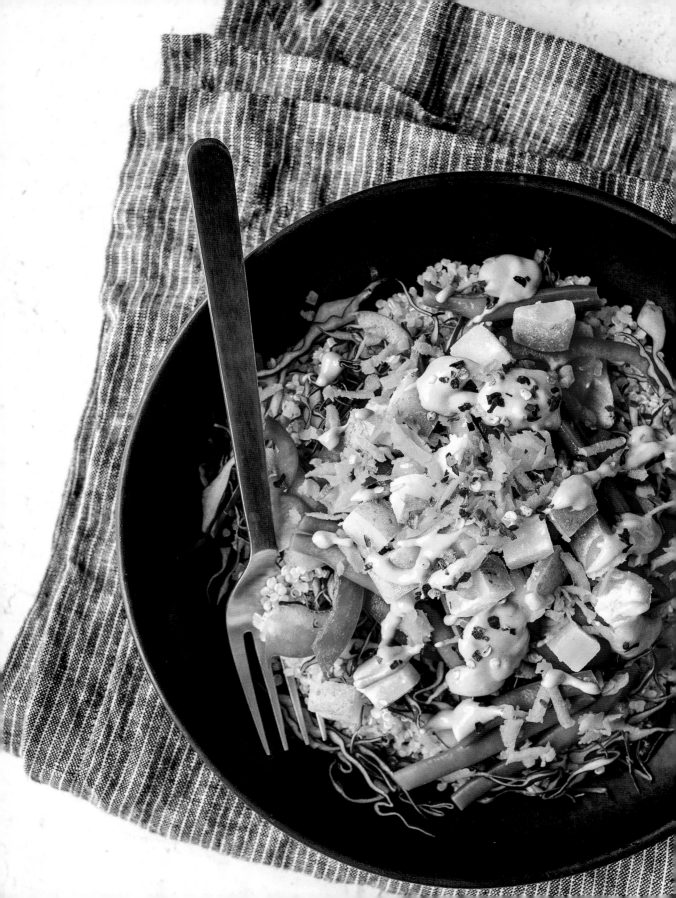

GADO-GADO QUINOA BOWL

9+ Plant Points

Serves 4

Gado-gado in Indonesian literally means "mix-mix." The expression comes from mixing the wide variety of vegetables with the nut butter dressing. Gado-gado is widely sold in Indonesia, with each region having its own unique spin on this classic that's considered one of the national dishes of Indonesia.

300 g small red potatoes, halved or diced, depending on the size

180 g uncooked quinoa or other short grain

300 g washed and trimmed green beans or pea sprouts

120 g almond butter or sunflower seed butter, oil on top stirred well

2 garlic cloves grated into a paste or 1 teaspoon dried garlic powder

1 tablespoon grated fresh ginger or ¼ teaspoon ground ginger

¼ teaspoon crushed red pepper flakes (optional)

3 tablespoons apple cider vinegar

2 tablespoons toasted sesame oil (optional)

¼ teaspoon salt

105 g shredded red cabbage

2 carrots, grated

1 red sweet pepper, seeded and thinly sliced

1. In a medium pan, place the potatoes and cover with water. Cover with a tight-fitting lid and bring to the boil. Once boiling, allow the potatoes to cook for about 15 minutes, or until a potato flakes easily when pierced by a fork.

2. Rinse the quinoa and add to a saucepan with 480 ml water. Cover with a tight-fitting lid and bring to the boil. Reduce the heat to low and allow to cook covered for 12 minutes, then remove from the heat and let stand for another 3 minutes. Fluff with a fork and set aside to slightly cool.

3. If using green beans, bring a small pan of water to a boil. While the water is boiling, make an ice bath in a medium bowl with ice and water to cover. Add the green beans to the boiling water and cook for 2 minutes, then immediately drain and place in the prepared ice bath for 3 minutes, then drain and set aside.

RECIPE CONTINUES

4. In a small bowl, prepare the sauce by whisking together the almond butter, garlic, ginger, red pepper flakes, if using, vinegar, and sesame oil, if using, salt. If the nut butter is too thick, heat it in a saucepan over low heat or blend it in the base of a small blender or food processor. Add hot water, 1 tablespoon at a time (up to 5 tablespoons), until the sauce has a pourable consistency.

5. To assemble, divide the quinoa among four bowls. Top with shredded cabbage, green beans, carrots, cooked potatoes, and sweet pepper. Serve with the nut butter sauce.

FF UNLEASHED:

If you are not restricting histamine, you can substitute 125 g peanut butter for other nut butters and 3 tablespoons rice vinegar for the apple cider vinegar.

SWEET POTATO SHAWARMA BOWL

8 Plant Points

Serves 4

It's the spices that matter. The Arabic name *shawarma* refers to the turning action of a vertical spit that was developed in Turkey several hundred years ago to roast meat. But when most of us think of shawarma, we think about the explosion of complex flavour from the spices. Turkey was once the bridge between East and West, and so the spice trade flowed through it. It's no wonder that this melting-pot country produced this incredible multicultural spice bomb.

1 small head cauliflower, chopped into bite-size pieces

2 medium sweet potatoes, cut into bite-size pieces

½ teaspoon salt

½ teaspoon freshly ground pink pepper

3 garlic cloves, crushed

1½ teaspoons ground cumin

1½ teaspoons sweet paprika

½ teaspoon ground cinnamon (optional)

¼ teaspoon ground ginger

¾ teaspoon dried oregano

½ teaspoon ground turmeric

Pinch cayenne pepper (optional)

Drizzle of olive oil or water

90 g quinoa or other gluten-free short grain

280 g shredded lettuce

120 g thinly sliced cucumber

75 g thinly sliced red onion

80 g tahini paste

1 tablespoon apple cider vinegar

1. Preheat the oven to 200°C. Line two large baking trays with parchment paper or non-stick silicone baking mats and set aside.

2. In a large bowl, place the cauliflower, sweet potato, salt, pink pepper, garlic, cumin, paprika, cinnamon, if using, ginger, oregano, turmeric, and cayenne, if using. Add a drizzle of olive oil to loosen the mixture, then toss together to combine.

3. Spread in a single layer on the prepared baking trays and roast for 25 minutes, or until the veggies are tender.

4. While the veggies are cooking, make the quinoa. Rinse and place the quinoa in a medium saucepan over medium heat along with 360 ml water. Bring to the boil, then reduce the heat to low and cover with a tight-fitting lid. Let cook for 12 minutes, then remove from the heat and let sit another 2 to 3 minutes to set. Fluff with a fork, then set aside to cool.

RECIPE CONTINUES

5. Divide the lettuce, cucumber, and red onion among four bowls.

6. In a small bowl, whisk together the tahini and vinegar along with a pinch of salt. Keep whisking, drizzling in water, a tablespoon at a time, until a creamy dressing forms. It's normal for the tahini to become hard before it thins out.

7. Add the shawarma veggies to the prepared bowls and drizzle with tahini dressing.

FF UNLEASHED:

If you are not restricting histamine, you can substitute 1 tablespoon freshly squeezed lemon juice for the apple cider vinegar, and smoked paprika for the sweet paprika.

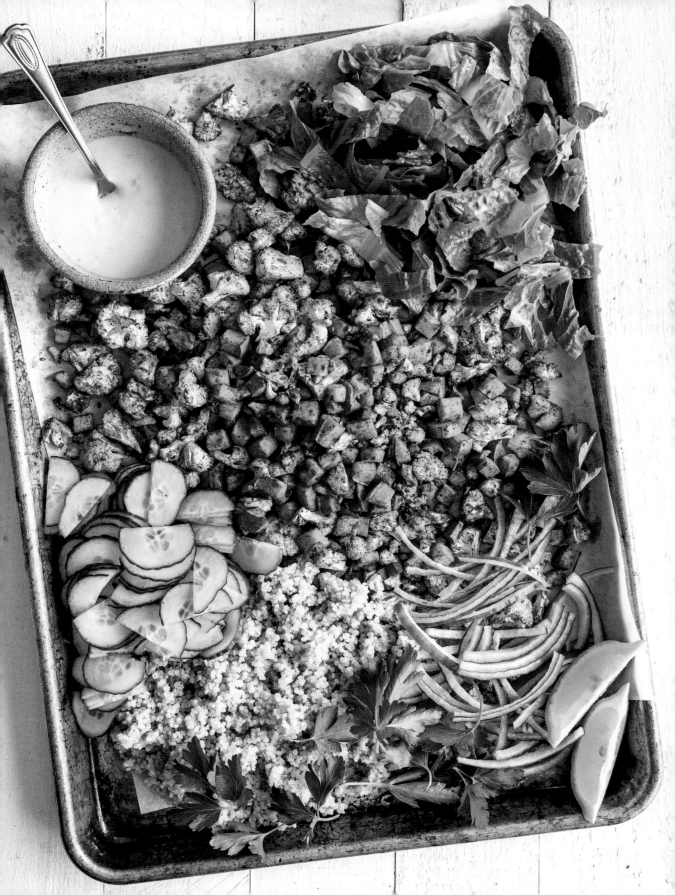

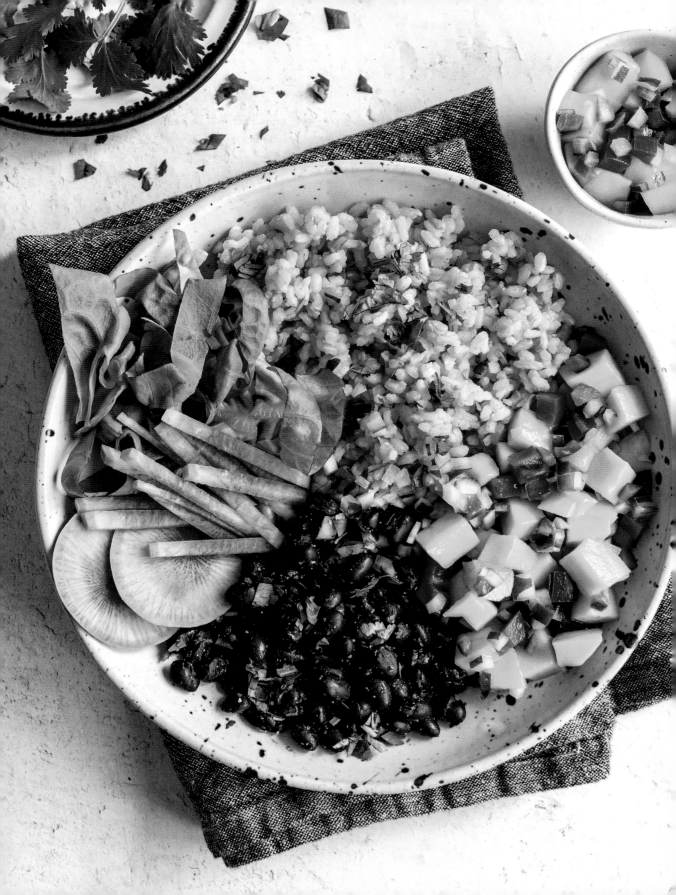

MANGO BURRITO BOWL

6+ Plant Points

Makes 4 bowls

Mango has been grown in India for more than four thousand years and is deeply rooted in Ayurvedic medicine, balancing all three doshas (or humours) and acting as an energizer. In ancient India, princes took pride in their mango gardens, and Ganesh, the Hindu elephant-headed god, is often shown holding a ripe mango. In other words, mango is celebrated among royalty, the divine, and us Fibre Fuellers. We hold good company.

190 g brown rice

½ teaspoon salt

¼ teaspoon paprika

330 g diced mango, about 2 mangoes

75 g seeded and diced red sweet pepper

35 g diced red onion

1 jalapeño, seeded and diced

1 teaspoon olive oil

Salt

450 g black beans, drained and rinsed

Pinch ground pink peppercorn

¼ teaspoon garlic powder

Supercharge It! (optional toppings):

Chopped red onion

Fresh chopped coriander

Chopped lettuce

Sliced radish

1. In a small pan set over high heat, place the rice with 480 ml water, the salt, and the paprika. Cover with a tight-fitting lid and bring to the boil. Once boiling, reduce the heat to low and simmer for 40 to 45 minutes, until the rice is tender and the water is absorbed. Turn off the heat, let sit for 5 minutes, then fluff with a fork.

2. While the rice is cooking, make the mango salsa and season the black beans. In a medium bowl, combine the mango, sweet pepper, red onion, and jalapeño. Toss with the olive oil and add salt to taste.

3. In a separate small bowl, combine the black beans, pink peppercorn, and garlic powder. Toss to combine and adjust the seasoning to taste.

4. Place equal amounts of rice in four bowls. Top with the mango salsa and black beans and any additional supercharged toppings.

FF UNLEASHED:

If you are not restricting histamine, you can substitute black peppercorns for pink peppercorns.

STUFFED SWEET POTATOES

6 Plant Points

Makes 4 sweet
potatoes

Sweet potatoes originate from South America, with the oldest carbon-dated remains coming from Peru ten thousand years ago. Sweet potato remains have also been identified in Polynesia about one thousand years ago. This is interesting because it suggests a connection between Polynesians and Native Americans *prior* to the arrival of Columbus in the Americas. A more recent study found genetic evidence connecting the Polynesians and Native Americans around 1200 AD at Easter Island—3,700 kilometres west of South America. One can speculate that the Native Americans must have loaded up their boats with sweet potatoes to make the voyage.

4 cooked sweet potatoes

2 teaspoons olive oil or Low-Histamine Biome Stock (page 159)

40 g diced red onion

50 g seeded and diced red sweet pepper

1 garlic clove, crushed

360 g cooked black beans

150 g frozen sweetcorn kernels

1 teaspoon ground cumin

1 teaspoon sweet paprika

¼ teaspoon salt

1. To cook the sweet potatoes, wash and dry them, then poke a few holes in the skin with a knife or a fork. Bake in a preheated oven at 200°C for 1 hour, or microwave for about 5 minutes, until the flesh is easily pierced with a fork.

2. In a large frying pan set over medium heat, heat the olive oil. Cook the onion for about 2 minutes, or until translucent. Add the sweet pepper and garlic and cook for another 2 to 3 minutes. Add the black beans, corn, cumin, paprika, and salt. Cook until the corn is thawed and the mixture is heated through.

3. Cut a slit into the top of each sweet potato to create a cavity, then top each with a quarter of the bean mixture and serve.

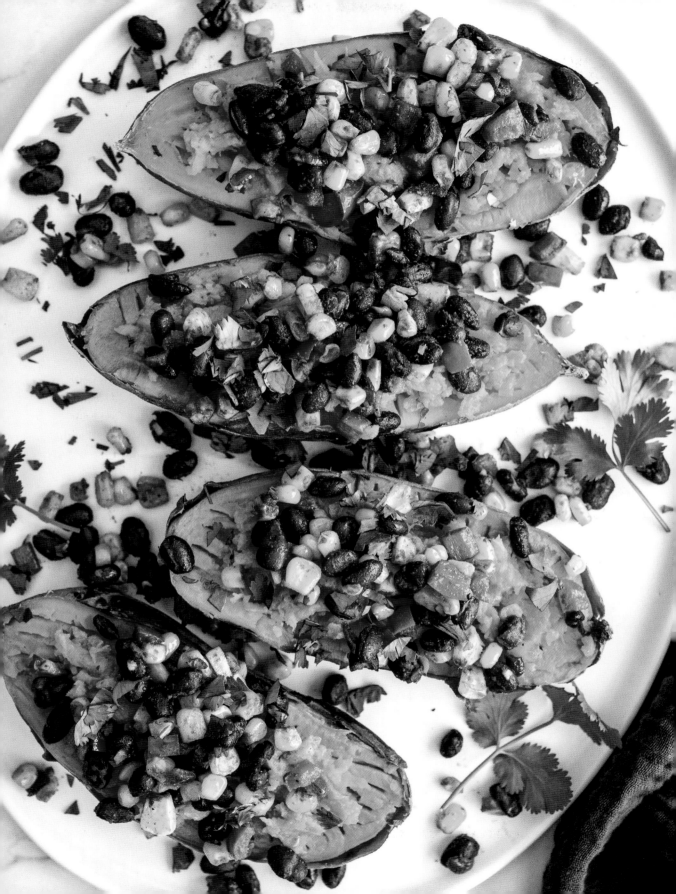

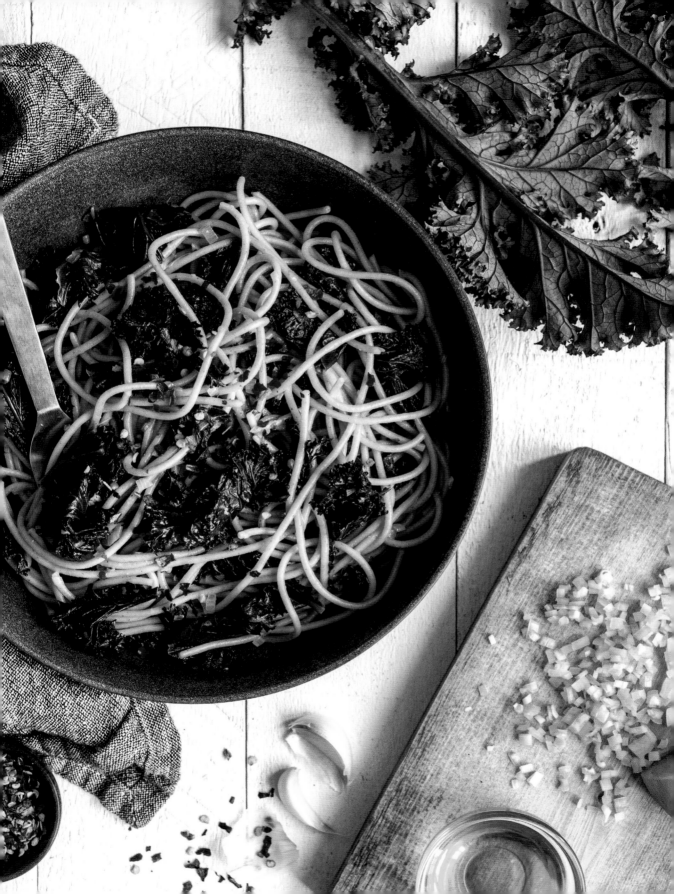

SIMPLE SPAGHETTI
with Garlicky Kale

3 Plant Points

Serves 4

Yes, it's a lot of kale, but it shrinks a ton when cooked. And consider this . . . You are getting almost half a kilo of the most nutrient-dense food that exists on the planet, and yet that entire half a kilo of food has just 100 calories. It's incredible. For an oil-free dish, use more stock.

P.S. You can use any type of green for this recipe. Swiss chard is also nice!

340 g spaghetti of choice

2 tablespoons olive oil or avocado oil

2 shallots, finely chopped

5 large garlic cloves, roughly chopped

½ teaspoon salt

Pinch ground pink peppercorn

450 g kale, stems and tough ribs removed

120 ml Low-Histamine Biome Stock (page 159)

1. Bring a large pan of salted water to the boil. Add the pasta, undercooking it by 1 to 2 minutes according to the packet directions (see Pro Tip for cooking gluten-free pasta). Drain, reserving 120 ml of the pasta water.

2. In a large frying pan set over medium heat, heat the olive oil. Add the shallots and cook for 2 to 3 minutes, then add the garlic, salt, and ground pink peppercorn. Cook for another 1 to 2 minutes, taking care not to burn the garlic. Add the kale and keep cooking until the kale is tender, about 5 more minutes.

3. Add the pasta to the kale frying pan along with the vegetable stock and a tablespoon of pasta water. Cook, tossing the entire time, until the pasta is tender and the sauce lightly coats the pasta. Add more pasta water as needed; you may need up to 120 ml total.

4. Season to taste, divide into bowls, and serve.

PRO TIP:

The undercooking method won't work for gluten-free pasta. For gluten-free pasta, cook to al dente according to the packet directions and toss with the greens, omitting the extra pasta water.

FF UNLEASHED:

If you are not restricting histamine, you can add crushed red pepper flakes to taste and substitute black peppercorns for pink peppercorns.

≫ *To view the 90 scientific references cited in this chapter, please visit www.theplantfedgut.com/cookbook.*

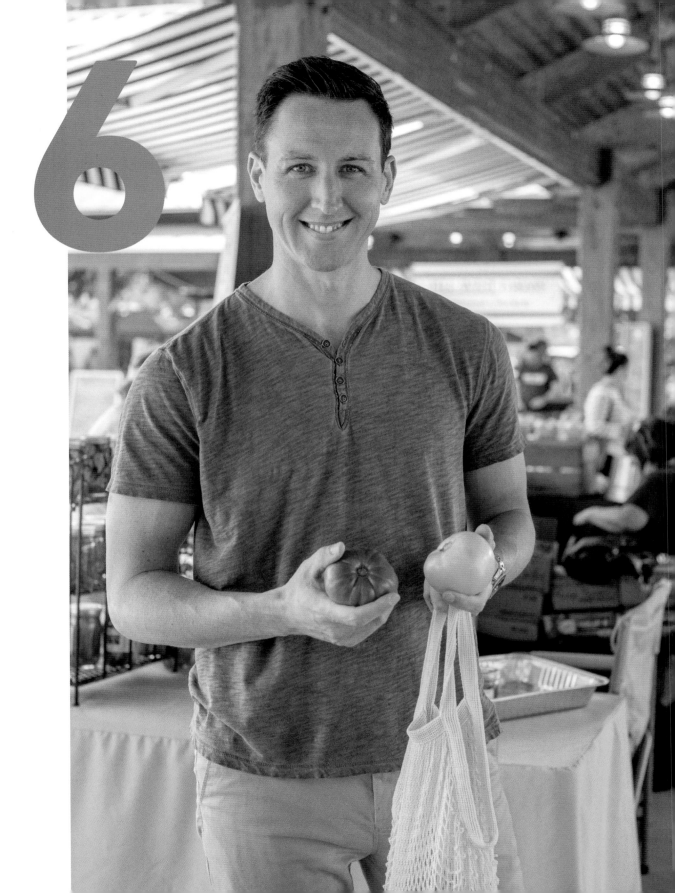

6

Sucrose, Salicylates, and Synthetic Substances (Oh My!)

The other food intolerances that you need to know about

In all cases of food sensitivity, there is a component of your food that is causing your symptoms, and these food elements could properly be described as chemicals. The chemicals can be a natural part of the food, like the FODMAPs that we learned about in Chapter 4 and the histamine and other biogenic amines that we learned about in Chapter 5. And then, of course, there are added food chemicals that are either synthetic or natural substances used by the food industry to preserve food and improve taste or appearance. We refer to these as additives.

So far I've focused your attention on FODMAPs and histamine because in my experience, these are the two most important food intolerances. But these aren't the only two, and so it's possible you have a different "what" behind your food intolerance.

With that in mind, I'd like to briefly cover a few of the other food intolerances with the intent that if you suspect after reading this chapter that you are experiencing problems with these, you'll know enough to take your first baby steps towards healing and seek the assistance of a health professional to get the proper testing and develop a treatment plan.

Sucrose Intolerance

Do you recognize the word "sucrose"? If you flip over a bag of the white granulated stuff we call table sugar and check the ingredients list, you'll find it as the lone ingredient. You may also recognize it from the myriads of processed foods that have it discreetly snuck in there to help you reach your bliss point, which is the food industry's way of creating products that trigger your reward system and turn you into a sugar junkie coming back for your fix. That's why you'll find 10 teaspoons of it in one 475 ml glass of Ocean Spray Cran-Lemonade Juice. Coming in hot!

Added sugar is clearly a problem, but sucrose itself is actually a natural part of many healthy foods. Beetroot, sweet potatoes, apples, and bananas are just a few of the foods that contain a significant amount of natural sucrose. Problems arise when the body can't break down sugar correctly, regardless of the source. Whether you eat an apple or drink a sugar beverage, the sucrose in your food is broken down by an enzyme in the small intestine called sucrase. If this enzyme is reduced, then the normal consumption of sucrose may be enough to trigger GI symptoms—diarrhoea, wind and bloating, abdominal discomfort.

There are some people born with a condition called congenital sucrase-isomaltase deficiency, or CSID. Historically it was thought that this was a rare disorder, affecting 0.2 per cent of the population. But more recent research has suggested that 2 to 9 per cent may be affected by this genetic disorder. We hear so much about coeliac disease and gluten, yet sucrose intolerance is far more common. Why aren't we talking more about sucrose intolerance? Part of the issue is that sucrose intolerance is relatively new on the scene.

The good news is that we have solid testing for this condition, so we don't need to speculate and we can fairly quickly size up whether or not there's a problem. The gold standard test is a small intestine biopsy with special testing for enzyme activity. I can tell you firsthand, this is not easy to get done because there are only a few labs that do it and it requires special processing. There's a hydrogen breath test that is fraught with false positives and false negatives, but thankfully there is also a more recently developed radiolabelled carbon-13 breath test that is non-invasive and performs well for detection of sucrase deficiency. And then there's the sucrose 4-4-4 challenge, which can be done easily at home to give you an idea as to whether or not sucrose intolerance may be an issue for you.

Take the 4-4-4 sucrose challenge!

The 4-4-4 challenge is rather simple. We're going to deliver a bolus of sucrose to your gut and see if it elicits symptoms. Before we do that, I want you to know that the point of the sugar challenge is simply to determine if you should have additional testing for sucrose intolerance. It is not intended to make the diagnosis by itself. If you already know that you're going to have extreme symptoms by doing this, please don't do it. In that case, consult with your GP to get confirmatory testing.

1. Stir 4 tablespoons sugar into 120 ml water.

2. Drink it on an empty stomach.

3. Monitor for the next four hours for symptoms that suggest sucrose intolerance. If present, check with your GP for confirmatory testing.

Although sucrose intolerance is only a small part of this book, I want you to know that it's a BIG part of my practice. What I mean is that I am thinking about sucrose intolerance as a possibility in every single patient who has wind, bloating, or chronic diarrhoea. If I have my way, 100 per cent of those patients get tested for sucrase deficiency. And guess what . . . I find a ton of it. About 15 per cent of my patients with wind, bloating, or chronic diarrhoea have sucrase deficiency as the cause. Again, this is far more common than coeliac disease.

If someone has been previously diagnosed with irritable bowel syndrome but they haven't been tested for sucrase deficiency, I'll give them that test at our first visit. I've had numerous patients who suffered for ten or more years with chronic digestive symptoms, bouncing from doctor to doctor trying to find a solution to their "IBS," only to discover that sucrose intolerance was the root of the problem. As I've said before, you have to know what you're treating before you can treat it properly.

I have to be up front—I am not a believer in a dietary approach to sucrose intolerance unless you have extremely mild symptoms. A low-sucrose diet is extremely restrictive, restrictive to the point that I worry about nutritional deficiencies and also harm to the gut microbiome. Remember, the single greatest predictor of a healthy gut microbiome is diversity, the opposite of restriction. The good news is that there is a safe, effective enzyme replacement for sucrase that can be used with meals. In people with CSID, 81 per cent using this enzyme were able to consume an unrestricted diet and remain symptom-free.

It's worth mentioning that if you do have CSID, you need to be aware that you may also struggle with digestion of starches found in rice, bread, pasta, root vegetables, legumes, and wholegrains. The sucrase enzyme replacement will fix the sucrase deficiency but not correct the difficulty with starches. This likely accounts for the 19 per cent who were not completely symptom-free while using the enzyme.

Dr. B's Advice

You can enhance the digestion of starches in your diet by spending more time chewing them. Your saliva contains enzymes designed to initiate digestion before the food even hits your stomach. About 30 per cent of starch digestion occurs in your mouth!

Salicylate Intolerance

Thirty-five hundred years ago in ancient Egypt it was a known practice to chew the bark of a willow tree for pain relief. Through the years you'll find a similar practice in ancient Sumer, Assyria, China, Europe, and among Native Americans. Fast-forward to nineteenth-century Europe and the active ingredient responsible for these medicinal effects, salicin, was identified and eventually chemically restructured by Bayer (formerly a dye manufacturer) as acetylsalicylic acid, which we commonly refer to today as aspirin. The origin story of modern pharmaceuticals and the most used medication in history started with one of my foundational principles—plants having healing properties.

Salicin is just one of many naturally occurring plant-based chemicals called salicylates that have anti-inflammatory properties similar to aspirin. They work by inhibiting cyclooxygenase, known as COX for short. COX inhibition reduces inflammation, reverses a fever, reduces blood clots, and treats pain. You can use aspirin or other nonsteroidal anti-inflammatory drugs (NSAIDs) to get this effect, but they increase your risk of intestinal ulcers, liver injury, and kidney failure while damaging your gut microbiota and potentially triggering inflammatory bowel disease. Or alternatively you can consume salicylate-rich foods, like asparagus, tomatoes and tomato products, apples, peaches, herbs and spices, coffee and tea, and get the benefits of reduced inflammation without making health and gut microbiota compromises in the process.

In people who have salicylate intolerance, however, these foods will trigger a pseudo-allergic reaction where the basophils and mast cells—the same ones we discussed in Chapter 5 as being relevant to histamine intolerance—get activated. What ensues sounds like an echo from the last chapter because the symptoms of salicylate intolerance mirror those of histamine intolerance—diarrhoea, abdominal discomfort, hives or rashes, asthma, running nose, headaches, fatigue, puffy eyes, brain fog, or ringing in the ears. In other words, if you suspect that you have histamine intolerance but then don't improve with a low-histamine diet, consider salicylate intolerance. We also need to bear in mind that there are people who have a true allergy to aspirin.

Unfortunately, there is no blood, breath, or stool test for salicylate intolerance. Typically, the best approach is to follow the GROWTH strategy and restrict salicylates, observe for improvement, and then work them back in to see the response. Taking aspirin with the intent of provoking symptoms is a possibility, but this should only be done under the guidance of a properly trained health professional.

Synthetic (and Natural) Substances

There are literally thousands of different food additives used throughout the food industry for various functions—food preservation, taste, texture, or appearance: preservatives, emulsifiers, flavours and flavour enhancers, firming agents, thickeners, and humectants. What the heck are humectants? (They're moisturizing agents. I had to look it up.)

Unfortunately, that means that there are thousands of different food chemicals that could be the driving force behind our symptoms and food intolerances. I don't say this to imply that food additives are automatically all bad. Some of them seem to be good, and some of them certainly are not. But my point is really about the absurd complexity of trying to sort out which specific food chemical is the issue when there are literally thousands of possibilities and they're always mixed together. It'd be easier if we consume them in isolation, but with very few exceptions, we do not.

I Absolutely Love My Coffee, but It's Not for Everyone.

I am the world's biggest lover of coffee and a huge fan of matcha green tea in the afternoon, but sadly, caffeine can worsen digestive symptoms in some. In some cases, there is a gene that predisposes to diarrhoea. In other cases, it can exacerbate anxiety, nervousness, or insomnia. If you suspect that caffeine may be connected to your symptoms, then it's time to take a break from the coffee, tea, cola soft drinks, chocolate, and energy drinks.

But here's what we can do: We can separate out the food intolerances that occur when we eat wholefoods from the food intolerances that occur when we eat ultra-processed foods. By wholefoods, I am referring to stuff that you could grow if I gave you a farm—fruits, vegetables, wholegrains, seeds, nuts, and legumes. There's no need for an ingredient list when you're describing real food. By contrast, ultra-processed foods are those where something starts as real food, and then gets subjected to a process of being sliced, diced, chopped, the fibre gets tossed in the rubbish, and in comes the preservatives, thickeners, colourants, and—gulp—humectants. If there are ingredients in the ingredient list that you can't identify or know how they are made, then you have an ultra-processed food on your hands, my friend. If it's literally impossible for you to make the food at home in your kitchen, you're dealing with an ultra-processed food. If it takes eighteen months for a team of food scientists to figure out how to create a food, that's also an ultra-processed food.

Making this distinction allows us to first identify the potential triggers of food intolerance that exist in wholefoods. So far we've focused on FODMAPs, histamine, and other biogenic amines, sucrose, and salicylates. All of these can be natural sources of food intolerance.

If You Haven't Heard of the New Alpha-Gal Syndrome, It's Time for a Chat.

There's a new diagnosis in town called alpha-gal syndrome in which people who were previously symptom-free start having hives, lip or throat swelling, abdominal pain, arthritis, or itching in response to eating red meat of any mammal—cow, pig, lamb, deer, rabbit, horse, or goat. You catch my drift. This definitely also includes organ meats (for those who are into that sort of thing) and for some will include milk, cheese and dairy products, lard, collagen, and gelatine-containing foods. Basically, anything derived from a mammal could trigger this reaction. It all starts with a tick bite. In the United States, the lone star tick is the number one cause of this disease. One day you're out for a hike, next thing you know a burger or even ice cream, gummy vitamins, or your collagen supplement is jacking you. I'm not an advocate for red meat consumption, so in general my position is that you're better off without it. That said, if you do consume red meat and you notice weird symptoms associated with it, you can have your doctor check a blood test for alpha-gal antibodies.

Food additives in some cases can also contribute to digestive symptoms like wind, bloating, abdominal pain, diarrhoea, or constipation. They have also been connected to extra-intestinal symptoms like rash, hives, eczema, headache, running nose, and postnasal drip. The list of additives associated with food intolerance is rather long, and likely to continue to grow in the future as we learn more. Here's where we are at the moment:

Food Chemical	Use	Common Food Sources
Sulphites	Preservative	Soft drinks, wine, beer, dried fruit, preserved potatoes, shrimp
Monosodium glutamate	Flavour (umami)	Chinese takeaway restaurants, canned vegetables/soups, processed meats, nutritional yeast
Benzoates	Preservative	Soft drinks, jams, chocolates, ice creams, pickles
Antioxidants (BHA, BHT)	Preservative	Oils, margarine
Carmine (red #4), Tartrazine (Yellow #5)	Food colouring	Cake mixes, pastries, soft drinks, hard sweets, yoghurt, ice lollies
Nitrates	Preservative	Processed meats
Propionates	Preservative	Breads
Sorbic acid	Preservative	Processed cheese slices

Let's break this down, because there is a lot to chew on. By no means am I suggesting that all foods containing these additives are inherently unhealthy. To be clear—I'm not! Here are four things that I AM claiming:

1. There are a minority of people who experience adverse symptoms when they consume these additives in normal amounts.

2. These additives are found in numerous ultra-processed foods in varying concentrations.

3. The widespread and various use of these additives makes it extremely difficult to isolate and identify which one is the causative agent of symptoms.

4. Therefore, it may be easier to do a trial with elimination of all ultra-processed foods up front and assess for symptom improvement rather than trying to isolate the additives individually.

With all that said, I feel compelled to share with you how I feel in general about these ultra-processed foods. First, transparency: I consume them. I do strive to limit my intake, but ultra-processed foods still end up in my diet. There are foods and beverages that I consume because I enjoy them, not because I expect that they're going to help me live longer with less disease. That's my choice, that's part of keeping it real and being human, and I don't feel guilty or upset with myself for it. I am all about progress over perfection.

I'm not here to set unrealistic expectations that no normal human can meet and then make you feel stress or guilt if you can't meet those unrealistic expectations. I'm all about setting goals you can actually accomplish and not wasting energy on imperfections. Perfect doesn't exist. Why would we strive towards something that doesn't exist? But I have to be honest with my concerns about diets that lean heavily on ultra-processed foods. I would be failing you as a medical doctor if I didn't speak up about what the science is showing us about these foods and their effect on human health.

In the United States, about 60 per cent of calories consumed come from ultra-processed foods. That disturbs me. There are at least ten thousand additives in our food supply, many of them approved through a regulatory loophole called GRAS—generally recognized as safe. Unfortunately, when a chemical is GRAS'd into our food supply, it is given a free pass into our diet with an assumption of safety but without proof. The vast majority of these additives have never had a human study of any variety prior to GRAS approval. None of them have had long-term human studies. Read that again. We simply don't know what they're going to do to us. They get introduced into a system that includes ten thousand other food additives, and then we get to try to sort out the mess after the problem already exists, rather than take the precautionary steps to understand what we're getting ourselves into before unleashing it in the food supply.

It's not a question of short-term safety. If these chemicals were unsafe in the short term, we'd actually figure it out very quickly. But safety thresholds established by our regulatory agencies are established using short-term data and mostly animal studies that have a poor track record of accurately translating to real-world humans. Literally a thousand years ago, Ibn Sina commented on the need to study humans rather than animals. There's a reason that legitimate scientists always look to verify animal study findings in human studies, but apparently our regulatory agencies don't see it that way.

Perhaps it's a desire to remove barriers to technology advancing the food industry. If we required long-term human studies, they would be prohibitively expensive and, obviously, take a long time to perform. But have we gone too far in removing the barriers? The majority of calories consumed in the United States now come from ultra-processed foods that have been linked in research studies to increased risk of obesity, heart disease (our number one killer), cancer (our number two killer), stroke (our number five killer), Alzheimer's disease (our number six killer), diabetes (our number seven killer), and chronic kidney disease (our number nine killer). Oh, and shorter life expectancy. That's no surprise, is it? When I wrote *Fibre Fuelled*, I shared two references to support my concerns regarding ultra-processed foods. Now I point to twenty-two studies, most of them published in the last two years.

These are more than just observational studies, although those studies are critical to understanding diseases that take years or decades to develop. We all accept that smoking causes lung cancer, but there's never been a randomized controlled trial of smoking and lung cancer. We needed epidemiology to discover that, just as we need epidemiology to better understand risk factors for heart disease, other cancers, stroke, Alzheimer's, diabetes, and chronic kidney disease. But we also need supporting evidence, which is also mounting. In fact, there are studies indicating that artificial sweeteners, polysorbate 80, carboxymethylcellulose, titanium dioxide, aluminosilicates, and sulphites are just a few of the additives that have negative effects on the gut microbiota. Those additives continue to exist in our food supply, and the rest of the additives remain largely untested, so we just don't know what they do. Meanwhile, the evidence continues to emerge with a clear message—a diet heavy in ultra-processed foods is bad for human health.

If you suspect that one of the additives found in ultra-processed foods may be causing a food intolerance, I think the solution is rather simple and obvious—eliminate the ultra-processed foods as much as possible. If a food intolerance to ultra-processed foods motivates you to reduce your intake of them, that's a blessing in disguise. That would be taking lemons and turning them into a tall, cold glass of lemonade on a hot summer day. Your gut microbes will be refreshed and thank you for it.

>> *To view the 53 scientific references cited in this chapter, please visit www.theplantfedgut.com/cookbook.*

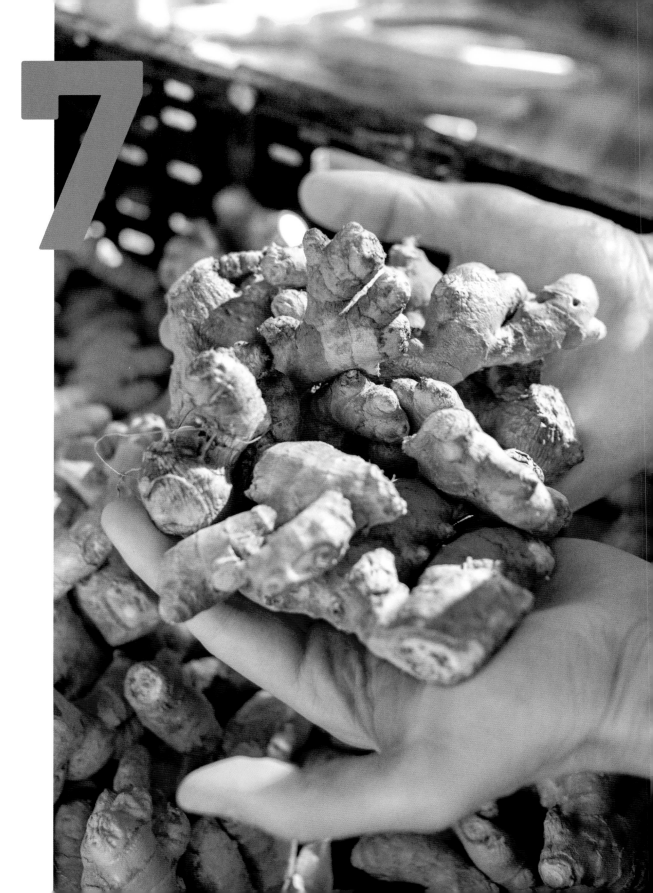

7

T | Train Your Gut

The method to repair and restore function to even the most decimated gut

I see many patients who have come to believe they aren't capable of consuming certain foods. That's almost certainly not true. The gut is forgiving. It is adaptable. If you're suffering from food intolerances that involve the gut microbiota, the GROWTH strategy is the method that you use to eat to grow your microbiome in all facets—biodiversity, digestive enzyme levels, and functional abilities. You have the ability to make it what you want it to be. But in order for it to work the way you want it to, you have to understand the rules of engagement. Jumping into a raw vegan or macrobiotic diet is not something I would ever recommend to someone suffering with digestive issues, yet I see people do it all the time. Then they fail, and they say that a plant-based diet doesn't work. That's simply not true. Whipping from fad diet to fad diet suggests confusion about the healing process. Taking things to an extreme, thinking that an extreme must be better, is not actually the way that your body works.

You Have to Understand the Process in Order to Properly Heal

If you pull out a microscope and take a look at the thirty-eight trillion microbes living inside you, you would discover a community where everyone plays a role. Each microbe has unique skills contributing to the greater whole. That greater whole is you, and those collective skills are the microbiome's contributions to your super-organism physiology—immunity, metabolism, hormones, brain function, gene expression, and, of course, digestive function.

The sum of the microbiome's constituent parts plays a massive role in your ability to digest food. You are a super-organism, but you lack the enzymes needed to digest complex carbohydrates like fibre, having just 17 glycoside hydrolase enzymes. Meanwhile, *Bacteroides thetaiotaomicron*, a single-celled organism, possesses 260 glycoside hydrolases in its genome alone. Your gut microbiome may contain up to 60,000 glycoside hydrolases in sum. Each one is a tool your microbes use to unpack your complex carbohydrates.

We need so many unique enzymes because there are so many unique plants to consume, and unpacking fibre is complicated. It requires a sequence of multiple enzymes, functioning in concert, to break down. For example, the breakdown of type I rhamnogalacturonan requires at least a dozen different enzymes, and then even more are needed to work on type II. Thankfully, nature is intelligent and has developed systems to do it for us. You don't really need to think, you just need to support your gut microbes and then get out of the way and let them go to work.

How do we support our gut microbes so that they will be ready, willing, and able to do their job in digesting our food? Quite simply, they need to be fed. If you feed your gut microbes, they are more than happy to take care of everything else for you. When they are fed, they grow stronger and are more powerfully represented. They bring with them the enzymes needed to help you unpack future meals. When you eat beans, you will have more microbes that are really good at digesting beans. The more you eat beans, the stronger they become.

But if they are not fed, you can't expect the same. They will grow weaker, become marginalized, and at some point become incapable of doing their job. This is particularly obvious when you ask them to step up and do more. If you haven't been eating beans, and then you pull out the five-bean chilli, you're going to be miserable. Why? Because your gut microbes weren't prepared for the amount of beans you consumed and weren't equipped with the proper enzymes to digest it.

What I'm describing is a process in which your gut and its functionality are conditioned by and proportional to your food choices. Eat more of one food and you will become better at processing that food. Eat less of that food, and you should expect that you won't be as capable at processing that food. Eat lots of different plants and you will gain abilities from . . . ALL OF THEM! The ability to condition our organs is a beautiful and celebrated part of being human.

When you practise something, you get better at it. Muscles can be trained. If you lift weights, you can lift heavier weights over time. If you run, you can run faster and farther over time. If you practise at sports, such as shooting free throws in basketball, you get better over time.

Adaptation is everywhere. The heart actually remodels itself in response to exercise: Larger chambers allow more blood volume while each squeeze becomes more efficient, resulting in more blood circulating with less effort. Our lungs adapt to exercise, too: larger lung volumes, stronger respiratory muscles, more blood vessels, and more alveoli to facilitate gas exchange. Think about that. Demand creates transformations—even in human anatomy.

Our brain is a muscle. It can be trained, too. Neuroplasticity means that the brain is anything but fixed; it can be adapted to our individual needs. Deaf individuals have enhanced visual capabilities. Blind individuals have enhanced auditory capabilities. People who have a stroke can regain function with physical therapy. We can learn to speed-read or practise and get better with the Rubik's cube.

We are capable of more than we realize. Things that seem impossible are actually possible if you're willing to put in the effort. Abebe Bikila ran an entire marathon in 2 hours and 15 minutes while barefoot. Karoline Meyer held her breath underwater for 18 minutes and 32 seconds after four months of training. Tom Amberry made 2,750 free throws in a row—at the age of seventy-one. SeungBeom Cho completed a Rubik's cube in 4.5 seconds—so fast that onlookers needed more than 4.5 seconds to process what had just happened.

The body is capable of amazing adaptations, but none of these people rolled out of bed with innate superhuman abilities and just did the task when prompted. Every single one invested effort and consistency into a rigorous training protocol to build themselves up to the point that they could do something that no one thought possible. Every single one had a plan, invested tremendous effort into that plan, and had to persevere through challenges and setbacks in order to develop the abilities that make them superhuman.

The gut is no different. It is a muscle. It can be trained. You can make it stronger. It is forgiving and adaptable. You can restore function that is lost and enhance function beyond what you thought you were capable of. You are entirely capable of having a superhuman gut if you're willing to commit yourself to the training protocol, invest the effort, and persevere through the challenges. That piece of broccoli that's had you terrified doesn't stand a chance.

But you don't just wake up one day and eat whatever the heck you want. Or decide that you're going to give the raw vegan diet a spin because you heard that was healthy, so you're just going to jump in. There is a process to training your gut, just as there is a process to training your muscles at the gym.

I'm going to be your personal gut trainer. Our goal is to train it to maximize your gut's function and strength. Let's look at a few scenarios to help us understand exactly how this works.

It's Your First Day at the Gym after You've Committed to Getting Stronger

I'm glad you're here! The future is bright, but it's important to pace yourself and recognize that all good things take time, patience, effort, and consistency. You don't heal your gut in one day or one meal. You heal your gut with consistency, repetition, having a plan, and staying committed to the process. It's easy to be excited and overly ambitious on your first day in the gym. Let's not make the mistake of exercising way beyond your abilities. At a minimum, that will leave you sore for a week. Or worse, you could hurt yourself and suffer a serious setback.

You Need to START LOW.

When you first start exercising your gut, stay within the thresholds you worked to identify during the first steps of the GROWTH process. That is critical information because we are defining exactly what "start low" means for you. Wherever the threshold for tolerance exists, you want to go below that. If you're not sure of the threshold, start with 1 teaspoon of the food in question.

It's also important to recognize that soreness is a normal part of the process. When the body initially starts to change, you're asking it to move in a different direction and do something that it's not yet adapted to or good at. Discomfort is to be expected when you ask your body to do something beyond its current capability. Don't be discouraged by some discomfort. See it for what it is—a normal part of the GROWTH process.

You've Been Consistently Going to the Gym and Your Goal Is to Build Muscle

Regular exercise enhances performance in a reproducible pattern. Our muscles do work, our body compensates for the increased work demand with muscular hypertrophy, and a few days later your muscles are slightly bigger and stronger. If you put them to work again, ratcheting up the demand ever so slightly, you will continue this growth phase. On the flip side, if the exercise stops, demand is reduced, the muscles atrophy, and function and ability are reduced.

This is the way it works in the gut, too. You need to exercise your gut. Every single food group is like working a different muscle. We want to work all the muscles so that the whole body grows stronger, not just a few limited muscles.

Building muscle still requires a plan. You don't just lift whatever you want and immediately jump to whatever your goal is. You need to work within your ability, push the limits of what you can do, and grow over time.

You Need to GO SLOW.

If you go too fast, you will hurt yourself. When it comes to meeting your goals, you're not looking at days or weeks. We're looking at months, in some cases years. But if you commit to that process and stick to the plan of ratcheting up ever so slightly over time, you will see the gains you desire. If you're not sure how much to increase a specific food that you're working on, try increasing it by 1 teaspoon every three days.

You Suffer a Setback and Get Hurt

There is a path of recovery that leads to restoring function and strengthening. But setbacks can happen when you're exercising a muscle, and this is true in the gut, too. The problem is that a setback dramatically reduces your ability, and you don't automatically bounce right back to where you were before. A few examples of setbacks include an infection that requires antibiotics, a flare-up of Crohn's disease or ulcerative colitis, or a traumatic event that has your stomach in knots. If you experience a setback, you'll need to recalibrate.

The process of recovery from injury usually doesn't take place at the gym. In many cases, you need a trained physical therapist to work with you. You return to the basics. If it's your shoulder that you hurt, you're no longer lifting weights over your head. Heck, you may not be able to lift your arm above your shoulder. But if you commit to the process, you can restore function and get your strength back.

You Need to START LOW and GO SLOW.

Recovery from injury takes time, and you'll need to be gentle and patient. Really, you are doing the same thing you did before the injury, except you'll likely need to start lower and go slower. This may require you to drop so low that it almost seems absurd. Anyone out there eating three chickpeas at a time? But this isn't any different than the person who goes from lifting 20 kilos over their head, injures their shoulder, and then needs to go back to small movements without any weight at all just to get their arm overhead.

But by trusting the process, that person goes from needing assistance to lift their arm, to lifting their arm unassisted, to lifting 2 kilos, 4 kilos, 6 kilos. This level of growth may take months! But that's how you work your way back at the gym, and eventually get back to cranking 22 kilos overhead. Start with 1 teaspoon of the food you're working on training your gut to tolerate and increase it by 1 teaspoon every 3 days. At this pace, you'll have a gut capable of rocking 7 teaspoons in about 3 weeks. If you need to slow it down, no problem. Instead of 3 days, wait 4 or 5 before ramping things up.

Are There Conditions in Which Training Your Gut Isn't Possible?

Of course, the GROWTH strategy doesn't work for every single food sensitivity. This goes back to our discussion of the genesis of the problem. There are medical conditions that won't allow you to condition your gut, or they will cause you to face limitations in restoring gut function. Here are a few of the particular scenarios I'm referring to:

1. **Coeliac disease:** From my perspective, there is no path to safely add gluten back into your life if you have coeliac disease, and therefore you should remain gluten-free permanently.

2. **Food allergies:** It's technically possible to heal and reverse food allergies in some cases, but it is complicated and dangerous and therefore requires a trained health professional to guide therapy. The GROWTH strategy is not intended to reverse food allergies.

3. **Genetic food intolerances:** You have to play the hand that you are dealt in life, and it's always in our interest to maximize it and do the best we can. That said, you don't get to choose the cards you're dealt. If you have a genetic cause for sucrase-isomaltase, lactase, or diamine oxidase (DAO) deficiency, then you will need to work around your limitations by moderating your intake of the intolerant foods. In this setting, the GROWTH strategy absolutely still makes sense; we are just limited in terms of what's possible.

4. **Irreversible chronic health issues:** If you have an irreversible chronic health issue—such as chronic pancreatitis or a gallbladder problem—you need to start by addressing that specific issue. That said, you can still apply the GROWTH strategy moving forward. It's just important to recognize that you will be held back by that health issue if it is not properly addressed.

So who is the GROWTH strategy for? Everyone suffering from food intolerances that involve the gut microbiota. The GROWTH strategy is the method that you use to eat to grow your microbiome in all facets—biodiversity, digestive enzyme levels, and functional abilities.

Six Tools to Help You Train Your Gut

Training your gut is about applying a system of principles to restore and enhance the capabilities of your digestive apparatus—and it never hurts to have extra tools in your toolbox during training! With that in mind, here are some strategies that I've found helpful in reducing food sensitivity. Don't try to do them all at once. Instead, start with whichever feels the most interesting to you. Master that one, and then you can come back to this list and consider the next one that seems most appealing, and so on.

1. Practise diaphragmatic breathing often. It is your friend and can be powerful

Digestion is an activity of the parasympathetic nervous system. Diaphragmatic breathing has been shown to activate the parasympathetic nervous system. No surprise, it has shown benefit for acid reflux and anxiety, and is believed beneficial for irritable bowel syndrome.

To do diaphragmatic breathing, choose a comfortable position, either sitting or lying flat. Relax your shoulders. Put one hand on your chest and the other on your stomach. Breathe in through your nose slowly over 4 seconds, allowing your stomach to do the work by moving out while keeping your chest relatively still. Hold for 2 seconds. Now purse your lips, press gently on your stomach, and exhale slowly for 4 seconds. Pause for 2 seconds before repeating the inhalation cycle. With each breath, allow the stress and anxiety to leave your body. Use breathwork as an opportunity to allow your entire body to slow down and enter into a more relaxed state. Do this for at least 8 breaths or up to 15 minutes. It can be done before and after meals and throughout the day for grounding and relaxation.

2. Take a moment of gratitude before meals

Saying a blessing prior to meals is a tradition in many cultures and homes, but it's one thing to say it and it's another to engage with it and mean it. One study found that taking a moment of gratitude was associated with improvements in healthy eating behaviour in adolescents and young adults.

Take a moment to say a prayer of gratitude or have a mindful moment where you focus on your food—the colours, textures, smells, and tastes. Be thankful that you have delicious food that nourishes your body. Not everyone is so lucky. Be grateful that the earth has generously provided you this food. It is the product of time, the sun and the soil, and effort from nature to make available food that nourishes your body and your gut microbes. Be thankful for your loved ones that you share this meal with. One of life's great pleasures is to socialize and share food with others.

3. Visualize the experience you want to have with your meal and manifest that intention

Establishing a concrete goal and then visualizing the path to success in that goal is a tried-and-true method used by professional athletes like Michael Phelps, Muhammad Ali, Lindsey Vonn, Tiger Woods, Novak Djokovic, Katie Ledecky, and many others. Whether it's athletic performance or digestive function, the idea is that you are creating the neural networks, or brain pathways, for your desired outcome. It's like a mental dress rehearsal. Practice makes perfect, even when the practice is only in your head.

Let's try one together. Imagine an experience where you have no fear of food, you have only joy and delight. Visualize the sight of the food, the smell. Imagine savouring the flavour and texture. Imagine what happens when you chew on it. How does it make you feel? Feel the warmth and satisfaction that come from filling your stomach with food, the happiness of delicious food. Live in this moment for a little; don't rush it. This is your destiny. This will be your new normal; it is just a matter of when it will happen.

Visualize an enlightened path to getting there. You are growing, you are empowered, and you are becoming stronger. Along this path you face challenges, but you can handle them, and your confidence surges as you rise above each one. Your ability is a ball of light that grows bigger and brighter as you continue down this path towards your ultimate destination.

As you come back to the present moment, allow yourself a moment to decompress. Simply observe your breathing and pay attention to your senses as they reconnect with the world around you. When you're ready, open your eyes and slowly reintroduce yourself to your outer world.

If you make this part of your daily routine, you will be amazed at how much improvement you will see in your life. You can literally heal yourself and manifest this reality by having a daily visualization practice.

Something important happens subconsciously when you visualize—you identify a specific goal. If you reflect on what you just did, you will see that in order to visualize the outcome and also the triumphant path of perseverance, you must inherently have a goal in mind. Let's bring that goal from the subconscious into the conscious and properly establish it—with an index card and a pen.

Write down your goal. Just one. Make it something concrete, with a clear definition of success. Also, make sure it is attainable. We don't want to set unrealistic goals. We want goals that are achievable so that we can achieve them, then line up the next one. Once you have this goal established, I want you to post it somewhere where you'll see it every day. I recommend the bathroom mirror. There's no missing it there.

Do me one last favour, while you're at it. Grab a second index card and your pen and write these two lines:

Progress over perfection.
—Dr. B

I want you to post this next to your goal. It's a simple way for me to be with you and remind you every day that I support you, that I want to see you succeed, and that if you adhere to our mantra you will get there. Anything is possible, and visual imagery can help enhance your success and manifest your intention into reality.

4. Slow your roll at mealtimes

We live in a fast-paced society in which mealtimes are a burden that stands in the way of our work or something else we're trying to accomplish. It isn't right, and it's messing up our digestion! Our body wasn't designed to digest food as an afterthought. And the idea of choosing foods because they're easier for us to scarf down is a short-term gain, long-term loss proposition because you are always compromising the quality of your food when you do that. You're also compromising your digestion. Instead, let's make time committed to eating and enjoying our food a priority. Making time for yourself and to enjoy one of life's greatest pleasures (food) is a form of self-care.

Chewing your food is the first step in digestion, and it needs to be taken seriously. In your mouth, food mixes with your oral microbiome and digestive enzymes in your saliva that break down carbohydrates and proteins. Thirty per cent of starch digestion takes place in your mouth. The act of chewing crushes and breaks apart the food, mixing it with microbes and digestive enzymes. What we're doing here is starting with large particles and breaking them down into smaller particles. That's what digestion is all about, folks!

If you imagine your digestive system as a factory line, each step prepares the food for the next step in a process of transformation that has an end result. Chewing your food is that important first step that future steps in the process build upon. If you barely chew your food, you're skipping the first step in the factory and hoping to get the same result in the end. Should you be surprised that you don't? Of course not. It's to be expected that mistakes from the beginning lead to more mistakes down the entire line. If you have digestive symptoms, you need to slow your roll and chew your food—thoroughly.

5. Enhance your mealtime experience with digestive teas

I'm a huge believer in having a warm, soothing beverage after meals to help calm and relax the digestive system. The concept is so straightforward and simple—teas taste good, and they make you feel good. Sure, from a scientific standpoint there are phytochemicals circulating in the tea that add flavour and have medicinal effects.

Ginger	Gingerol	Reduces nausea
Peppermint	Menthol	Relaxes intestinal smooth muscle
Fennel	Trans-anethole	Stimulates motility
Chamomile	α-Bisabolol	Relaxes intestinal smooth muscle

You could make any of these teas individually, based upon your taste preference or digestive needs, but I have also included my Digestive Bliss Tea (page 287), which combines all four. It's like the Avengers—great individually, but unbelievable when working as a team.

Generally, I consider the best time to drink these teas is after the meal. That being said, I fully support an intuitive approach when it comes to introducing digestive teas. If you drink them before or during meals, and find that that works for you, I am with it 100 per cent.

6. Go for a walk after meals

Have you ever overeaten to the point of abdominal discomfort, and you basically have two choices—throw on the tracksuit bottoms and lie on the couch making groaning noises for the next hour, or throw on the athletic shoes and go for a light walk for thirty minutes and feel energized, lighter, and less bloated? I love tracksuit bottoms as much as anyone, but it's a bit masochistic to drag out your misery on the couch, even if the trackie bottoms are super comfortable.

There's a physiologic basis for taking a walk after meals. Gastric emptying increases with exercise, even light walking, compared to rest. Just mild exercise is needed to improve intestinal gas clearance and improve bloating. A thirty-minute walk can reduce colon transit time and improve constipation. A short walk after a meal is also good for your metabolism—regulating blood sugar, lowering blood pressure, reducing blood lipids, and burning intra-abdominal fat. Not only are these risk factors for heart disease, but they've also been correlated with dietary inflammation. Is it too good to be true? No! It's the way we were wired. We are not sedentary creatures.

Despite everything I've said, there are some people who will find that exercise actually aggravates their symptoms. No worries, just take a little time after the meal before you head out, and slow your walking speed a little.

The Role of Supplements and Medications

Optimal healthcare blends together the best of diet, lifestyle, supplements, medications, and procedures. To take the best from each is to accept the best that exists without imposing arbitrary limitations. To shun or refuse one is to place limits on your ability to prevent and treat disease, and for that reason it is inherently an inferior choice. I believe that food comes first, but that there is definitely a role for supplements and medications. When the best approach for my patient is to include supplements or medications in the treatment plan, I include them. As for which ones, it really depends on the condition that you are trying to treat, and it is a topic that goes beyond the scope of this book. Follow me on social media and subscribe to my email list to get routine updates on the strategies that I use to help my patients.

The One Thing That's More Important Than Diet, Lifestyle, Pills, or Procedures

I'm of the belief that having the grit to see something to completion is the key to success in all arenas, including our own health. You can be blessed with innate talent or "healthy genes," but those are finite resources that run out at some point. Hard work can take you far and allow you to exceed the limitations of your talent or genes, but only if you stick with it long enough to allow it to happen. At some point, we all face challenges. The going gets tough . . . If diversity of plants is the single greatest predictor of gut health, how you respond to challenges is the single greatest predictor of ultimate success. If you quit, progress is halted and you start to lose ground towards your goal. But if you just won't quit under any circumstances, I can assure you that you will get what you want at some point. It's only a matter of time in that case.

This is true for our health. Even if you're healthy, at some point you will face challenges. It can come in many forms, including a reluctance or unwillingness to make the changes necessary to get there. Change is never easy; it's a challenge in its own right because it requires adaptation. I want you to commit to having the grit and the audacity to stick with it until you get what you want. Whether it is exercising at the gym, learning a new diet or lifestyle, or training your gut, you know that adaptation is possible, it makes you stronger, and persistence is how you make it happen time and again until you accomplish your goals.

>> *To view the 33 scientific references cited in this chapter, please visit www.theplantfedgut.com/cookbook.*

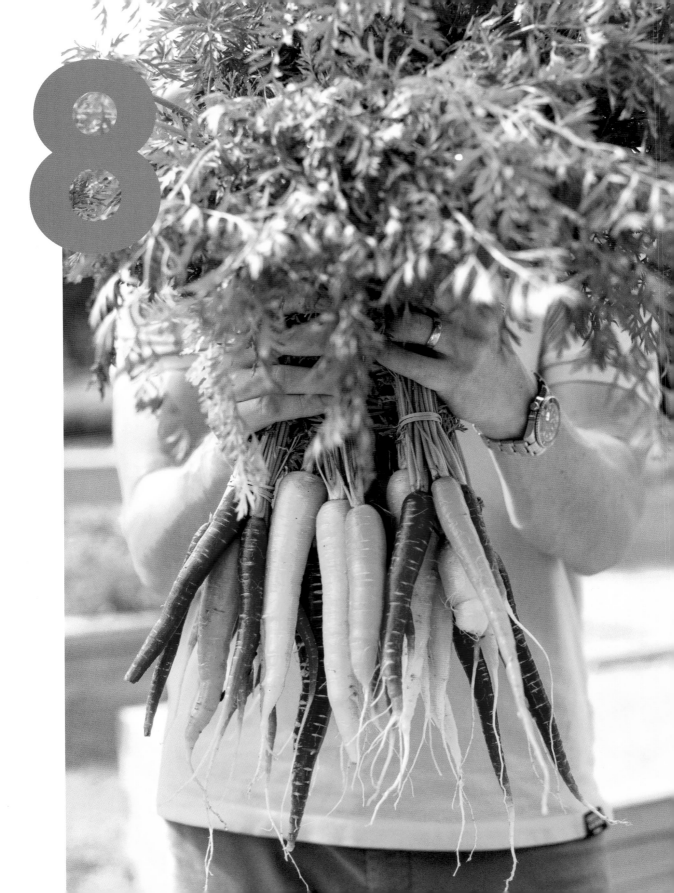

H | Holistic Healing

Your gut is the micro and to heal it we need to tend to the macro

In medicine, we fractionate the body into systems so that we can develop expertise. But there's a problem—this is not how the world works! Everything is interconnected. Relationships are complicated. Nothing takes place in isolation, even though that's how we study and try to understand it.

But there's good news. We can use this to our advantage. We can recognize that in our interconnected world, all choices have a ripple effect like a stone being thrown into water. If we're smart about it, we can recognize that by elevating organs other than the gut we can indirectly achieve our goal of optimizing digestive function. It's called rising the tide on human health. When you improve the health in one part of the body, you are simultaneously improving the health in other parts, too, due to these interconnections. This is why we need to look at the person as a whole and not as a group of fractionated parts. This is why ignoring the health of parts outside the digestive system is a mistake that can hold us back. This is why we need to heal the whole person and watch that tide of human health rise for optimal results throughout.

Strategies for Healing the Gut without a Fork or a Plate

Food isn't the only way to train your gut. You can make it stronger without putting food in your mouth, which is a beautiful thing when you're not feeling well. Here are some of the strategies that, by taking care of the whole person, you can use to elevate the health of your gut.

Give Your Gut Microbes a Rest

Some of us spend eighteen hours per day in a postprandial state, actively digesting food that we've consumed in the last few hours, meaning our gut microbes remain hard at work. Recent research indicates that a twelve-hour fast is sufficient to induce changes in the gut microbiota that are beneficial. Therefore, make it a daily goal to stop late-night snacking and limit your intake to water only for a period of twelve hours.

Does Coffee Affect the Gut Microbiome?

Yes, coffee does in fact alter the microbiome and end the twelve-plus-hour fast. In research from my friends Drs. Tim Spector and Sarah Berry, they found that coffee consumption was associated with growth of *Lawsonibacter asaccharolyticus*, a butyrate-producing microbe. That's a win for coffee consumers but also why we limit our intake to water only while fasting.

It's Not Just Calories, Macronutrients, and Micronutrients . . . Timing Matters!

You could eat the exact same food at two different times in the day and get two different metabolic outcomes. We are most insulin sensitive in the morning and become progressively more insulin resistant as the day goes on. The timing of our food is important because our body, our hormones, and our gut microbes are trained to function on a twenty-four-hour rhythm that is synchronized with the rise and fall of the sun. The rather simple takeaways here are to shift more of your calories to earlier in the day, have an early light dinner, and limit your intake in the evening.

Physical Fitness Actually Translates into Gut Fitness

Research has shown us that exercise training alters the composition and functional capacity of the gut microbiota regardless of the food you eat. Translation: You can improve your gut health through exercise. Be cautious not to go overboard, as high-intensity exercise can actually exacerbate digestive issues. A great option to consider is yoga, which combines movement, stretching, weight bearing, and mindfulness. No surprise, research suggests that yoga is nearly as effective as the low FODMAP diet for irritable bowel syndrome.

Here are five simple stretches that can be part of your daily routine and can also be used around meals to help reduce digestive distress:

Cobbler pose: Sit tall with a long spine. Bend your knees and bring the soles of your feet together as your knees fall to either side. Draw your feet as close to your body as is comfortable and either hang on to your feet or reach your hands out onto the floor in front of you. Take at least six deep breaths in this position.

Seated twist: Sit cross-legged and tall with a long spine. Gently twist to one side, bringing one hand behind you and the other to rest on your opposite knee. Take at least six deep, slow breaths before switching to the other side.

Spinal twists: Lie flat on your back. Bring both knees to your chest while untucking your tailbone. Form a "T" with your arms and slowly let both of your legs fall to one side. Gaze over your opposite shoulder. Take six breaths before switching to the other side.

Happy baby: Lie flat on your back and bend your knees toward your chest at a 90-degree angle. Face the soles of your feet toward the ceiling. If you can, grab and hold the outside of your feet. Spread your knees apart. Gently rock side to side, inhaling and exhaling for at least six breaths.

Legs up the wall: Start by sitting on the floor with one hip close to the wall. Swing your legs up the wall as you simultaneously lie back on the floor. Take at least six deep breaths, focusing on using your diaphragm for the breaths.

Your Gut Heals and Grows Stronger When You Sleep

A new study showed us that gut microbiota diversity increases with increased sleep duration and better sleep quality. Ever have something on your mind that wakes you up at two in the morning? In the study, sleep interruption was associated with reduced microbiota diversity, the point being that sleep is extremely low-hanging fruit and can help support a healthy gut. It's important to be disciplined and go to bed early enough to get at least seven and ideally eight hours of sleep.

Head for Greener Pastures

Time spent outdoors and in greener environments has been shown to improve mental health and general feelings of wellness, in addition to reduced risk of attention deficit disorder among children. In an intervention study with preschool-age children, scheduled time outdoors yielded beneficial changes in the gut microbiota, increased serotonin levels in the stool, a reduction of their sense of stress, and a decrease of the frequency of angry outbursts. Kids aren't the only ones who need time outdoors! A recent study of adults found that dipping their hands into a mix of soil and plant-based material on a daily basis led to increased gut microbial diversity over two weeks. Opt for outdoor hobbies or schedule outdoor time for a healthy gut and to reduce your angry outbursts.

Put Down Your Phone and Reconnect with Real Humans

We often focus on risk factors for disease like smoking or obesity and completely ignore human connectivity, yet research says that having strong human relationships is actually *more* important for longevity. Perhaps it defies your expectations, but it shows the importance of being social to human health. Think about it—the easiest way to torture someone is to isolate them. It turns out that one of the perks of human connection is that it makes you more connected to your gut microbes. In a recent study, researchers found that spouses share microbes more so than siblings, that the sharing was not due to dietary factors, and that this only occurred in those who reported feeling connected to their spouse. The sharing of microbes did not happen among spouses who were less connected. Furthermore, married couples had greater microbiome diversity compared to people who lived alone, with the greatest diversity seen among couples who felt strongly connected to their spouse. Fascinating, right?

The Echoes of Trauma Persist in the Subconscious Until They Are Dealt With

In my clinic, I often meet people who have tried it all. They've been to numerous doctors and tried seemingly every diet and medication out there. They've done everything they've been asked to do—eat clean, sleep, exercise, meditate. Yet, despite their investment in their health, they continue to suffer with digestive symptoms.

I've learned that what's often missing is an acknowledgment of how the past informs the present. We are not robots, we are humans. We have life experiences that can leave us wounded.

These wounds come in many forms, and they all impact our digestion. We know that physical, emotional, and sexual abuse during childhood are associated with increased risk of irritable bowel syndrome as an adult. In fact, physical punishment of any variety, an unhealthy relationship with a primary caregiver, losing a parent, witnessing violence, or living with someone with mental or psychiatric illness may lead to IBS. Things that many of us have experienced—the loss of a loved one, a car accident, divorce or traumatic breakup, a house fire or natural disaster—have been connected to the manifestation of symptoms in our gut as well. Post-traumatic stress disorder (PTSD) is a powerful risk factor for IBS.

I've seen this pattern for years. The most challenging digestive disorders are found in those with a prior history of trauma. The intensity of the prior trauma is often proportional to the intensity of the digestive issues. My mentor and friend, Dr. Douglas Drossman, pioneered this research more than thirty years ago. We continue to evolve in our understanding.

Just recently a study of children adopted from orphanages or foster care before age two—meaning before the formation of memories—showed that they had increased prevalence of digestive disorders and anxiety compared to healthy controls. Gut microbiome analysis revealed lower gut microbiome diversity and distinct gut microbial patterns. Functional brain imaging showed altered brain activity patterns, particularly in brain regions well known to be implicated in emotional functioning. These alterations in brain activity correlated to changes in the gut microbes.

While we continue to learn more, there is one simple fact that we already know to be true—your gut can only be as healthy as your emotional state. We expect that wounds will heal with time, but that's not always true. Dr. Drossman taught me that when patients are not responding to medicine and seem impossible to treat, it's important to take a thorough trauma and abuse history. This requires trust and takes time. But it's also the key to healing. If there are emotional wounds, we have to acknowledge their existence and create a plan to address them.

I know that these conversations can be difficult and even distressing. But the best healing in my career hasn't been fixing guts—it's been helping patients get the help they need to heal their emotional wounds, and then watching their "impossible" gut health problem disappear. If this resonates with you, when you feel ready, and at a pace where you can maintain control, I encourage you to seek the support of a health professional who can help you find coping strategies to heal life experiences that negatively impact your life. I suggest trying cognitive behavioural therapy, psychodynamic therapy, exposure therapy, or hypnotherapy.

Food Avoidance: When Your Relationship with Food Is on the Rocks

You're in a relationship with your food and sometimes it's not a great or fulfilling one.

There are a number of ways that this can happen. You might associate a traumatic experience with food, such as a choking episode or a case of food poisoning. Or you might be a "picky eater," which we often see in children who develop an aversion to certain tastes, smells, or textures. It can be chronic symptoms that make you neurotic and fearful of your food. Or it can be an unhealthy, disordered relationship that we develop with our food that may include:

- Fear or anxiety provoked by food
- Avoidance of specific foods that are deemed problematic
- Emotional eating with feelings of shame or guilt
- Using food to cope with stress
- Obsession with "eating healthy," being thin, and how you look in the mirror
- Aggressive exercise combined with food restriction
- The feeling that you need to "burn off" every calorie that goes in your mouth
- Rigid rules and rituals like calorie counting, macros, eat this/not that

- A feeling of loss of control around food, including compulsive eating habits
- Chronic weight fluctuations
- Judging others on their eating pattern

You don't need to have an eating disorder to have disordered eating. What I mean is that there are specific conditions that we have defined as eating disorders: anorexia nervosa, bulimia nervosa, avoidant/restrictive food intake disorder (ARFID), and binge eating disorder, just to name a few. There are eight total eating disorders identified in the most recent version of the *Diagnostic and Statistical Manual of Mental Disorders* (*DSM-5*). But the reality is that there is a spectrum for unhealthy food relationships that spans from mild food fear or anxiety all the way up to anorexia or bulimia. Most people who have a toxic relationship with their food do not meet the criteria for an eating disorder, but that doesn't mean they are not dealing with a real problem. Regardless of whether you meet the criteria for one of these diagnoses, if your relationship with food is unhealthy, then a pattern of disordered eating exists and is an added challenge that needs to be dealt with on your healing journey.

Unfortunately, when we create a separation between ourselves and our food, it can spiral out of control. Ivan Pavlov showed us in 1897 that he could train his dogs to salivate when he rang a bell. We can experience this, too—a specific food rings like the bell, and the response that you've learned is queasiness, discomfort, or anxiety. Our ability to associate specific foods with illness was evolved to protect us from eating toxic foods back in the day when we lived in a cave. Times have changed, but modern culture is pumping us up with food fear that promotes unhealthy food-symptom associations.

There are also several generations of us who were raised on the oversimplified and generally incorrect principle that "if food causes symptoms, then that food is bad and it must be eliminated." Or that certain foods contain toxins that are harming us and the solution to our problems is progressive restriction. The internet has taken these concepts and put them on steroids, taking unhealthy ideas and throwing them in our face every time we open an app.

Food is more than just chemistry. It's more than digestive juices and enzymes interacting with macro- and micronutrients. Food is complex. We are complex. And there is a lot more to our interaction with food than reducing it to chemical reactions. I want you to hear this, so I'm going to shout it out for the people in the back—

Our Emotional Relationship with Food Plays a Massive Role in Whether We Find Pleasure or Experience Pain When We Eat.

In other words, there is a psychological element to food sensitivity. It can amplify our experience—both positive and negative. It can also alter our digestion or even create new symptoms. You can optimize your microbiome and eat all the right foods, but if your emotional relationship with food is unhealthy, then you will never experience the full pleasure that's on that dish. I want you to have awareness of the importance of psychology in our relationship with food, because it's an important and required step for proper digestion. If we want you to enjoy your food, we can't just fix the microbiome. We need to heal your relationship with food, too.

First and Foremost, Be Compassionate to Yourself

Believe that you're worthy, that you deserve it. But also know that you have the stamina and grit to persevere through challenges. Setting the proper mindset is important to your success. We like to pretend that life is about victory and defeat. The hype makes it feel like each choice is life or death and that we should feel guilty when we don't make the choice that we've been told to or are supposed to. Folks, that is hogwash.

We make around 35,000 choices every single day. Over 200 of those choices are food choices. Sorry, but no one in the history of humanity has ever nailed all 35,000/200. The numbers suggest that even if we get it right most of the time, we're going to be getting it wrong many, many times each day. If every misstep is a bee-sting, how are we going to feel at the end of the day?

Let's be real. Perfect doesn't exist. It's a figment of the human imagination, presented as an attainable goal in marketing campaigns, media, and diet culture. It's so silly. Imperfect humans are what we all are, and it's our imperfection that makes us fun and interesting. We're all making choices that reflect our unique personality. Why are we demonizing the imperfection that is inevitable?

I say forget about perfect. Focus on progress. Progress is attainable. It's realistic. It's your own personal measure, not a comparison to someone else. And it's what matters!

Let's look at the big picture. We have this bucket, and we're going to add water to it. There will definitely be some water in that bucket every day, reflecting our success. Every day, there is success worth celebrating, we have to remember that. Some days we're going to look down at the bucket and see that there's not as much water in it. That's okay. There's still water in the bucket. You still get to drink. And you will come back tomorrow and have another chance to add water to the bucket.

So as you embark on this journey, I hope you find the GROWTH strategy to be helpful and a compass that guides you to a better place in terms of your overall health. But remember, while you're walking down that path, that this is a journey and not a sprint. It has highs and lows, which are part of the human experience. Be good to yourself. Allow compassion and forgiveness for your imperfections. Celebrate your successes at the end of the day because each day brings successes. And hold true to our shared philosophy for GROWTH: progress over perfection.

>> *To view the 29 scientific references cited in this chapter, please visit www.theplantfedgut.com/cookbook.*

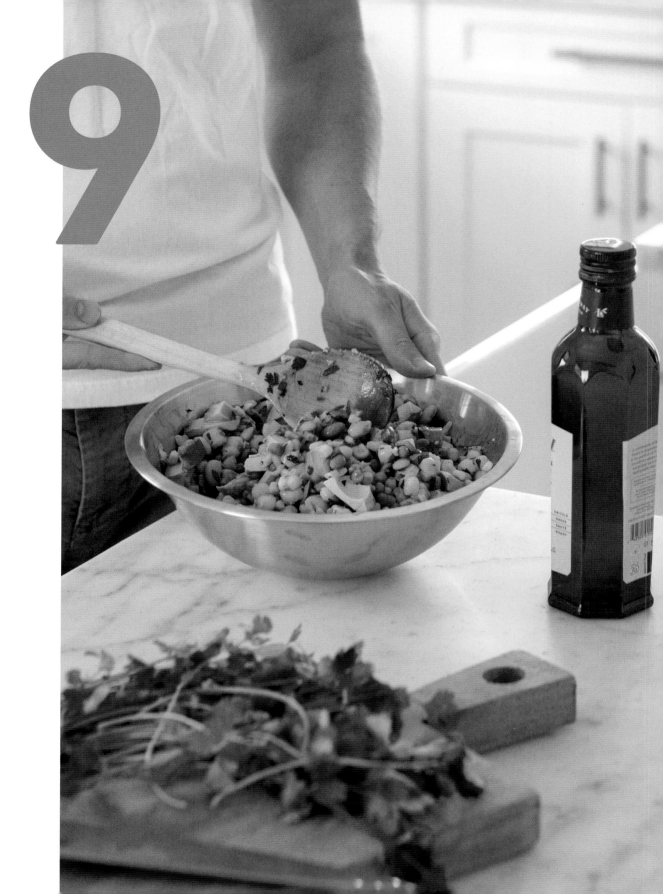

9

Fibre Fuelled
Unleashed

Collect your plant points and take the stage as a Fibre Fuelled rock star

There's a plant party going down in this chapter, and you're the guest of honour! It's time for us to enjoy plants in all their glory—the vibrant colours, fresh aromas, delectable flavours, and varied textures. Diversity is delicious!

Many different paths could lead you here. If you have no digestive issues, get your rear in gear and enjoy some delicious plants! But if you have food intolerances, you should have a good idea from the GROWTH strategy what your intolerances are, and the principles of going low and slow, so go at your own pace. If you're interested in details on which ingredients are high FODMAP or histamine, head to my website (www.theplantfedgut.com/cookbook), where you'll find that and lots of other resources.

No matter your path, we stand together united in our desire to support a diverse gut microbiota to enhance gut function, and to reap the benefits on our digestion, metabolism, immune system, hormones, mood, and brain health. That's what being *Fibre Fuelled* is all about.

Take Your Plant Diversity to the Next Level by Collecting Your Plant Points

Remember that our Golden Rule is to max out plant-based diversity. Every plant has its own unique blend of vitamins, minerals, phytochemicals, polyphenols, fibre, and protein. Perfectly balanced and packaged by nature, each plant has something positive to offer to your health. A biodiverse diet filled with as many fruits, vegetables, wholegrains, seeds, nuts, and legumes as possible fulfils the energy needs of a wider variety of microbes. In other words, a biodiverse, plant-based diet translates into a biodiverse gut, which is a healthier ecosystem. This isn't just a theory. The American Gut Project found that the diversity of plants in our diet was the most powerful predictor of a healthy gut microbiome. The healthiest guts were found in those consuming *more than thirty* different plant varieties in a week.

If diversity of plants is what we want, how are we going to make sure we get it? Well, a biodiverse diet starts with a biodiverse plate or bowl—every meal is an opportunity to feed our gut bugs the variety they crave. This is not meant to be a burden or an obligation. As I'm sure you've noticed by now, I'm not a big fan of applying pressure or stress to mealtimes. Instead, I believe that food truly is one of life's greatest pleasures. It's meant to be enjoyed and celebrated.

When I think of joy and fun, I think of games with friends and family. I have fond memories of long summer nights playing Ghost in the Graveyard as a kid. Or intense Monopoly games with my cousins. Now we have a family tradition of playing Charades before we exchange gifts with friends and family on Christmas Eve. Games are a wonderful way to connect with one another and have a shared moment.

That's why I devised the Plant Points game, which I first introduced in *Fibre Fuelled*. To play, you assign one Plant Point for every unique plant in your meal and add up your points. By collecting Plant Points, you have a fun way to be motivated to ratchet up your plant diversity with every meal. The end result is more biodiversity on your plate or in your bowl, which ultimately fuels a healthy gut microbiota.

The goal is to nourish your gut microbes with an adequate amount of plant fibre so that they can thrive and grow. Now, you don't get 21 Plant Points by simply eating a slice of bread that touts 21 wholegrains. To keep it honest, each plant should approximate a serving size. A standard serving size is typically 25 g of nuts, half a potato, 80 g of leafy greens, 1 medium tomato or piece of fruit, 1 slice of wholegrain bread, 2 tablespoons of nut butter, or 80 g of vegetables, wholegrains, or legumes. I give these as a general rule, but I haven't been too rigid about the Plant Points I've assigned to the recipes in this chapter.

Being Fibre Fuelled is not a diet or a rigid protocol; it is a lifestyle designed to heal you from the inside out. This is less about the rules and more about maxing out the diversity of plants in our diet.

Collecting Plant Points is meant to be fun. If you're fixated on the rules, you're probably missing out on the fun. For those wondering, I count fresh herbs and dried fruits but don't count plant milk or dried herbs. They're tricky, and you may beg to differ, but in determining whether to award Plant Points my north star is whether there is an adequate amount of plant fibre to feed the gut microbes. Plant milk has the fibre removed, while dried herbs are used in such trivial amounts. It seems inappropriate to give 5 Plant Points for a sprinkle of Italian seasoning, and then equate that to a complex, vibrant salad that includes five different veggies. Hence no Plant Points for dried herbs. But no matter how you approach it, just remember to have fun and get as much diversity onto your plate as possible.

Over the past few years, I've been amazed by how many of you have grabbed this concept and run with it. Nearly every day I get tagged in a post or a story on Instagram where someone is celebrating how many Plant Points they have on their plate. I've also had messages pouring in from around the world where people have shared how their pursuit of Plant Points has been transformative. Families that hang a white board in the kitchen to motivate their children to devour plants and collect their Plant Points. Friends or partners competing against one another to see who can get more Plant Points. Influencers and private Facebook groups creating Plant Point Challenges.

In *Fibre Fuelled*, I introduced the idea of collecting Plant Points for a week to determine your plant-based rock star status. This time, the goal is to see how many Plant Points you can rack up at each meal so that every time you sit down to eat, you can challenge yourself. Let's get going, and start crushing those Plant Points!

Plant Points (within one meal)	Rock Star Status
0–4	Rock Rookie
5–9	Rock Artist
10–14	Rock Star
15–19	Rock Legend
20 or more!	Rock God

When your kids ask why you're standing on the chair playing an absolutely vicious air guitar, you can let them know, "20 Plant Points! Dr. B says I'm a Rock God!" Perhaps you've always wanted your kids to think you're cool. Congratulations, the moment has arrived. Make sure to tag me @theguthealthmd in all your plant-devouring glory, and DEFINITELY tag me when you catch a shot of your kids, your boss, or your grandma playing the air guitar! A rock star is a rock star, it doesn't matter the age. (See Mick Jagger.)

Breakfast Unleashed

An Ode to Avocado Toast
  Summer Avocado Toast
  Avocado 'Shroom Toast
  Eggy Avocado Toast

Carrot Lox

Harissa White Bean Toast

Buckwheat Vegetable Crepes

Biome Stock Unleashed

Biome Stock Unleashed

Chickenless
Biome Stock

Fancy French
Biome Stock

Tuscan Biome Stock

Asian Biome Stock

Soups and Sandwiches Unleashed

Spicy Peanut Stew

Biome Stock Pho

Nashville Not Chicken

Vegetable Ceviche

Tofu Bánh Mì

Tofu Peanut Satay

Tempeh Bacon BLTA with
Celeriac Fries

Celeriac Fries

Hearty Mains Unleashed

Garlicky Kale

Paella

Easy Caprese Pasta

Where's the Beef?
Steak Plate
    Portobello Steaks
    Homemade Steak Sauce
    Mashed Potatoes

Herbed Potato Salad

Pozole

Very Veggie Indian Curry

Creamy Cajun Bowl

Sweet Potato and Okra Bowl

Tuscan Flatbread

Taking Your Sweet Potato Game
to the Next Level!
    Harissa Style
    Crispy Chickpeas
    Great Greek
    Tex-Mex

Beverages Unleashed

Herbal Infusions
    Digestive Bliss Tea
    Peppermint Tea
    Ginger Turmeric
      Lemon Tea
    Chamomile Tea
    Fennel Tea

Summertime Coolers
    Ginger Lemonade
    Turmeric Orange Cooler
    Matcha Honeydew Cooler

Sweets Unleashed

Peanut Butter Date Cookies

Mexican Hot Chocolate Brownies

Cookie Milk

Chocolate Cookie Milk

Crispy Dark Chocolate Bites

The Snickers Bites That Made You Freak
Out, So Now I'm Quadrupling Down
    Snickers Bites
    Simple and Sweet Date Bites
    Pomegranate Date Bites
    Snickers Ice Cream Bites

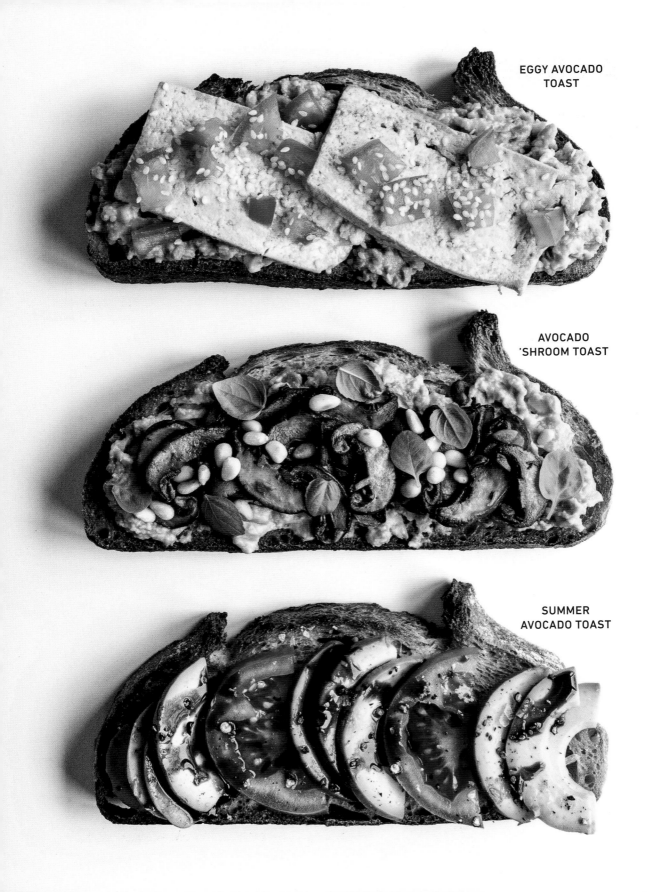

EGGY AVOCADO TOAST

AVOCADO 'SHROOM TOAST

SUMMER AVOCADO TOAST

AN ODE TO AVOCADO TOAST

Here we have three variations on one of my all-time favourite breakfasts—avocado toast. There's a lot to love. First, avo toast is easy. Toast some bread, transfer the avo on top, and mash it down. Boom! Done. Second, avo toast is flexible. We're giving you three options, but you can go whatever direction you like. I enjoy a savoury, acidic avo toast with balsamic vinegar, garlic, and Maldon sea salt. But you can have it whatever way suits your fancy. Finally, avocado toast is good for you! Avocados are high in fibre and incredibly healthy for the gut microbiota. In a randomized controlled trial, avocado consumption increased microbial diversity and enhanced the growth of short-chain-fatty-acid-producing microbes like *Faecalibacterium* and *Lachnospira*. Gimme all the avocado toast!

RECIPE CONTINUES

There's nothing worse than being excited for avo toast and then cutting open a brown avocado. Here are a few tips:

- Look at the avocado to assess where it is in its life cycle. Hard, bright green avocados are still 4 to 7 days away from being ripe. Dark green, almost black avocados that are firm with a slight flex when squeezed are ripe and ready to go. Black avocados that are mushy, dry, and wrinkled are past their prime. Use them now and salvage what you can.

- Try removing the brown stem for some added intel. If the stem is stubborn and won't budge, then the avocado isn't ripe. If you remove the stem to reveal a green nub, then the avocado is ripe and ready to go. But if the nub is brown, then the avocado may be past its prime.

- If you want to accelerate ripening and get it ready in the next 1 to 2 days, place the avocado in a paper bag with 1 or 2 bananas. Once the avocado is ripe, place it in the refrigerator until you're ready to consume it. Avocado flesh turns brown on exposure to air, but an acid such as lemon juice or lime juice can maintain the attractive pale green colour.

SUMMER AVOCADO TOAST

3+ Plant Points

Serves 2

I'm in love with those luscious slices of summertime tomatoes over a perfectly ripe avocado with a few accoutrements to round it out.

2 slices sourdough bread, or homemade sourdough bread (page 317)

½ large ripe avocado

4 slices good-quality tomatoes

Balsamic vinegar

Pinch flaky salt (I like Maldon)

Freshly cracked black pepper

Supercharge It! (optional toppings):

Sprouts

Crushed garlic

Extra-virgin olive oil

Fresh basil

Rocket

Sauerkraut

Toast the bread, then spread the avocado on top. Layer on the tomatoes and drizzle a little balsamic vinegar along with a generous pinch of flaky salt and cracked black pepper. Add optional toppings of your choice.

AVOCADO 'SHROOM TOAST

5+ Plant Points

Serves 2

This is more of a fork and knife type of avocado toast. 'Shrooms are technically not plants; they're fungi. But they're an excellent source of prebiotic polysaccharides like β- and α-glucans and chitin that feed our gut microbes and facilitate the production of short-chain fatty acids. So they're clearly worthy of being +1 Plant Point. To take this recipe to the next level, add a slice or two of the Eggy Avocado Toast (opposite).

1 teaspoon olive oil or vegetable stock

225 g button or chestnut mushrooms, stems removed and thinly sliced

Salt

2 garlic cloves, crushed

2 large slices sourdough bread, or homemade sourdough bread (page 317)

1 large ripe avocado

1 teaspoon freshly squeezed lemon juice

Freshly ground black pepper

Supercharge It! (optional toppings):

Toasted pine nuts

Tahini drizzle

Chopped fresh basil

1. In a large frying pan set over medium heat, heat the olive oil. Add the mushrooms and a pinch of salt and cook for 8 to 10 minutes, until the mushrooms start to brown and the liquid has evaporated. Stir in the crushed garlic and cook another minute or two, until warmed through.

2. Toast the sourdough bread. While the bread is toasting, mash the avocado with the lemon juice and a generous pinch of salt and pepper, then spread onto the toast.

3. Add the warm mushrooms and garnish with supercharged toppings.

EGGY AVOCADO TOAST

3+ Plant Points

Serves 2

Simple, fibre- and protein-packed, healthy fats, satiating. This is your *Fibre Fuelled* version of avocado toast with egg, only no eggs are consumed or required. Combine it with Garlicky Kale and everything bagel seasoning and thank me later.

115 g firm tofu, pressed and sliced into 4 thin slices

¼ teaspoon kala namak black salt (optional, for egg-like taste)

¼ teaspoon ground turmeric

1 teaspoon soy sauce

1 teaspoon nutritional yeast

Cooking spray, for oiling the frying pan

2 slices sourdough bread, or homemade sourdough bread (page 317)

½ large ripe avocado

Supercharge It! (optional toppings):

Garlicky Kale (page 259)

Everything bagel seasoning

Sliced fresh tomato

Sesame seeds

Sauerkraut

1. Place the tofu in a wide baking dish. In a small bowl, whisk together the salt, if using, turmeric, soy sauce, nutritional yeast, and 60 ml water. Pour the marinade over the tofu and let sit for at least 15 minutes, flipping halfway through.

2. When ready to cook, lightly spray a medium frying pan and place over medium heat. Remove the tofu, shaking off as much excess marinade as possible. Cook for 3 to 4 minutes per side in the prepared frying pan, until golden brown.

3. While the tofu is cooking, toast the bread, then spread with the avocado. Top with tofu eggs and supercharged toppings of your choice.

CARROT LOX

2+ Plant Points

Serves 4

The perfect addition to toasted sourdough bread or bagels piled high with your favourite toppings. The oil really helps give this a traditional oily fish taste, but you can omit it if desired. A pinch of kelp powder in the marinade will also give it a fishy taste. Leftover kelp powder is great on baked tofu for no-fishy fingers!

4 large carrots, rinsed

65 g salt, for coating

3 teaspoons olive oil

⅛ teaspoon lemon zest

1 tablespoon freshly squeezed lemon juice

¼ teaspoon smoked paprika

Freshly ground black pepper

Pinch kelp powder (optional)

Supercharge It! (optional ingredients):

Sourdough bread or bagels

Dollop of avocado or dairy-free cream cheese

Chopped dill

Spring and/or red onions

Pickled onions

Capers

Jalapeño and/or tomato slices

Onion sprouts

1. Preheat the oven to 200°C.

2. Place the carrots on a piece of aluminium foil large enough to wrap the carrots, then sprinkle with the salt. Fold the foil around the carrots, tucking in the edges to make a packet, then place in the oven and bake for 50 to 70 minutes, until the carrots are easily pierced with a fork. Larger carrots will take longer, though take care not to overcook them to mush. Alternatively, line the bottom of a small baking dish with parchment paper, then cover with a thin layer of salt. Add the carrots, then sprinkle more salt on top. Cook as directed. This step may be done a day ahead of time.

3. While the carrots are cooking, whisk together the olive oil, lemon zest, lemon juice, paprika, pepper, and kelp powder, if using.

4. Once the carrots are cool enough to handle, rub off the excess salt and pat dry. The carrot skin should have come off with the salt, but if it didn't, then gently rub or peel it off. Using a sharp knife (or a sharp peeler), slice the carrot into long strips as thinly as possible.

5. Add the carrot strips to the marinade, tossing gently until the strips are coated. Let marinate for at least 2 hours, or overnight in the refrigerator. The carrot lox will keep in the fridge for a few days and tastes best at room temperature.

6. Serve it on toasted bagels or sourdough bread with a generous dollop of avocado or plain dairy-free cream cheese. Get creative with your supercharge options! There are so many great choices on this one—dill, capers, sliced jalapeños, tomato slices. You can have onions four ways—spring, red, pickled, and sprouted.

HARISSA WHITE BEAN TOAST

5+ Plant Points

Serves 2

"Harasa" is the Arabic word for "to pound," and if you pound red hot chilli peppers you get harissa, a Tunisian hot chilli paste that I'm obsessed with. But this is more than flavour. Red hot chilli peppers may be longevity foods. In a large population-based prospective study encompassing 273,877 person-years of follow-up, people who consumed red hot chilli peppers had a 13 per cent reduced risk of death during the study.

1 teaspoon olive oil or stock

1 large garlic clove, crushed

270 g canned white beans or chickpeas, drained and rinsed

1 to 2 teaspoons harissa paste

1 to 2 tablespoons tahini or plain non-dairy yoghurt

Juice of 1 lime

Pinch salt

2 slices sourdough bread, or homemade sourdough bread (page 317)

Supercharge It! (optional toppings):

Crushed red pepper flakes

Sprouts

Fresh flat-leaf parsley

1. Heat the oil in a medium frying pan over medium heat. Add the garlic and cook for 30 seconds, stirring, until just fragrant.

2. Add the beans and cook for a few minutes, until warmed and slightly crisp on the edges. Add the harissa paste, tahini, lime juice, and salt. Reduce the heat to low and let warm, adding in more harissa for spice, lime for tang, or tahini for creaminess as desired.

3. Toast the bread and spoon the warmed harissa beans on top. Garnish with supercharged toppings as desired.

BUCKWHEAT VEGETABLE CREPES

5+ Plant Points

Makes 2 or 3 crepes

We love these for a savoury weekend breakfast or brunch. If you like traditional stuffed omelettes, then you'll love these crepes. It's 100 per cent plant-based food that's not trying to be anything it's not. For best results, use a non-stick pan lightly coated with cooking spray or a very thin layer of olive oil to just coat the pan.

90 g plain flour

90 g buckwheat flour

1 teaspoon baking powder

1 tablespoon ground flaxseed

¼ teaspoon garlic powder

360 ml unsweetened almond milk (or other unsweetened non-dairy milk of choice), plus more if needed

¼ teaspoon salt

Olive oil or vegetable stock, for sautéing

1 shallot

75 g seeded and chopped red sweet pepper

100 g sliced button or chestnut mushrooms

90 g chopped courgette

Freshly ground black pepper

Cooking spray or olive oil, for oiling the frying pan

60 ml cashew cream

Fresh flat-leaf parsley, microgreens, and/or sprouts, for garnish

1. Whisk together the flours, baking powder, flaxseed, garlic powder, almond milk, and salt until a smooth batter forms. It should be the same consistency as pancake batter. If too thick, add in more milk.

2. Heat a large frying pan over medium heat and coat with a thin layer of olive oil. Add the shallot, sweet pepper, mushrooms, and courgette along with a pinch of salt and pepper and cook for 10 minutes, until soft. Season to taste, adding more salt or pepper as needed. Set aside.

3. Heat a large non-stick frying pan over medium heat and lightly oil it using either cooking spray or a very thin layer of olive oil.

4. Add a third to a half of the crepe batter (depending on the size of your pan) and tilt the frying pan to gently spread the mixture out to the edges as much as possible. Cook until set on the bottom, about 3 minutes, then flip and cook another 2 to 3 minutes until set. Repeat with the rest of the batter.

5. To serve, dollop cashew cream on the crepes, then top with the cooked vegetable mixture and fresh parsley, microgreens, and/or sprouts for serving.

PRO TIP:

To make cashew cream, blend together 30 g raw cashews, 60 ml water, ½ tablespoon freshly squeezed lemon juice, ¼ teaspoon chopped garlic, and a pinch of salt until very creamy and smooth. As a quick alternative, substitute in dairy-free cream cheese.

The gut-nourishing stock your body actually needs—Biome Stock!

When I started writing *Fibre Fuelled* in 2018, I was very motivated to correct the misinformation that was rampant (and still is) in the gut health space. One of the biggest trends in gut health was bone stock, hyped up with promises of improving gut health, food intolerances, allergies, joint health, inflammation, immunity, sleep, weight loss . . . The list goes on. Surely, with all these haughty health claims there must be strong evidence to back up the benefits of bone stock, so brace yourself for the evidence that bone stock is good for gut health and food intolerances . . . Wait for it . . . Okay, I'm done. There's none. Not a single study. But there *is* research suggesting that toxic heavy metals in the bones can leach into the stock. While we're at it, there's zero evidence that collagen is beneficial for gut health, either, but there *is* evidence that bone stock doesn't have as much of the collagen peptides as everyone thought.

I have no doubt that people feel better when sipping bone stock. But does that have anything to do with the bones? Or is it that drinking a warm, electrolyte-rich clear liquid is easy and soothing for the gut? Honestly, the most redeeming things about bone stock are the things you get from the plants—polyphenols, phytochemicals, prebiotic fibre. Yes, soluble fibre from the plants will dissolve into the stock and come along for the ride. But that has nothing to do with the bones.

This is why I created Biome Stock, the signature recipe of a *Fibre Fuelled* lifestyle that I introduced in my first book. Yes, I said it. Biome Stock is the signature recipe. Why? Because I am with you in your quest to have a stock that nourishes your gut, makes you feel warm and cozy inside. But I want it to be something that actually nourishes and delivers as promised. With that in mind, I have amplified our original Biome Stock recipe, delivering seven versions of it. This time around there is Low FODMAP Biome Stock (page 85), Low-Histamine Biome Stock (page 159), and opposite you will find Biome Stock Unleashed plus four fun epicurean versions.

You can use a slow cooker or an Instant Pot to make your Biome Stock—we're giving you instructions for both.

Why No Plant Points for Biome Stock? Doesn't That Defeat the Purpose?

As we discussed earlier in this chapter, we assign Plant Points for the consumption of whole or minimally processed foods that feed your microbes their complete spectrum of dietary fibre. Since we are removing the plants at the end to keep our recipe as clear stock, we are not giving Plant Points for Biome Stock. Bummer? Not really. It doesn't change its status as a super-healthy food. Now, some of you have reached out to ask me what to do with the vegetables from the Biome Stock recipe. Biome Stock effortlessly transforms into nourishing vegetable soup if you finely chop up the veggies at the end and add them back in. Then you can start counting your Plant Points!

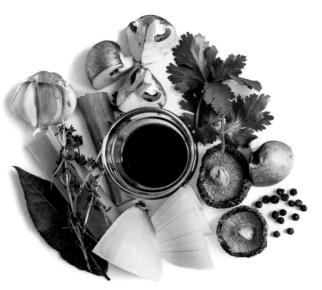

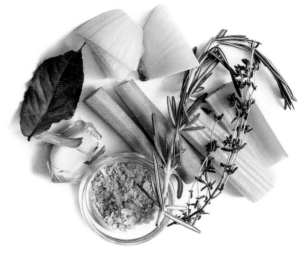

BIOME STOCK UNLEASHED

Makes 1 litre

You can enjoy this one as is, with a spoonful of miso stirred in while warm, or over rice noodles, tofu, and spring onions for a simple bowl of comfort.

2 celery sticks

225 g button mushrooms, quartered

1 onion, quartered

2 sprigs thyme

3 garlic cloves, crushed

6 peppercorns (or cracked black pepper if that's all you have)

1 bay leaf

7 g dried shiitake mushrooms

1 tablespoon low-sodium tamari or liquid aminos

In a large pan, place the celery, button mushrooms, onion, thyme, garlic, peppercorns, bay leaf, shiitake mushrooms, and tamari with 1.4 litres water. Bring to the boil, then reduce the heat to medium-low and simmer for 45 to 60 minutes, until reduced. Strain and use as desired.

CHICKENLESS BIOME STOCK

Makes 1 litre

This one is delicious as a warm sipper, or with your favourite chickenless soup. You can make it salt-free, or add in salt as desired. You can also use tamari or liquid aminos (just note this will darken the stock).

2 carrots, chopped into thirds

2 celery sticks, chopped into thirds

1 onion, quartered

1 sprig fresh rosemary or ½ teaspoon dried

2 sprigs thyme

3 garlic cloves, smashed

1 bay leaf

1 tablespoon nutritional yeast

Salt (optional)

In a large pan, place the carrots, celery, onion, rosemary, thyme, garlic, bay leaf, nutritional yeast, and salt, if using, with 1.4 litres water. Bring to the boil, then reduce the heat to medium-low and simmer for 45 to 60 minutes, until reduced. Strain and use as desired.

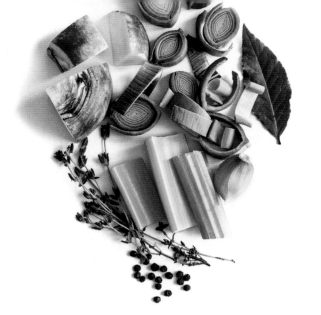

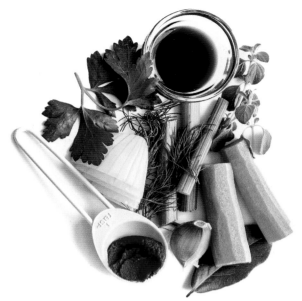

FANCY FRENCH BIOME STOCK

Makes 1 litre

A taste of France! The leeks, turnips, fresh herbs, and peppercorns will make you feel like you're sipping soup at a Parisian café. You can make this salt-free, or add in salt as desired. You can also use tamari or liquid aminos (but note this will darken the stock).

1 leek, white and green parts, roughly chopped

1 turnip, quartered

2 celery sticks, chopped into thirds

4 thyme sprigs

4 or 5 fresh flat-leaf parsley sprigs

3 garlic cloves, smashed

6 peppercorns (or crushed black pepper)

1 bay leaf

Salt (optional)

In a large pan, place the leek, turnip, celery, thyme, parsley, garlic, peppercorns, bay leaf, and salt, if using, with 1.4 litres water. Bring to the boil, then reduce the heat to medium-low and simmer for 45 to 60 minutes, until reduced. Strain and use as desired.

TUSCAN BIOME STOCK

Makes 1 litre

Simple ingredients and big flavours define this iconic Italian region. This one is also delicious as a base for minestrone soup—add in your favourite beans, frozen bag of mixed vegetables, and cooked short pasta.

2 fennel bulb, chopped into thirds

1 onion, quartered

3 garlic cloves, smashed

1 bay leaf

2 carrots

3 sprigs oregano

2 teaspoons tomato paste

4 sprigs fresh flat-leaf parsley

1 tablespoon low-sodium tamari or liquid aminos

In a large pan, place the fennel, onion, garlic, bay leaf, carrots, oregano, tomato paste, parsley, and tamari with 1.4 litres water. Bring to the boil, then reduce the heat to medium-low and simmer for 45 to 60 minutes, until reduced. Strain and use as desired.

ASIAN BIOME STOCK

Makes 1 litre

Ginger, spring onions, coriander, and miso flavours merge in a celebration of Eastern cuisine. This one is great as is, or with extra sliced spring onions, diced tofu, and more miso!

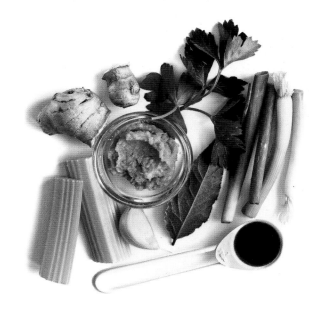

3 spring onions (white and green parts), chopped into thirds

7.5 cm piece fresh ginger, thinly sliced

3 celery sticks, chopped into thirds

4 garlic cloves, smashed

4 sprigs coriander

1 bay leaf

1 tablespoon low-sodium tamari

2 teaspoons miso paste

In a large pan, place the spring onions, ginger slices, celery, garlic, coriander, bay leaf, and tamari with 1.4 litres water. Bring to the boil, then reduce the heat to medium-low and simmer for 45 to 60 minutes, until reduced. Strain, return to the pot, and whisk in the miso.

PRO TIP:

Don't throw away the veggies! For all of these sippers, you can save the leftover veggies for another stock (freeze them) or finely chop them and add them back to the soup for a veggie soup. When you're done, they make great compost or food for a pet, if you're not going to eat them yourself!

Making Biome Stock in Your Slow Cooker or Instant Pot

Slow cooker directions (for all of these sippers): Place all of the ingredients in the base of a slow cooker and cook on low for 6 hours. Strain and use as desired.

Instant Pot directions (for all of these sippers): Place all of the ingredients in the base of an Instant Pot and cook on high pressure for 30 minutes, then naturally release for 10 minutes and quick release to remove any remaining pressure. Strain and use as desired.

SPICY PEANUT STEW

9 Plant Points

Serves 4

Hot peppers contain capsaicin, the spicy element evolved to protect peppers from being eaten. Ummm, yeah—that didn't work out so well in hindsight . . . Many of us humans are attracted to it. Capsaicin works by binding onto the nerves in the mouth and tongue that detect pain from high-temperature sources, tricking our brain into sensing burning heat. Capsaicin has beneficial effects for obesity, diabetes, and inflammatory disorders, and recent evidence suggests that the beneficial effects may be due to altering the gut microbiome and gut barrier. I love this recipe served with cooked brown rice and extra crushed peanuts on top.

1 tablespoon olive oil or Biome Stock Unleashed (page 239)

1 yellow or white onion, finely diced

390 g peeled and cubed sweet potato

½ teaspoon salt

½ teaspoon freshly ground black pepper

4 large garlic cloves, crushed

1 tablespoon finely grated fresh ginger

1 jalapeño, seeded and finely chopped

1 teaspoon ground cumin

60 ml tomato paste

480 ml vegetable stock or Biome Stock Unleashed (page 239)

480 g can fire-roasted chopped tomatoes

165 g smooth peanut butter

400 ml can light coconut milk (substitute almond milk for less creamy results)

400 g can chickpeas, rinsed and drained

1 teaspoon freshly squeezed lime juice

Hot sauce, to taste

Chopped peanuts, for garnish

Cooked rice, for serving (optional)

1. Heat the olive oil in a large pan over medium heat. Add the onion and cook for 5 minutes, until softened.

2. Add the sweet potato, salt, pepper, garlic, ginger, jalapeño, and ground cumin and cook for 5 minutes, stirring often. If the sweet potato sticks, add a little stock.

3. Add the tomato paste and cook another 2 to 3 minutes, until fragrant and toasted. Add the stock and chopped tomatoes and bring to the boil, then reduce the heat to a low simmer and cook for 20 to 25 minutes, until the sweet potatoes are tender.

4. Stir in the peanut butter, coconut milk, and chickpeas. Simmer another 25 minutes, until thickened, stirring occasionally. Add the lime juice and a dash of hot sauce, and season to taste. (For a thinner stew, add more stock.)

5. Garnish with chopped peanuts and serve with cooked rice, if desired.

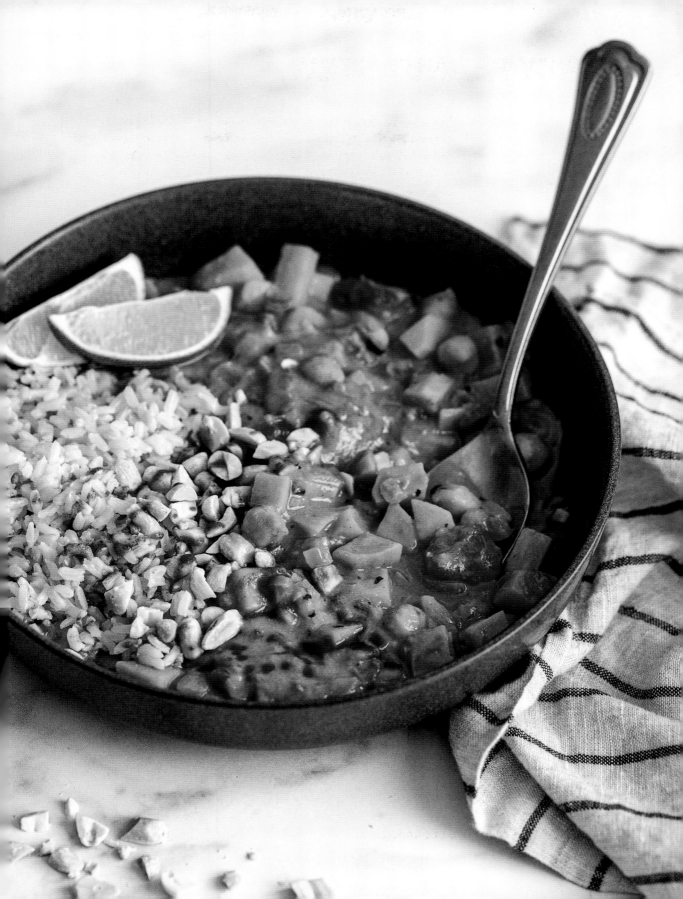

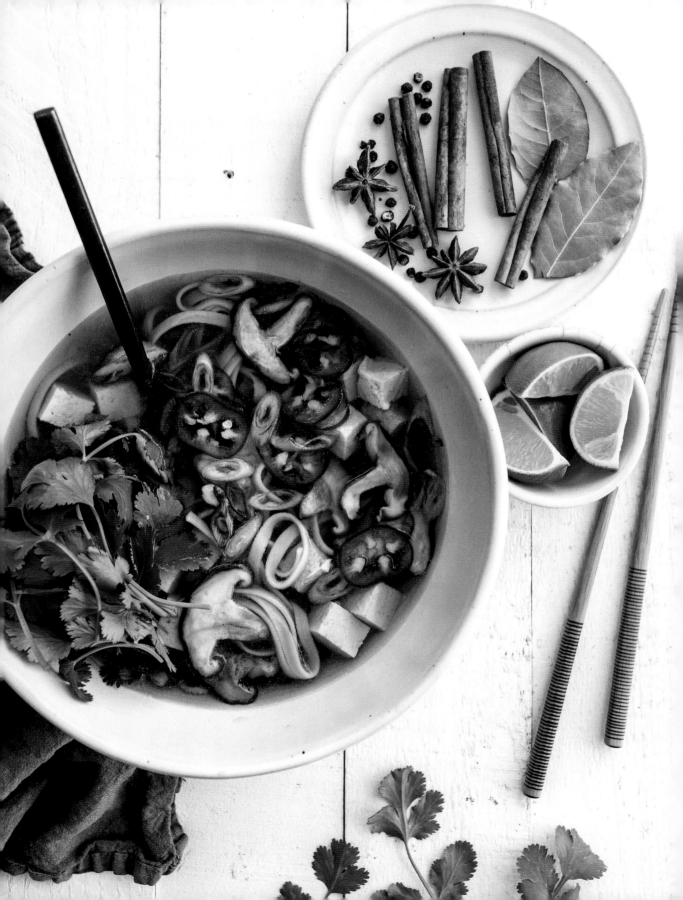

BIOME STOCK PHO

6+ Plant Points

Serves 4

When you nail a Vietnamese pho recipe, it's pretty hard to beat. There's a richness to the stock. Sweet, just slightly too salty, with undertones of cinnamon and star anise swirling on the tongue. The beauty is that you can have the decadence and complexity of pho, but simultaneously nourish your body with shiitakes instead of beef. Traditional pho has a hearty mouthfeel, but you can leave out the extra oil in this recipe if you'd like by charring the onions and ginger in the oven and sautéing the mushrooms, tofu, and greens in a little stock.

2 teaspoons avocado or olive oil, plus more to drizzle in the pan

1 large white onion, halved

10 cm piece fresh ginger, halved lengthwise

225 g dried rice noodles, brown rice preferred

3 garlic cloves, smashed

Two 7.5 cm cinnamon sticks

4 whole cloves

5 star anise

2 cardamom pods

1 tablespoon whole black peppercorns

1 tablespoon whole coriander seeds

28 g dried shiitake mushrooms

2 litres Biome Stock Unleashed (page 239) or other vegetable stock

1 teaspoon 100% maple syrup

2 teaspoons rice wine vinegar or white vinegar

1 to 2 teaspoons low-sodium tamari or soy sauce

225 g thinly sliced fresh shiitake mushrooms

225 g pressed extra-firm tofu, cubed

2 baby pak choi, halved and sliced

Supercharge It! (optional toppings):

Bean, onion and/or broccoli sprouts

Fresh mint, basil, and/or coriander

Thinly sliced spring onions (green parts only) and/or jalapeño peppers

Lime wedges

RECIPE CONTINUES

1. Heat a large, heavy-bottomed pan over medium heat and lightly drizzle with oil. Add the onion and ginger cut-side down and cook, pressing down, until the exposed sides are lightly charred, 5 to 6 minutes. Remove and set aside.

2. While the onion is cooking, prep the noodles and cook according to the packet directions. Drain, rinse with cold water, and set aside.

3. In the same heavy-bottomed pot, add the garlic, cinnamon, cloves, star anise, cardamom, peppercorns, and coriander seeds and let toast for 1 minute, stirring often, until fragrant. Add the charred onion and ginger along with the dried shiitake mushrooms and Biome Stock.

4. Reduce the heat to low, cover with a tight-fitting lid, and let simmer for at least 45 minutes. Strain out the solids, then add in the maple syrup, vinegar, and tamari. Taste, adjusting seasonings as needed.

5. While the stock is in the last 10 minutes or so of simmering, heat the 2 teaspoons avocado oil over medium heat in a large non-stick frying pan and add in the sliced shiitakes. Cook for about 5 minutes, stirring often, until the mushrooms are golden. Add in the tofu cubes and pak choi and cook another 3 to 5 minutes, until the tofu is lightly seared on the outside and the pak choi has wilted.

6. Divide the tofu, mushrooms, pak choi, and rice noodles into four bowls and top with hot stock. Garnish with toppings of your choice.

NASHVILLE NOT CHICKEN

1 Plant Point

Serves 4

If you love spicy food as much as I do, then your heart is probably racing with excitement to see this recipe. Hot Chicken is a Nashville food trend where the chicken is coated in spices, fried, then covered in more hot, spicy oil. Our take—it's not about the chicken or even the oil. It's about the heat. So we're bringing the heat with as low an amount of oil as possible, and the chickens are still dancing. Serve alongside sourdough bread and plenty of pickles. It's also amazing chopped on your favourite salad or with Herbed Potato Salad (page 268).

Cooking spray, for oiling the baking tray (optional)

450 g extra-firm tofu, drained and pressed

6 tablespoons corn flour, arrowroot starch, or tapioca starch

60 ml unsweetened soy milk or almond milk

85 g panko-style bread crumbs

1½ teaspoons smoked paprika

¼ teaspoon cayenne pepper

½ teaspoon salt

¼ teaspoon freshly ground black pepper

3 tablespoons avocado oil or other neutral oil, plus more to drizzle over tofu if wanting a crispier texture

1 to 2 tablespoons cayenne pepper

1 tablespoon date syrup or 100% maple syrup

½ teaspoon garlic powder

1. Preheat the oven to 220°C. Line a rimmed baking tray with parchment paper or a silicone baking mat or lightly oil with cooking spray; set aside.

2. Cut the tofu into 1 cm planks by slicing the tofu block into 6 slices width-wise, then slice each of those into 3 slices lengthwise. Or, you can tear into nugget-size pieces.

3. In a shallow bowl, place the corn flour. In another shallow bowl, place the milk. In a third shallow bowl, mix together the bread crumbs, ½ teaspoon of the paprika, ¼ teaspoon of the cayenne, the salt, and black pepper.

4. Lightly dip each piece of tofu into the corn flour, then the milk, then roll in the bread crumb mixture, pressing to stick to each side. Place the finished tofu onto the baking tray and continue with the rest of the tofu. There should be enough bread crumbs, but depending on how much you coat them, you may need to add more.

RECIPE CONTINUES

5. Bake for 25 minutes, then flip and bake for another 10 minutes, until nice and crispy. For crispier not-chicken, you can lightly drizzle on oil or cooking spray after flipping.

6. While the tofu is cooking, in a small bowl or measuring cup, whisk together the avocado oil, the remaining paprika, remaining cayenne, the date syrup, and the garlic powder.
Pour over the crispy tofu fingers and serve immediately.

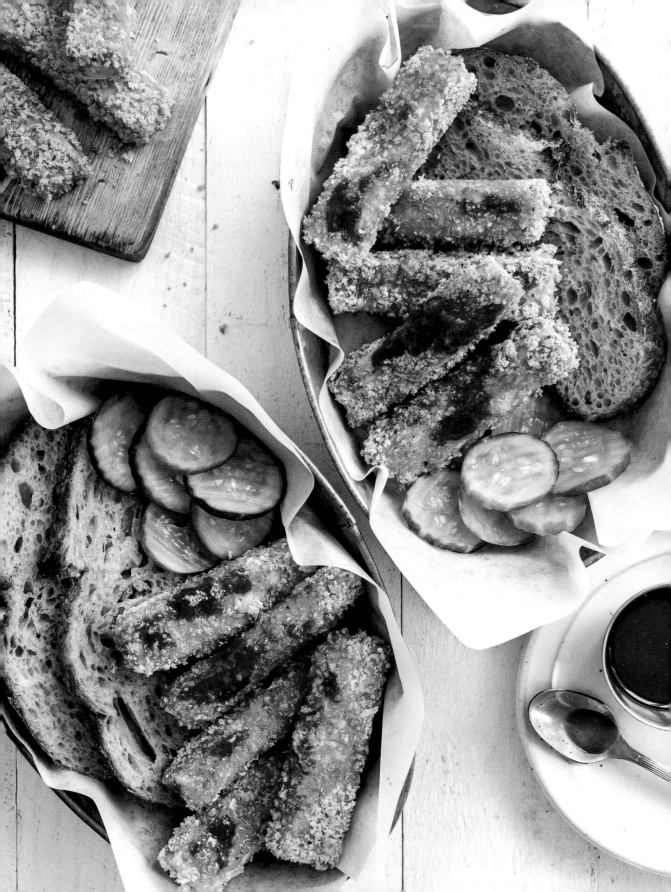

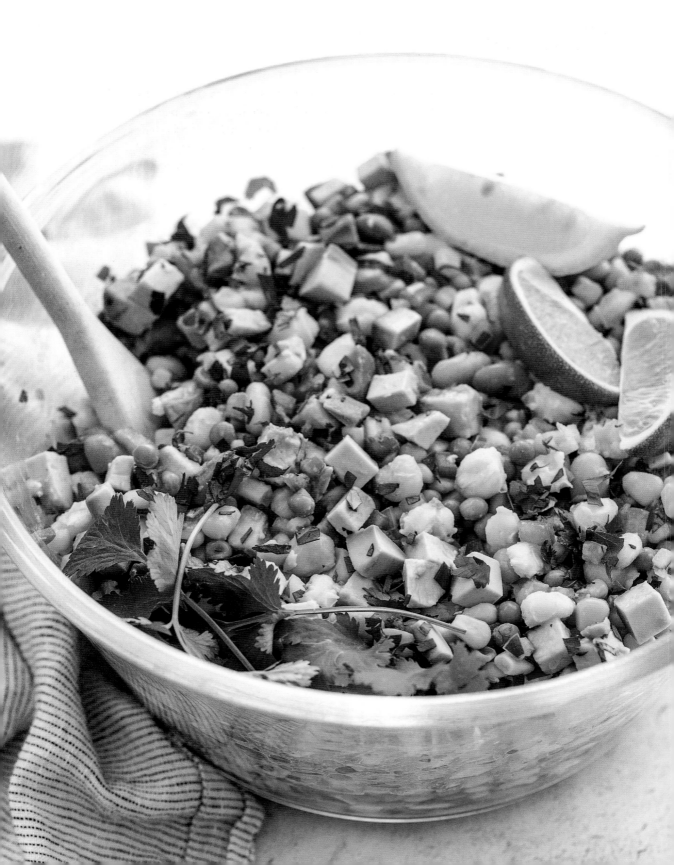

VEGETABLE CEVICHE

11 Plant Points

Makes 2 kg

Leave the fish in the ocean and reach for hominy grits to create this tangy, citrussy salad that's delicious on its own, scooped onto your favourite green salad, or yes, served with baked tortilla chips. Hominy is low in calories and high in fibre, and the process of creating hominy from corn releases the B vitamins. This recipe tastes great cold or at room temperature.

80 ml freshly squeezed lemon juice

120 ml freshly squeezed lime juice

150 g finely chopped red onion

1 red sweet pepper, seeded and finely chopped

One 400 g can pinto beans, drained and rinsed

One 400 g can yellow hominy, drained and rinsed

One 400 g can white hominy, drained and rinsed

One 400 g can very sweet young peas, drained and rinsed

One 400 g can sweetcorn, drained and rinsed

One 400 g can white beans, drained and rinsed

10 g finely chopped coriander

Salt and freshly ground black pepper

2 large ripe avocados, diced

Extra-virgin olive oil, for drizzling (optional)

1. In a large bowl, place the lemon juice and lime juice and add in the red onion. Let sit for 5 minutes to quickly pickle; this process takes some of the bite out of the raw red onion.

2. Add in the sweet pepper, pinto beans, yellow hominy, white hominy, peas, sweetcorn, white beans, and coriander. Toss, adding in a few pinches of salt and freshly ground black pepper to taste.

3. Right before serving, fold in the avocado. If desired, drizzle with good-quality extra-virgin olive oil.

PRO TIP:

If making ahead of time, add in the avocado right before serving. For a more decadent salad, drizzle on high-quality extra-virgin olive oil and Maldon sea salt right before serving. (I'm obsessed with Maldon sea salt.) In the UK, you may have to source your hominy online.

TOFU BÁNH MÌ

8+ Plant Points

Makes 4 sandwiches

This staple of Vietnamese cuisine exemplifies food fusion—it combines native Vietnamese flavours with French baguette to produce a savoury and delicious plant-based submarine sandwich.

1 small carrot, sliced into thin matchsticks

1 small cucumber, peeled, seeded, and sliced into matchsticks

½ to 1 jalapeño, seeded and thinly sliced (depending on preferred spice level)

80 ml white wine vinegar

80 ml rice vinegar

¼ teaspoon salt

One 400 g block extra-firm tofu, drained and pressed

3 tablespoons low-sodium tamari, liquid aminos, or soy sauce

Zest and juice of 1 lime

2½ teaspoons grated fresh ginger

2 large garlic cloves, crushed

1½ tablespoons finely chopped lemongrass

Cooking spray, for oiling the non-stick frying pan

Sriracha Mayo (see Pro Tip)

4 baguette pieces, sliced in half

Supercharge It! (optional toppings):

Sliced jalapeños

Fresh coriander sprigs

1. In a shallow bowl, place the carrot, cucumber, and jalapeño, then cover with the vinegars and salt. Set aside to quickly pickle while you prepare the rest of the ingredients.

2. Slice the tofu into thin slabs. In a separate shallow bowl, whisk together the tamari, lime juice, ginger, garlic, and lemongrass. Add the tofu and coat, turning to cover. Let marinate for 10 to 15 minutes.

3. When ready to cook, lightly oil a non-stick frying pan with cooking spray. Add the tofu and cook for 3 to 4 minutes per side, until golden brown and crispy.

4. Lightly spread the Sriracha Mayo on the sliced baguette pieces, then stuff with the tofu, pickled veggies, and supercharged toppings of choice.

PRO TIP:

To make Sriracha Mayo: Soak 60 g raw cashews in water for at least 1 hour, then drain and rinse. Alternatively, cover raw cashews with boiling water and quick soak for 10 minutes. In the base of a high-speed blender, blend together the cashews with 60 ml water, 1 tablespoon lime juice, ½ teaspoon salt, 1 teaspoon maple syrup, 2 teaspoons low-sodium tamari or soy sauce, and 1 tablespoon sriracha until creamy and smooth.

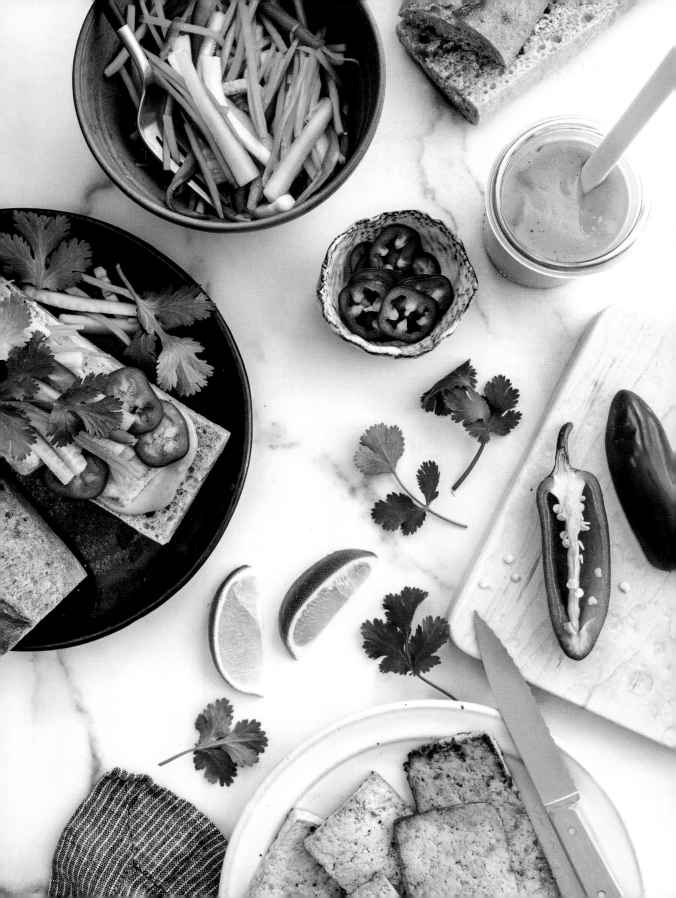

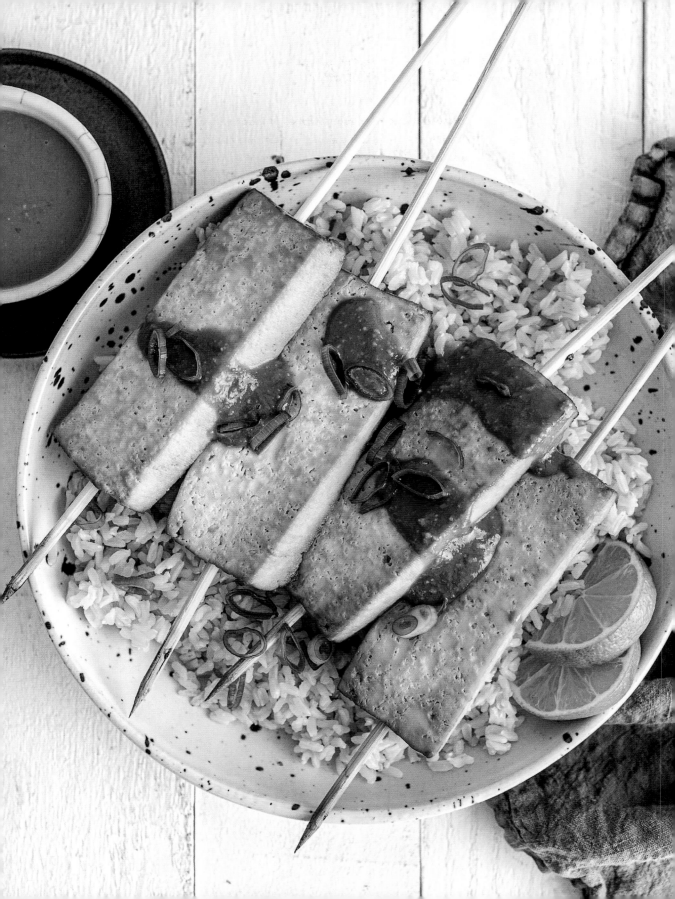

TOFU PEANUT SATAY

5 Plant Points

Serves 4

Satay is one of the national dishes of Indonesia and a popular street food. Traditionally it is a grilled protein on a bamboo skewer served with a sauce, with the classic sauce being peanut-based. Serve this one with steamed rice and steamed pak choi for a bowl or insert it into Tofu Bánh Mì (page 252) as an alternative protein.

450 g extra-firm tofu, drained and pressed

2 large garlic cloves, crushed

3 tablespoons plus 60 ml low-sodium tamari

3 tablespoons 100% pineapple juice

80 g smooth peanut butter

2 tablespoons rice vinegar

1 tablespoon freshly squeezed lime juice

½ teaspoon grated fresh ginger, plus more to taste

1 teaspoon chilli garlic sauce, plus more to taste

1 tablespoon date syrup or 100% maple syrup (optional)

1. Cut the tofu into strips thick enough to thread onto a skewer.

2. In a shallow bowl, whisk together the garlic, 3 tablespoons tamari, and the pineapple juice. Add the tofu to coat. Let marinate for at least 30 minutes, flipping halfway through. If using skewers, add the tofu to them now.

3. While the tofu is marinating, make the sauce. In a separate small bowl, whisk together the remaining 60 ml tamari, the peanut butter, vinegar, lime juice, ginger, and chilli garlic sauce. Season to taste, adding more lime juice for a brighter sauce, more chilli garlic sauce for spice, and date syrup for a sweeter sauce, if using.

4. Preheat the oven to 200°C. Place the tofu on a parchment paper-lined baking tray or non-stick silicone baking mat and bake for 30 to 40 minutes, flipping halfway through, until the tofu is golden brown and firm.

5. Remove from the oven and serve with satay sauce.

PRO TIP:

For a richer satay sauce, omit the lime juice until just before serving and heat in a medium saucepan over low heat with 120 ml canned coconut milk and 1 to 2 teaspoons red curry paste. Stir in the lime juice right before serving.

TEMPEH BACON BLTA
with Celeriac Fries

5+ Plant Points

Makes 4 sandwiches
with fries

Tempeh is made with fermented whole soybeans. It's extremely versatile and takes on the flavours that you assign to it with marinades. It's also incredibly healthy, packed with protein and prebiotic fibre and the phytochemical isoflavones that are known to have metabolic and hormonal benefits. It's all a win, especially when the tempeh is a vehicle for big flavours.

225 g tempeh

60 ml low-sodium tamari or soy sauce

¼ teaspoon ground cumin

⅛ teaspoon smoked paprika

60 ml apple cider vinegar

2 teaspoons 100% maple syrup or date syrup

Cooking spray, for oiling the baking tray (optional)

8 sourdough or wholegrain bread slices

1 large ripe avocado

8 crisp lettuce leaves

4 thick slices of ripe tomato

Celeriac Fries (page 258)

1. Slice the tempeh into thin, short strips. Place in a large, shallow bowl and set aside.

2. In a small bowl, whisk together the tamari, cumin, paprika, vinegar, and maple syrup. Pour over the tempeh and marinate for at least 30 minutes, turning once.

3. When ready to cook, preheat the oven to 175°C. Line a large baking tray with parchment paper or a non-stick baking mat or lightly spray with cooking spray, if using.

4. Place the marinated strips on the baking tray, leaving a little room in between each piece. Bake for 15 to 18 minutes, until lightly browned, flipping halfway through. Alternatively, for crispier bacon, you can panfry in a single layer for 3 to 4 minutes per side, until golden and crispy.

5. To assemble each sandwich, toast the bread and spread each of 4 slices with a quarter of the avocado, then layer with 2 lettuce leaves, a tomato slice, and cooked bacon. Top with the remaining bread slices. Serve with Celeriac Fries.

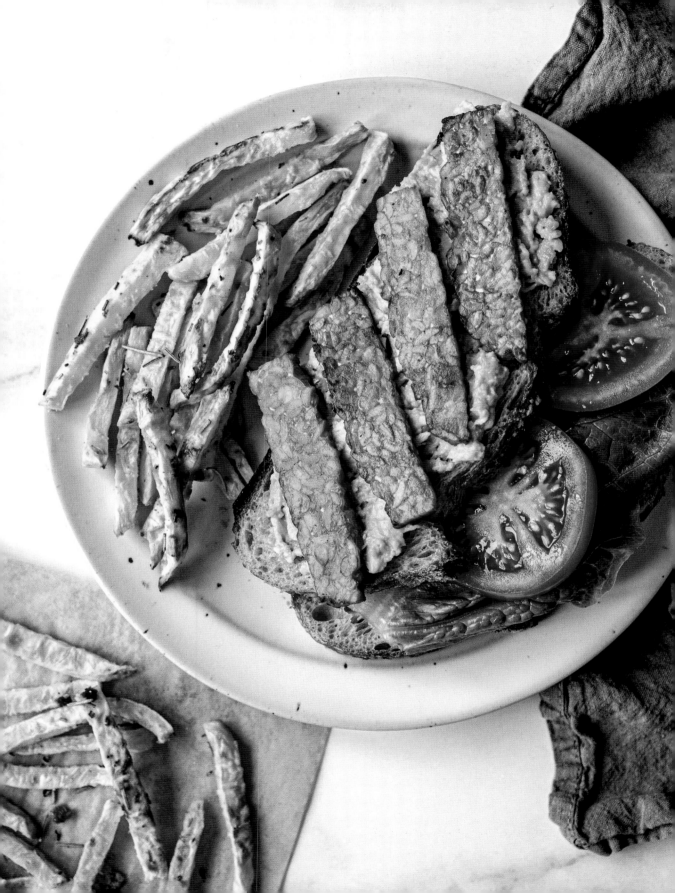

CELERIAC FRIES

1 Plant Point

Serves 4

One of the biggest secrets of the vegetable world, celeriac is a root vegetable with shoots that has a subtle, celery-like flavour, with nutty overtones.

1 large or 2 small celeriac

1 teaspoon garlic powder

1 teaspoon dried rosemary

½ teaspoon onion powder

½ teaspoon salt

½ teaspoon freshly ground black pepper

Olive oil, for drizzling

1. Preheat the oven to 200°C. Line a baking tray with parchment paper or a non-stick baking mat. Set aside.

2. Bring a pan of water to the boil over medium heat.

3. Peel the celeriac and slice into thick fry shapes, approximately 7 mm. Add the celeriac to the boiling water and cook for 3 minutes, then drain and pat dry.

4. Place the celariac on the baking tray and sprinkle with garlic powder, rosemary, onion powder, salt, and pepper. Drizzle with olive oil, then use your hands to massage the seasoning into the celeriac. Spread in an even layer on the baking tray, then bake for 30 to 35 minutes, until tender on the inside and slightly crispy on the outside.

PRO TIP:

The olive oil helps these crisp up like fries, but you can also use an air fryer. You can also cook them in stock—they'll have a less crisp outside.

GARLICKY KALE

2 Plant Points

Serves 4

This is a flexible, delicious side dish that pairs well with Eggy Avocado Toast (page 233), Where's the Beef? Steak Plate (page 265), or whatever dish you want to complement with a side of delicious, nutritious greens.

1 tablespoon olive oil or 2 tablespoons stock

4 garlic cloves, crushed

2 bunches cavolo nero or other kale, stems removed and sliced into thin ribbons

Salt and freshly ground black pepper

1. In a large frying pan set over medium heat, heat the oil or stock. Add the garlic and cook, stirring, about 30 seconds, until fragrant, taking care not to burn the garlic.

2. Add the kale and 2 tablespoons water or vegetable stock. Cover with a tight-fitting lid and let the kale steam for 2 minutes.

3. Remove the lid and season with the salt and pepper. Cook, tossing, for 3 to 5 minutes more, until the kale is tender.

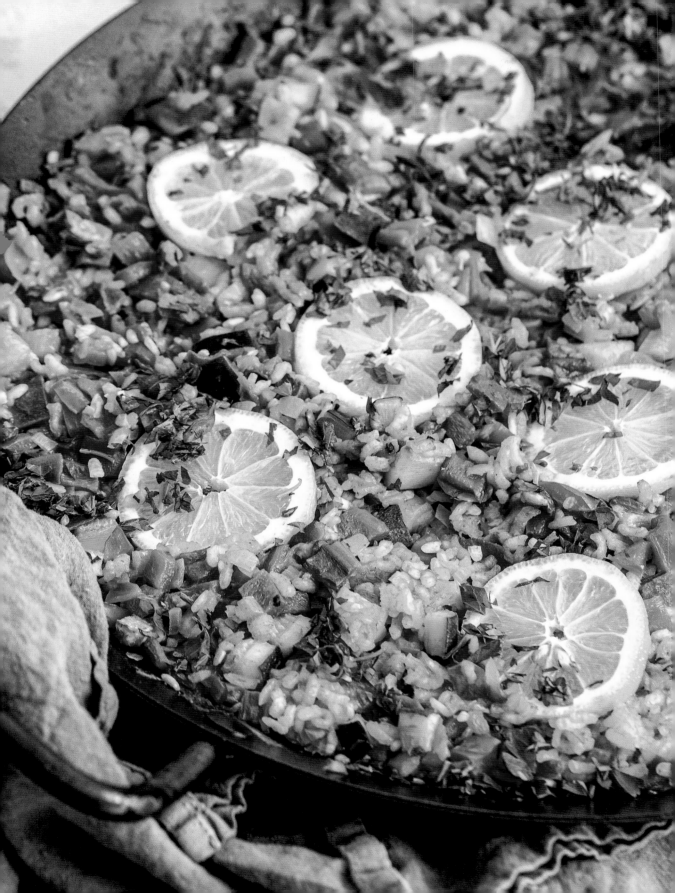

PAELLA

9 Plant Points

Serves 4

Saffron is a bulbous perennial plant in the iris family that blooms in the autumn. Harvest takes place over two weeks and the flowers are hand-picked before dawn, before they open for the day. It requires more than six thousand flowers and over twelve hours of labour to create just 30 grams of saffron, hence the nickname "red gold." In this recipe, the musky, piney saffron is complemented by the earthy, smoky paprika and garlicky sweetness. It's a taste of heaven.

1 tablespoon olive oil or vegetable stock

1 medium yellow or white onion, finely chopped

1 jarred roasted red pepper, chopped

1 red sweet pepper, seeded and chopped

1 medium courgette, chopped

2 garlic cloves, crushed

2 tomatoes, seeded and chopped

1 pinch saffron threads

1 teaspoon smoked paprika

⅛ teaspoon cayenne pepper

220 g short-grain rice (Arborio, Japanese sushi rice, Bomba rice)

600 ml Biome Stock Unleashed (page 239) or vegetable stock

10 g fresh flat-leaf parsley, finely chopped

1 lemon, sliced

1. In a paella pan or a large, shallow frying pan, heat the olive oil over medium heat. Add the onion, roasted red pepper, and sweet pepper to the pan and cook for about 10 minutes, until brown and reduced.

2. Add the courgette, garlic, tomato, saffron, paprika, and cayenne and cook over medium heat, stirring occasionally, for another 10 minutes, until the vegetables are soft.

3. Add the rice and stock and stir once to combine, then shake the pan to evenly distribute the rice and vegetables. Reduce the heat to medium-low and let simmer for 22 to 25 minutes. Check for most of the liquid to be absorbed and the rice at the top to be nearly tender. If for some reason your rice is still not cooked, add 60 ml more water or stock and continue cooking (can also finish cooking in the oven; see Pro Tip).

4. Remove the pan from the heat and cover with a tight-fitting lid or foil, then place a tea towel over the lid to rest for 5 minutes (this allows the rice to finish steaming). Garnish with fresh parsley and lemon slices.

PRO TIP:

Once the rice is mixed in, resist the urge to stir it again in order to allow a crispy crust to form at the bottom, called a *socarrat*. Depending on the size of your pan or burners on the hob, you may need to finish this in the oven. Cover with foil, then finish in a 175°C oven, until the rice is cooked through.

EASY CAPRESE PASTA

4+ Plant Points

Serves 4

A new spin on a classic flavour profile. Caprese melds tomatoes, basil, and mozzarella—an Italian paragon echoing the colours of their flag. But here comes the Tofu Feta . . . any scepticism will be replaced with enthusiasm and satisfaction.

450 g whole cherry tomatoes

1 tablespoon olive oil

½ teaspoon salt

¼ teaspoon freshly ground black pepper

Pinch crushed red pepper flakes (optional)

3 garlic cloves, crushed

340 g wholewheat farfalle, penne, rigatoni, or other short pasta of choice

½ batch Homemade Tofu Feta (page 84)

10 g torn fresh basil

½ teaspoon balsamic vinegar

1. Preheat the oven to 200°C.

2. In an ovenproof baking dish, place the cherry tomatoes and drizzle with olive oil, salt, black pepper, and red pepper flakes, if using. Bake for 20 minutes, then stir in the garlic. Place back in the oven and cook for another 5 minutes, or until the tomatoes start to "burst" and are easily squashed with the back of a spoon. Remove from the oven and stir, gently breaking up the tomatoes to create a sauce.

3. While the tomatoes are cooking, bring a large pan of water to a boil and add the pasta. Cook until al dente according to the packet directions. Drain, reserving 2 tablespoons of pasta water, and return the pasta to the warm pot.

4. Add the tomatoes to the pasta along with 1 tablespoon of pasta water and stir to combine. Stir in the tofu feta, basil, and vinegar and serve immediately. If the sauce is too thick, add in the remaining tablespoon of pasta water to thin.

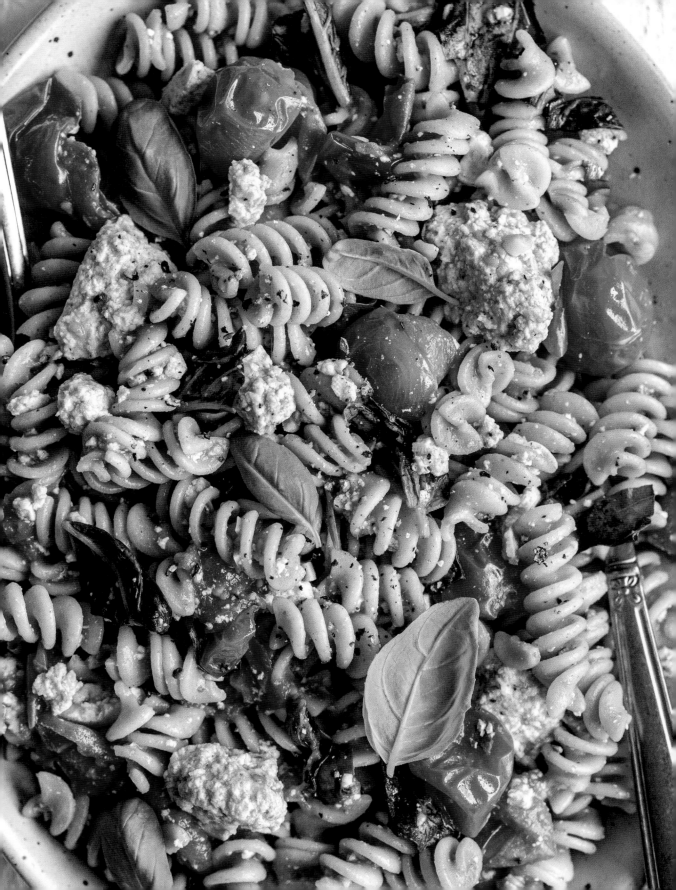

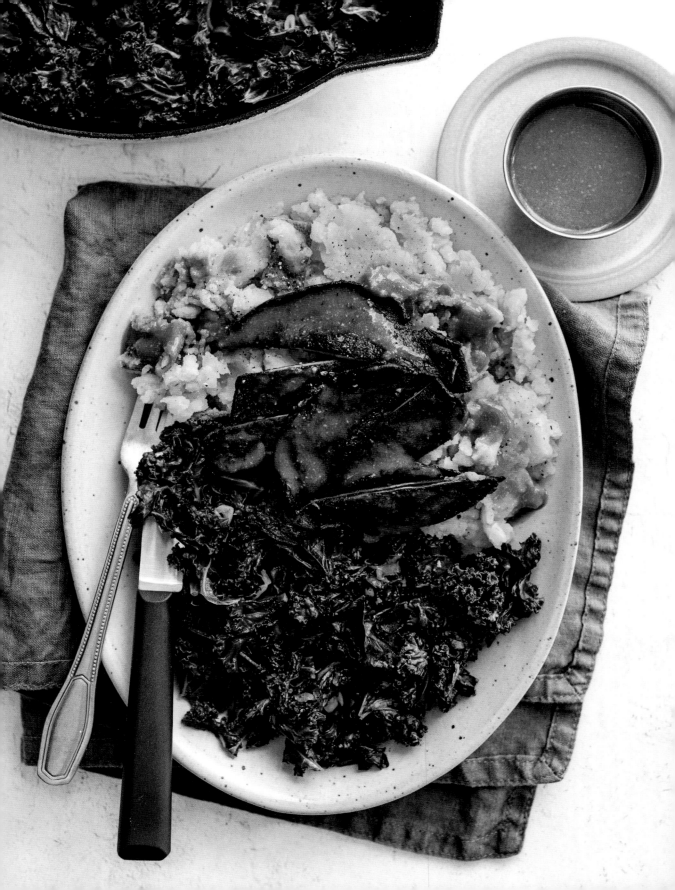

WHERE'S THE BEEF? STEAK PLATE

Serves 4

This dish captures everything you love about a traditional steak-and-potatoes meal—firing up the grill, the smoky, savoury flavour, steak sauce (and mashed potatoes to clean up the extra sauce!). We have all of it . . . But where's the beef? Trust me, you won't miss it. And the cows will be mooing your name with gratitude.

This is not just one recipe, it's a series. It's meant to create an entire table spread, an experience to share with family and friends. We're lining up the options, and you get to choose your own adventure at the dinner table.

Want classic steakhouse vibes? Slather that mushroom in homemade steak sauce. Want an Argentinian steakhouse experience? Smother the mushrooms and potatoes in our Quick Coriander Chimichurri Sauce (see page 170). Will it be mashed potatoes or potato salad? And will you opt to have the Garlicky Kale (see page 193), too? Honestly, you can't go wrong and you will be happy.

RECIPE CONTINUES

PORTOBELLO STEAKS

1 Plant Point
Makes 8 steaks/4 servings

This recipe is inspired by the Steak Plate from Plant Restaurant in Asheville, North Carolina. You can also use the steak as a sandwich filling or alongside your favourite pasta.

8 portobello mushrooms, stems removed and gills cleaned (optional, for a cleaner-looking "steak")

3 tablespoons BBQ Rub (recipe below)

Olive oil

240 ml shop-bought BBQ sauce

80 ml water or stock

BBQ Rub (see Pro Tip)

1 tablespoon salt

1 tablespoon smoked paprika

2 teaspoons black pepper

2 teaspoons garlic powder

1 teaspoon onion powder

¼ teaspoon dried oregano

½ teaspoon chipotle powder

1 batch Homemade Steak Sauce (opposite)

1. Clean the mushrooms and pat dry. Preheat the oven to 200°C. Line a baking tray with a non-stick mat or parchment paper and set aside.

2. Make the BBQ Rub: Combine all ingredients in an airtight container. (This will keep in the cupboard for 6 months.)

3. Heat a thin layer of olive oil in a large cast-iron frying pan over medium-high heat. Add the mushrooms, then place another heavy pot on top to help press the mushrooms into the pan. The additional pot helps the mushrooms to release their juices and become crispy. After 5 minutes, remove the pot, flip the mushrooms, and repeat for another 5 minutes, or until the mushrooms are thin and starting to crisp on the edges. You will likely need to do this in batches if using all 8 mushrooms.

4. Remove the heavy pot and sprinkle 1½ tablespoons of the BBQ rub over the mushrooms, using tongs to press in as much seasoning as possible. Flip, then repeat with the remaining 1½ tablespoons of the BBQ rub. Cook another few minutes per side, letting the rub sear into the mushrooms.

5. While the mushrooms are cooking, place the BBQ sauce and water into a large, shallow bowl and whisk to combine. To be clear, this is BBQ sauce that you purchase from the shop (choose your favourite), not the steak sauce that you will use on top. Remove the frying pan from the heat and, using tongs, place the mushrooms into the BBQ bowl, turning to evenly coat.

6. Place the mushrooms on the prepared baking tray, shaking off as much excess sauce as possible. Bake for 12 minutes, flipping halfway through. You can also finish the mushrooms on the grill instead of baking: Grill for 8 to 10 minutes, until lightly charred on the edges and juicy in the middle.

7. Remove, let sit for a few minutes, then thinly slice into strips.

PRO TIP:

If you don't have the time or ingredients to make the homemade BBQ Rub, simply mix together ½ teaspoon each smoked paprika, salt, onion powder, and garlic powder.

HOMEMADE STEAK SAUCE

Makes about 200ml

The sauce is a flavour amplifier. You take a delicious Portobello Steak and add a whole new dimension with this steak sauce. Feel free to use it elsewhere as well, like on grilled tofu or tempeh cubes.

60 ml balsamic vinegar	¼ teaspoon coarse sea salt
2 tablespoons vegan Worcestershire sauce	¼ teaspoon freshly ground black pepper
3 tablespoons ketchup	Pinch cayenne pepper
1 tablespoon Dijon mustard	1 large garlic clove, smashed
2 tablespoons raisins	Juice of 1 orange (about 3 tablespoons)
¼ teaspoon celery seed	

1. In a medium saucepan set over medium heat, place 60 ml water, the vinegar, Worcestershire sauce, ketchup, mustard, raisins, celery seed, salt, black pepper, cayenne, and garlic. Bring to the boil, then reduce the heat and simmer for 10 minutes, stirring occasionally.

2. Add in half of the orange juice, then simmer for another 5 minutes. Strain using a fine-mesh strainer (or remove the raisins) and place back in the saucepan. Add in the remaining orange juice, then season to taste with salt and black pepper. The sauce will continue to develop as it cools and thickens. For a thicker sauce, continue to cook over low heat until the desired thickness is achieved.

3. Store in the fridge for 1 week; leftovers can also be frozen, then thawed, heated, and cooled for next use.

PRO TIP:

The steak sauce gets better over time. It's a great thing to make a day in advance and store in the fridge.

MASHED POTATOES

1 Plant Point

Serves 4

White potatoes are an excellent source of resistant starch, which technically is not fibre but behaves exactly the same way (prebiotic) so it might as well be. Each time you heat then cool the potatoes, you increase the production of resistant starch. Just a little kitchen hack with your gut microbes in mind.

2 large King Edward potatoes	Salt and freshly ground black pepper, to taste
120 to 240 ml vegetable stock or Biome Stock Unleashed (page 239)	

1. Cut the potatoes into chunks, place in a pan, and cover with water. Bring to the boil, then reduce the heat to medium and cook for 15 to 20 minutes, until the potatoes are soft and easily pierced with a fork.

2. Drain the potatoes and place back into the pan off the heat. Add in 120 ml vegetable stock and mash the potatoes to the desired consistency, adding more of the vegetable stock as needed. Season to taste with salt and pepper.

HERBED POTATO SALAD

5+ Plant Points

Serves 4

A good herbed potato salad is hard to beat and extremely versatile as a complement to other summertime dishes.

680 g small red potatoes, scrubbed

Salt

10 g fresh flat-leaf parsley

25 g thinly sliced spring onions (white and green parts)

2 tablespoons freshly squeezed lemon juice

1½ teaspoons Dijon mustard

1 garlic clove, chopped

Freshly ground black pepper

60 ml olive oil or stock

Supercharge It! (optional toppings):

Halved tomatoes

More sliced spring onions (white and green parts)

More chopped herbs

1. In a large stockpot, place the potatoes and a generous pinch of salt and cover with water by 5 cm. Bring to the boil, then reduce the heat to low and simmer for 5 to 8 minutes, until the potatoes are just tender, taking care not to overcook them.

2. Drain, reserving 2 tablespoons of cooking water, then let the potatoes cool and slice them into ½ cm slices.

3. Place the parsley, spring onions, lemon juice, mustard, garlic, another pinch of salt, and a pinch of pepper in the base of a food processor and pulse 7 or 8 times until roughly chopped. With the motor running, drizzle in the reserved cooking water and olive oil to make a creamy sauce, stopping to scrape down the sides as needed.

4. Taste, adding in more salt, lemon juice, mustard, parsley, or spring onion as desired. Pour the sauce on top of the potatoes and gently fold in, taking care not to crush the potatoes. Enjoy it cold or at room temperature.

PRO TIP:

This is a traditional potato salad made with parsley, but you can also substitute in coriander or basil for a fresh twist.

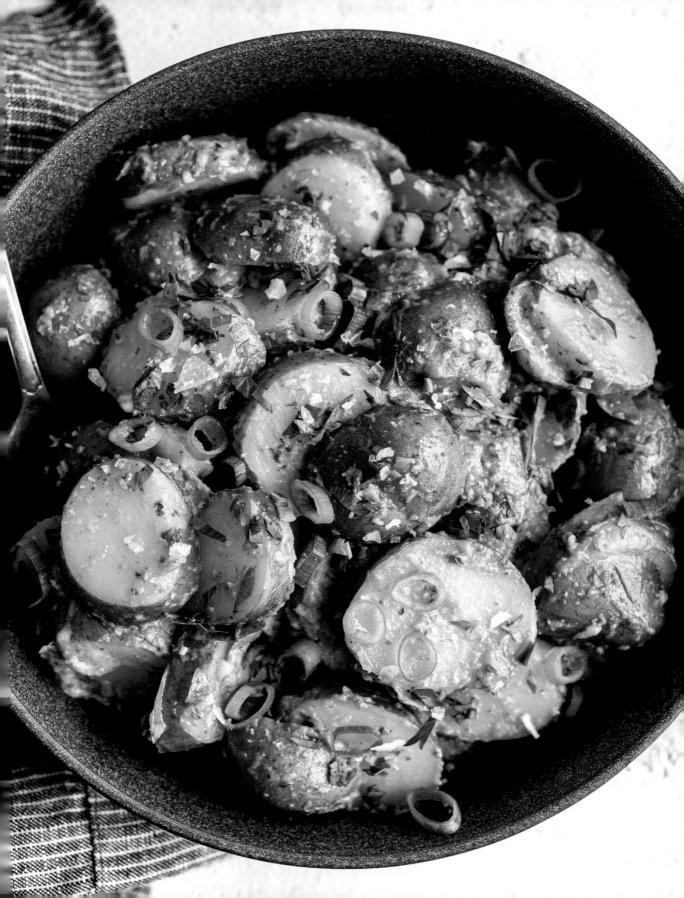

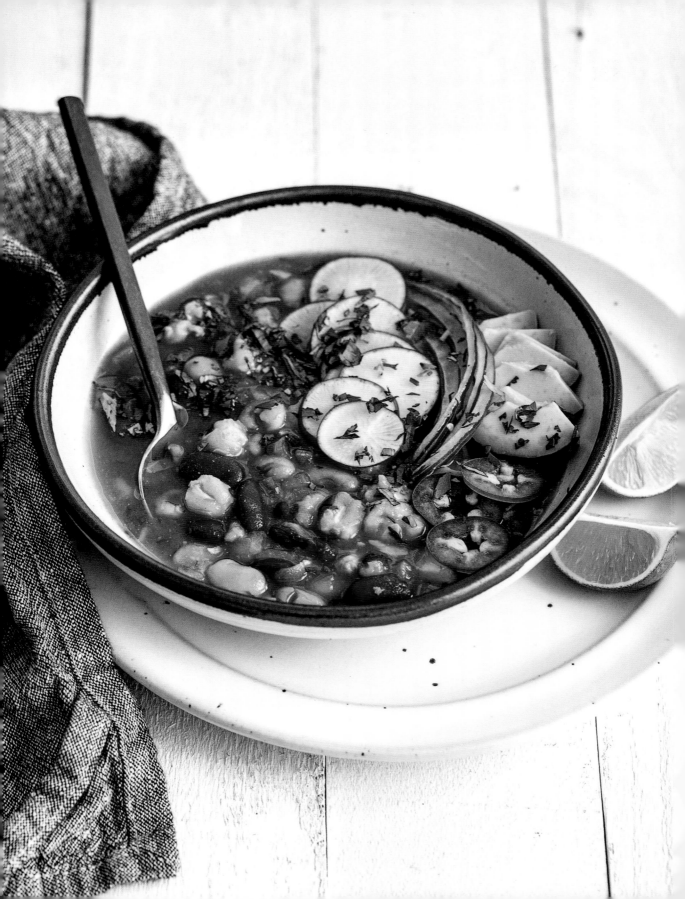

POZOLE

9+ Plant Points

Serves 6

Hominy is the main ingredient in pozole, a traditional Mexican stew. It's made from soaking dried corn in an alkaline solution, which enhances its nutritional value.

3 or 4 dried guajillo chilli peppers or dried ancho chillis

1 litre vegetable stock or Biome Stock Unleashed (page 239)

1 large white or yellow onion, finely chopped

Salt

4 garlic cloves, crushed

1 tablespoon ground cumin

120 ml tomato paste

2 bay leaves

Two 400 g cans pinto beans, rinsed and drained

One 400 g can kidney beans, rinsed and drained

One 400 g can hominy, rinsed and drained

10 ml chopped coriander

Juice of 1 lime

Supercharge It! (optional toppings):

Chopped avocado

Thinly sliced radish and/or jalapeño peppers

Finely chopped red onion

Shredded green cabbage

1. Remove the stems from the chilli peppers and rinse to remove as many seeds as possible, then pat dry.

2. Heat a large stockpot over medium heat. Add the chillies and toast for 30 seconds or so, pressing them down with a spatula or tongs, then flipping them and toasting for another 30 seconds, taking care not to burn them. Remove the chillies and set aside.

3. Add 60 ml of the vegetable stock into the warm pot, then add the onion and a pinch of salt. Cook, stirring often, for 5 minutes, until the onions are soft and tender. Add the garlic and cumin and cook for 1 minute while stirring. Add the tomato paste and cook for another minute while stirring.

4. Add the toasted chilli peppers, bay leaves, pinto beans, kidney beans, hominy, the remaining 940 ml stock, and 240 ml water. Add salt to taste. Bring to a low boil, then reduce the heat to low and let simmer for about 45 minutes. The mixture should reduce and thicken considerably. If needed, add more water.

5. Remove the chilli peppers and bay leaves. Stir in the coriander and lime juice. Add more salt, lime juice, and supercharged toppings, if desired.

PRO TIP:

This recipe freezes great, and can easily be halved for smaller portions. In the UK, you may have to source your hominy online.

VERY VEGGIE INDIAN CURRY

10 Plant Points

Serves 4

Although many versions of garam masala exist, the foundation is generally a mix of cumin, turmeric, chilli, ginger, and garlic. If you don't have all of the spices, I've made recommended adjustments.

3 teaspoons extra-virgin olive oil or vegetable stock

300 g cauliflower florets, about half a large head of cauliflower

3 medium Maris Piper potatoes, cubed

3 medium carrots, chopped

1 medium onion, chopped

1 teaspoon cumin seeds

2 garlic cloves, crushed

1 tablespoon grated fresh ginger

1 teaspoon ground turmeric

¼ teaspoon cayenne pepper (optional), or to taste

½ teaspoon garam masala, or more curry powder

1 teaspoon yellow curry powder

½ teaspoon ground coriander (optional)

½ teaspoon salt

¼ teaspoon freshly ground black pepper

170 g frozen green peas

240 ml Biome Stock Unleashed (page 239) or vegetable stock

240 ml coconut milk, or more stock

½ teaspoon lemon zest

1 tablespoon freshly squeezed lemon juice

400 g cooked brown rice, for serving

Chopped fresh coriander, for serving

1. In a large frying pan set over medium heat, heat 2 teaspoons of the olive oil. Add the cauliflower, potatoes, carrots, and onion.

2. Sauté for about 7 minutes, or until the vegetables begin to brown. If the mixture starts to stick, add a splash of vegetable stock to reduce sticking.

3. Push the mixture to the side of the pan, then add in the remaining teaspoon olive oil and the cumin seeds. Allow to crackle for about a minute, until fragrant, then stir into the vegetable mixture and add in the garlic and ginger and cook an additional minute, taking care not to burn the mixture.

4. Mix in the turmeric, cayenne, if using, garam masala, yellow curry powder, ground coriander, if using, salt, and pepper. Add the peas and the stock and cook for an additional 5 to 10 minutes, stirring often, until the vegetables are tender-crisp.

5. Add the coconut milk and cook for another few minutes, until warmed through. Add in the lemon zest and juice, then taste, adding more salt and pepper as desired.

6. Serve over cooked brown rice and garnish with chopped coriander.

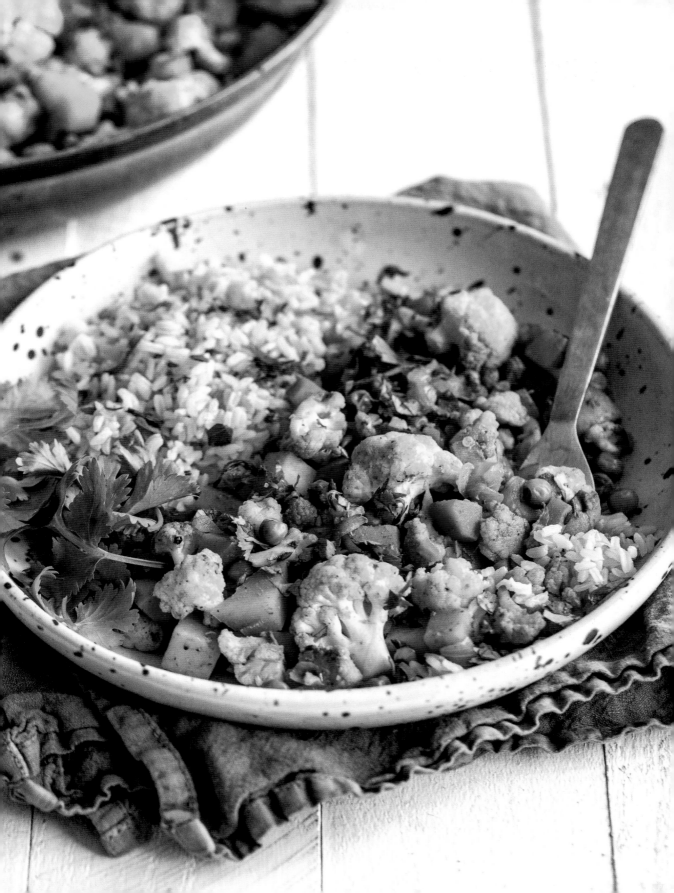

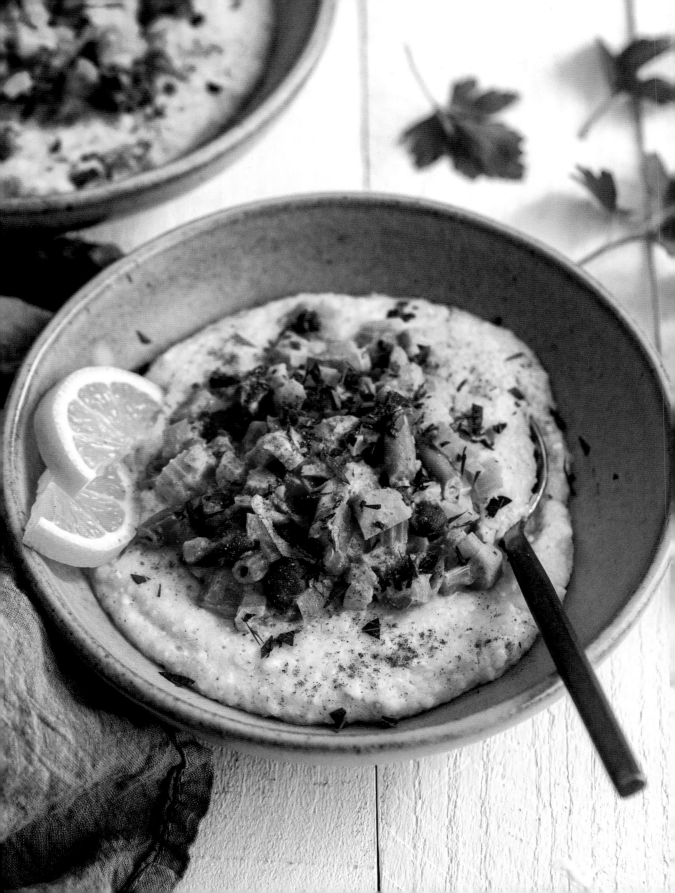

CREAMY CAJUN BOWL

11+ Plant Points

Serves 4

The holy trinity in Cajun and Louisiana Creole cuisine is a trio of ingredients generally used in combination—celery, onions, and sweet peppers. They form the base for several of the classic dishes in the regional cuisines of Louisiana such as gumbo, jambalaya, and étouffée. The trinity is really an evolution of French mirepoix, which includes onions, carrots, and celery. For our Creamy Cajun Bowl, we're bringing you both the holy trinity and the French mirepoix to deliver an explosion of flavour and a diversity of plants that will have you doing a fais-dodo and shouting, "Ça c'est bon!"

240 ml vegetable stock or Biome Stock Unleashed (page 239)

1 medium white or yellow onion, chopped

1 sweet pepper, seeded and chopped

100 g chopped celery

130 g chopped carrots

360 g chopped tomatoes

½ teaspoon salt

300 ml non-dairy, unsweetened milk of choice

1 tablespoon nutritional yeast

160 g quick-cooking grits

2 tablespoons Cajun seasoning (see Pro Tip)

150 g frozen green beans

One 400 g can kidney beans, drained and rinsed

60 g cashews

1 teaspoon freshly squeezed lemon juice

**Supercharge It!
(optional toppings):**

Chopped fresh flat-leaf parsley

Lemon wedges

1. In a stockpot or an enamelled cast iron casserole dish set over medium heat, heat 60 ml of the vegetable stock. Add the onion, sweet pepper, celery, carrots, and tomatoes along with a pinch of salt and cook for 10 to 15 minutes, until the vegetables are softened and reduced, adding in a splash of water or stock as needed.

2. While the vegetables are cooking, make the grits. In a medium saucepan set over medium heat, heat 2 cups of water with the non-dairy milk, nutritional yeast, and salt. Bring to a low boil, then slowly whisk the grits in as you add them to the pot. Keep whisking as you pour so the grits don't clump. Reduce the heat to low and simmer for 10 to 15 minutes, depending on packet instructions, until they are thick and creamy.

3. Stir in 1 tablespoon of the Cajun seasoning, the green beans, and kidney beans to the cooked vegetable mixture and let simmer over medium-low heat for another 5 to 10 minutes.

RECIPE CONTINUES

4. While the vegetables are cooking, in the base of a blender or food processor, place the cashews, lemon juice, the remaining 180 ml stock, and the remaining tablespoon Cajun seasoning and purée until very creamy and smooth, scraping down the sides as needed. Depending on the strength of your blender, you may need to add in an additional splash or two of stock. Stir 120 ml of the cashew mixture into the cooked grits and the rest into the cooked vegetables. Reduce the heat to low.

5. When ready to serve, divide the grits among four bowls and top with the Cajun mixture. Garnish with chopped parsley and lemon wedges, as desired.

PRO TIP:

To make homemade Cajun seasoning, mix together 2 teaspoons smoked paprika, ¼ teaspoon salt, ½ teaspoon garlic powder, ½ teaspoon freshly ground black pepper, ½ teaspoon onion powder, ½ teaspoon dried oregano, ¼ teaspoon cayenne, and ¼ teaspoon dried thyme.

SWEET POTATO AND OKRA BOWL

Serves 4 to 6

Our home—Charleston, South Carolina—is a charming coastal city in the South that is the home of the Gullah people and their African American history and food traditions. Centuries ago, the enslaved West African ancestors of the Gullah brought rice, okra, and cowpeas to the area. Broad beans, corn, and tomatoes were already native to the region. Spring and turnip greens and yams were also staples in the kitchens of people who were enslaved. As you can see, food and history are inseparable in Charleston. These recipes are inspired by Gullah traditions. Enjoy a table abundantly filled with delicious dishes!

Beans and Greens
5 Plant Points

180 g dried black-eyed peas, soaked overnight and rinsed (or 540 g cooked black-eyed peas)

1 white or yellow onion, finely diced

1 green sweet pepper, seeded and diced

600 ml Biome Stock Unleashed (page 239) or vegetable stock

6 garlic cloves, diced

2 bay leaves

1 teaspoon vegan Worcestershire sauce

Hot sauce, as desired

Salt

1 teaspoon low-sodium tamari, soy sauce, or liquid aminos

½ teaspoon smoked paprika

¼ teaspoon crushed red pepper flakes (optional)

450 g spring greens, stems removed and sliced into very thin ribbons

1 teaspoon apple cider vinegar

Candied Sweet Potatoes
2 Plant Points

570 g sweet potatoes, peeled and cut into 4 cm pieces

2 to 3 tablespoons 100% maple syrup

2 tablespoons Biome Stock Unleashed (page 239) or vegetable stock

2 teaspoons freshly squeezed lemon juice

½ teaspoon salt

Freshly ground black pepper

Baked Okra
1 Plant Point

450 g okra, rinsed and patted dry

1 to 2 teaspoons avocado oil or olive oil

¼ teaspoon garlic powder

¼ teaspoon salt

⅛ teaspoon cayenne pepper

¼ teaspoon smoked paprika

Freshly ground black pepper

Shop-bought BBQ sauce, for serving

RECIPE CONTINUES

1. In a large pot, place the soaked and drained black-eyed peas, onion, green pepper, 80 ml of the stock, 2 garlic cloves, and the bay leaves. Bring to the boil, then reduce the heat to low and cook for 45 to 50 minutes, until the beans are tender but not mushy. If using cooked beans, simmer over low heat for 10 to 15 minutes, until heated through. Stir in the Worcestershire sauce and season with hot sauce and salt.

2. While the beans are cooking, make the candied sweet potatoes. Preheat the oven to 200°C. Arrange the sweet potatoes in a single layer in a 22 × 13 cm casserole dish. In a small bowl or measuring cup, whisk together 1 tablespoon of the maple syrup, the stock, lemon juice, salt, and pepper. Pour over the sweet potatoes, tossing well to coat all of the pieces. Lightly tent with foil or cover with an ovenproof lid and bake for 25 minutes. Uncover, stir, and cook again until very tender, about 30 minutes, stirring occasionally. Remove and stir in 1 tablespoon of the maple syrup. Keep covered until serving.

3. Make the baked okra. Trim the okra by removing the stem ends and tips, then slice in half lengthwise. Place in a large bowl and cover with the avocado oil, garlic powder, salt, cayenne, paprika, and pepper. Rub well, coating the okra as much as possible. Place the okra in a single layer on a rimmed baking tray and roast for 20 minutes, stirring halfway through, until lightly browned and tender.

4. In a large frying pan, place the remaining 120 ml stock, the remaining 4 garlic cloves, tamari, smoked paprika, and red pepper flakes, if using, and bring to the boil. Add the spring greens, reduce the heat to medium-low, and cook for 10 to 15 minutes, stirring occasionally. Add the vinegar and season to taste with salt, pepper, or more hot sauce. Keep warm over low heat.

5. To serve, pile the cooked beans and greens, candied sweet potatoes, and crispy okra. Drizzle with BBQ sauce and more hot sauce.

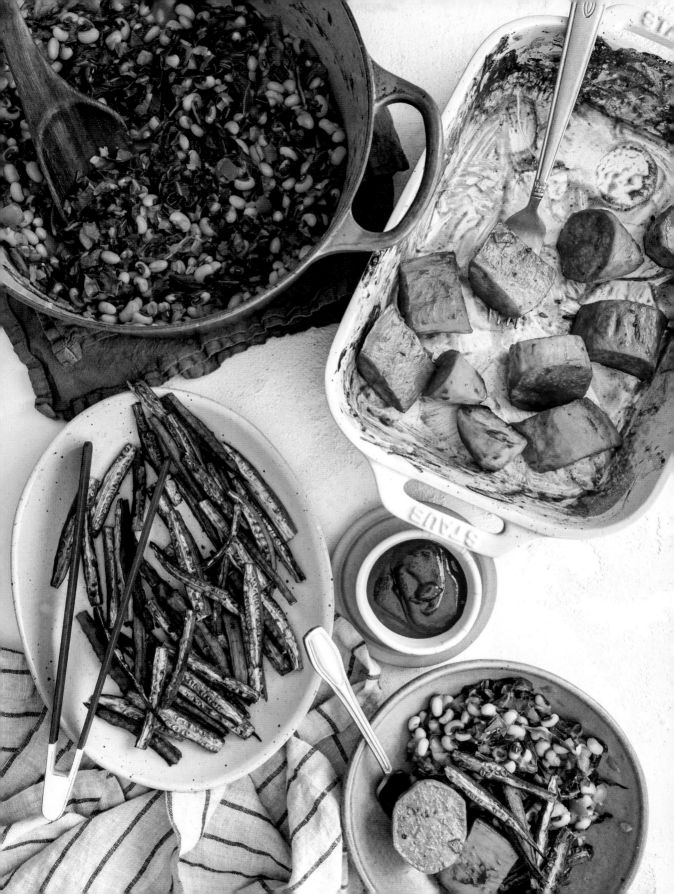

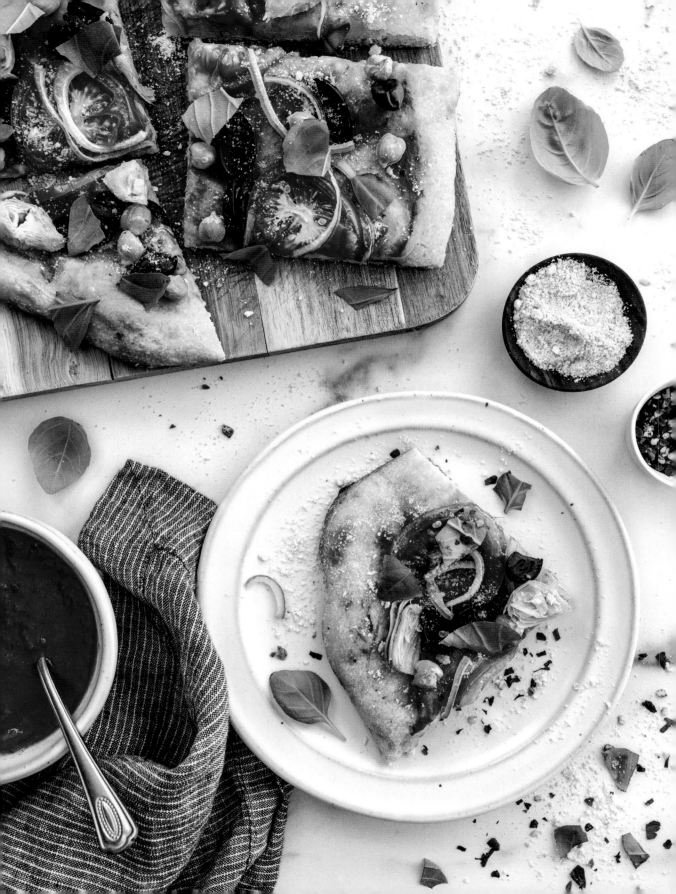

TUSCAN FLATBREAD

6+ Plant Points

Serves 4

Everyone loves pizza, but most of us don't love the food hangover, the digestive issues, or the excessive calories from saturated fat. How about some healthy substitutions? Bye cheese, hello Cashew Parm. Hasta la vista white flour crust, hola Sourdough Pizza Crust. You can have pizza your way—delicious AND nutritious.

1 prepared wholewheat pizza dough or 1 recipe Sourdough Pizza Crust (page 325)

80 ml pizza sauce

1 medium tomato, thinly sliced

85 g sliced canned or bottled artichoke hearts

35 g halved black olives (about 12 olives)

40 g cooked chickpeas, drained and rinsed if canned

40 g thinly sliced red onion

Crushed red pepper flakes (optional)

Pinch flaky sea salt (optional)

Olive oil, to brush on (optional)

30 g Cashew Parm (see Pro Tip)

Handful torn basil

1. Preheat the oven to 230°C.

2. Gently stretch the dough and place on a pizza stone lightly dusted with cornmeal or lined with parchment paper, or on a large rectangular baking tray. Place in the oven to parbake for 7 to 8 minutes, until just lightly golden.

3. Gently remove from the oven and place on a heatproof surface or hob. Spread the pizza sauce evenly on top using the back of a spoon, making circular motions to evenly distribute the sauce, then top with the sliced tomato, artichoke hearts, halved black olives, chickpeas, and red onion. If desired, sprinkle with red pepper flakes and a small pinch of flaky sea salt. For a more golden crust, brush with a little olive oil.

4. Place back in the oven and cook for another 10 to 12 minutes. Remove and sprinkle generously with the Cashew Parm. Let cool for 5 minutes, then sprinkle with basil. Slice and serve.

PRO TIP:

To make Cashew Parm, place 60 g raw cashews, 20 g slivered almonds (or almonds with skins off), 3 tablespoons nutritional yeast, 1 tablespoon garlic powder, and a pinch of salt in the base of a blender or food processor. Blend until very finely powdered.

TAKING YOUR SWEET POTATO GAME TO THE NEXT LEVEL!

You think you know sweet potatoes, but do you? Did you know that sweet potatoes are actually roots, whereas regular potatoes are underground stems? Or that the plant grows best in warm temperatures, which partially explains why North Carolina is the largest producer of sweet potatoes in the United States? Or that the dietary fibre found in sweet potatoes has been shown in research to be beneficial to your gut microbes and facilitate the production of short-chain fatty acids? There's so much love in these tubers that we decided to give you four different ways to enjoy them. But, as usual, you should look for ways to make these recipes your own by adding in the superchargers and cranking up the Plant Points.

Here are some tips to properly handle your sweet potatoes:

- The ideal sweet potato should be smooth and firm, with no soft spots or bruising.

- Sweet potatoes should only be washed right before cooking because moisture promotes spoilage.

- Unwashed sweet potatoes can store well for weeks or even months in a dry, cool, dark place.

- But not in your fridge! Storing sweet potatoes in a refrigerator causes an off-taste and a hard core in the centre. Remember, they like warmer temperatures!

RECIPE CONTINUES

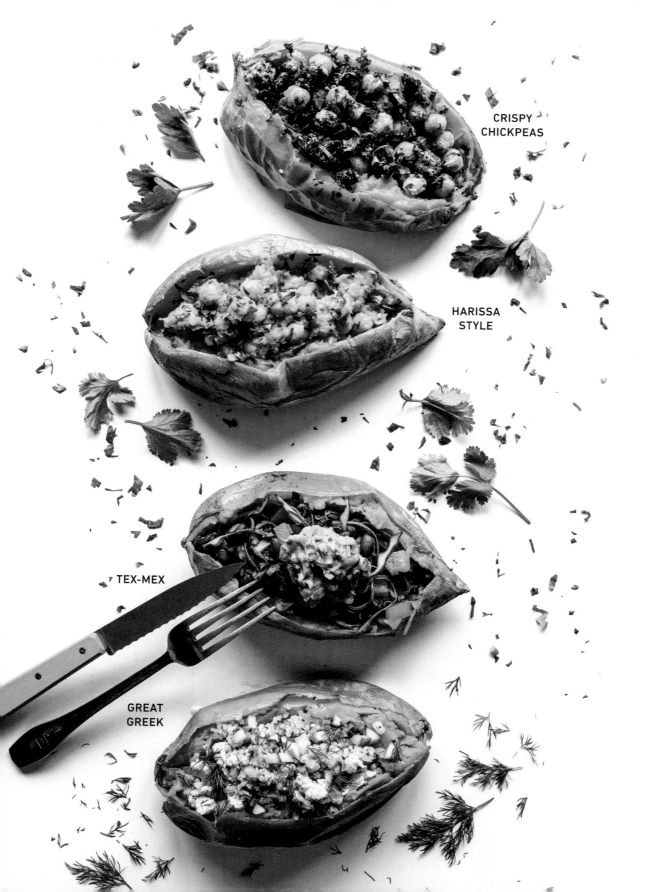

CRISPY
CHICKPEAS

HARISSA
STYLE

TEX-MEX

GREAT
GREEK

HARISSA STYLE

6 Plant Points
Serves 4

4 large sweet potatoes, scrubbed

One 400 g can chickpeas, drained and rinsed

2 tablespoons tahini

2 to 3 teaspoons harissa paste

2 to 3 tablespoons freshly squeezed lime juice

Olive oil, for drizzling (optional)

Fresh coriander, for topping (optional)

1. Preheat the oven to 200°C. Using the tines of a fork, prick a few holes in the potatoes and place on a rimmed baking tray in the oven. Cook for 45 to 50 minutes, until the potatoes are just tender.

2. While the potatoes are cooking, in a small bowl, combine the chickpeas, tahini, harissa paste, and lime juice. Gently mash some of the chickpeas into the tahini.

3. Remove the sweet potatoes from the oven, slice open, and remove about half of the filling. Add the filling into the chickpea mixture, stir together, then scoop back into the sweet potatoes.

4. If desired, drizzle with a little olive oil, then place back in the oven and cook another 5 to 10 minutes, until warmed through. Remove and garnish with fresh coriander, if desired.

CRISPY CHICKPEAS

6 Plant Points
Serves 4

4 large sweet potatoes, scrubbed

280 g torn kale leaves

One 400 g can chickpeas, drained and rinsed

1 to 2 teaspoons olive oil

¼ teaspoon ground cumin

¼ teaspoon smoked paprika

2 tablespoons tahini

2 tablespoons freshly squeezed lemon juice

¼ teaspoon crushed red pepper flakes (optional)

10 g freshly chopped flat-leaf parsley

Salt and freshly ground pepper

1. Preheat the oven to 200°C. Using the tines of a fork, prick a few holes in the potatoes and place on a rimmed baking tray in the oven. Cook for 45 to 50 minutes, until the potatoes are just tender.

2. Place the kale and chickpeas in a large bowl and drizzle with the olive oil. Add the cumin and paprika and rub together with your hands to coat the kale and beans. Place in a single layer on a baking sheet and bake for 10 minutes, or until the kale is crispy. Remove and place back in the bowl along with the tahini, lemon juice, red pepper flakes, if using, and parsley. Season to taste with salt and pepper.

3. Remove the potatoes, then slice in half, taking care not to cut all the way through. Massage the outside of the potato to fluff the centre, season with a sprinkle of salt and pepper, and top with the crispy chickpea and kale mixture.

SWEET POTATO BAR
GREAT GREEK

7 Plant Points

Serves 4

4 large sweet potatoes, scrubbed

185 g cooked quinoa

3 tablespoons fresh dill

½ batch Homemade Tofu Feta (page 84)

2 tablespoons finely chopped red onion

2 to 3 tablespoons tahini

2 to 3 tablespoons freshly squeezed lemon juice

Salt and freshly ground black pepper, to taste

1. Preheat the oven to 200°C. Using the tines of a fork, prick a few holes in the potatoes and place on a rimmed baking tray in the oven. Cook for 45 to 50 minutes, until the potatoes are just tender.

2. While the potatoes are cooking, in a small bowl, toss together the quinoa, dill, tofu feta, red onion, tahini, and lemon juice. Season to taste, adding salt, pepper, or more tahini for creaminess and lemon juice for tang, as desired.

3. Remove the potatoes, then slice in half, taking care not to cut all the way through. Massage the outside of the potato to fluff the centre, season with a sprinkle of salt and pepper, and top with the quinoa mixture.

SWEET POTATO BAR
TEX-MEX

9 Plant Points

Serves 4

4 large sweet potatoes, scrubbed

280 g finely shredded red cabbage

One 400 g can black beans, drained and rinsed

60 ml plus 2 tablespoons freshly squeezed lime juice

1 sweet pepper, seeded and diced

10 g chopped coriander

Salt and freshly ground black pepper

2 ripe avocados

40 g finely chopped red onion

1 jalapeño, seeded and finely chopped

1. Preheat the oven to 200°C. Using the tines of a fork, prick a few holes in the potatoes and place on a rimmed baking tray in the oven. Cook for 45 to 50 minutes, until the potatoes are just tender.

2. While the potatoes are cooking, make the slaw. Place the red cabbage, black beans, 60 ml lime juice, sweet pepper, and half of the chopped coriander in a large bowl. Toss together until well combined, then season with salt and pepper.

3. Make the guacamole by placing the avocados in a separate bowl, then gently mashing with a fork. Add in the remaining chopped coriander, red onion, jalapeño, and remaining 2 tablespoons of lime juice. Mix well, then season to taste with salt and pepper.

4. Remove the potatoes, then slice in half, taking care not to cut all the way through. Massage the outside of the potato to fluff the centre, season with a sprinkle of salt and pepper, and top with the slaw and guacamole.

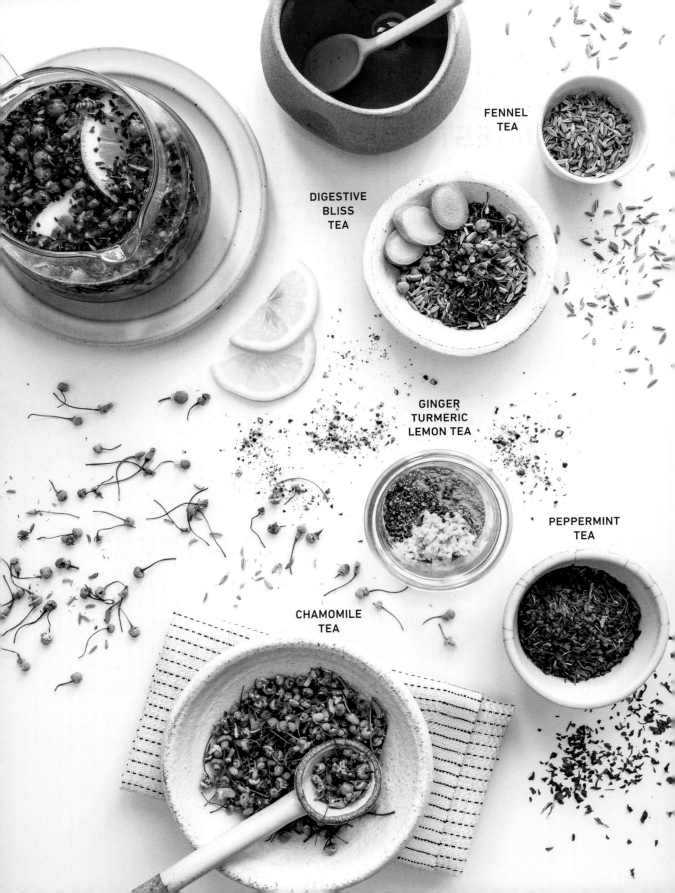

FENNEL
TEA

DIGESTIVE
BLISS
TEA

GINGER
TURMERIC
LEMON TEA

PEPPERMINT
TEA

CHAMOMILE
TEA

HERBAL INFUSIONS ARE NATURE'S MEDICINE FOR DIGESTIVE DISTRESS

In Chapter 7 | Train Your Gut on page 213, I mentioned how Digestive Bliss Tea can be a tool used to soothe mealtime symptoms. I'm a huge fan! The components making up Digestive Bliss Tea are good for you AND they help to soothe an upset gut. Each one has its own unique medicinal properties: peppermint reduces spasms, chamomile is soothing and relaxing, fennel reduces wind and diarrhoea, and ginger targets queasiness or nausea. You can use any or all of the recipes below in combination as a part of your strategy to improve your symptoms. Make them a routine part of your mealtime ritual! Your gut microbes will be grateful for the polyphenols and phytochemicals while you settle into a relaxing herbal tea.

DIGESTIVE BLISS TEA

Serves 1

This is the holy grail of digestive tea! Here, the superhero herbs for your gut come together to create the ultimate team. Feel free to make this recipe your own and adjust as needed. For example, peppermint can make acid reflux worse, so if that is a concern, you may want to omit the peppermint.

1 teaspoon dried peppermint leaves

1 teaspoon dried chamomile flowers

½ teaspoon lightly crushed fennel seeds

Three or four ½ cm thick slices fresh ginger

Slice fresh lemon, if you have it

240 ml just-boiling water

Sweetener (optional)

In a small teapot or large mug, place the peppermint, chamomile, fennel, ginger, and lemon and pour boiling water over the top. Cover and steep for 10 minutes. Strain, then return the contents to the mug to sip and enjoy. Sweeten as desired.

PRO TIP:

You can use either fresh ginger or dried pieces (not powder). If using ground ginger, reduce the amount to 1 to 2 teaspoons dried ginger.

PEPPERMINT TEA

Serves 1

Peppermint relaxes your intestines, soothes spasms, and as a result may benefit wind, bloating, and indigestion. In a systematic review and meta-analysis of placebo-controlled clinical trials, peppermint was found to be beneficial for irritable bowel syndrome symptoms and abdominal pain.

1 tablespoon dried peppermint leaves

350 ml boiling water

Sweetener (optional)

In a large mug, place the peppermint leaves and cover with boiling water and let steep for 3 to 5 minutes. Strain using a fine-mesh strainer. Add sweetener, if desired.

GINGER TURMERIC LEMON TEA

Serves 1

This tea reduces nausea, inflammation, and pain. Both ginger and turmeric come from the plant rhizome, a stem that grows underground and produces shoots off its sides, similar to a root system. Both have powerful phytochemicals—ginger has gingerol and turmeric has curcumin. And both have been repeatedly shown to be beneficial to the gut microbiota. Add a little date syrup or maple syrup if desired for sweetness.

1 teaspoon ground turmeric	¼ teaspoon freshly ground black pepper
Juice of ½ large lemon	Sweetener (optional)
1 teaspoon grated fresh ginger	350 ml boiling water

In a large mug, whisk together the turmeric, lemon juice, ginger, pepper, and sweetener, if using. Slowly whisk in the boiling water.

CHAMOMILE TEA

Serves 1

Chamomile reduces stress and inflammation, creates relaxation, and improves sleep. In one study, drinking chamomile tea every day for two weeks led to changes in the metabolites present in the urine that in part explained the beneficial effects of chamomile. Interestingly, when the study participants stopped drinking the chamomile tea, they still found that the effects persisted for several weeks. This implies that the change is caused by a lasting shift in gut microbe metabolism caused by chamomile ingestion.

1 tablespoon dried chamomile flowers	350 ml boiling water
	Sweetener (optional)

In a large mug, place the chamomile flowers and cover with boiling water. Let steep for 3 to 5 minutes. Strain using a fine-mesh strainer. Add sweetener, if desired.

FENNEL TEA

Serves 1

Fennel reduces flatulence and upset stomach, helps balance both diarrhoea and constipation, and improves breath. What's not to like? Fennel seeds are traditionally chewed after meals in India. The major component of fennel oil seeds is anethole, which happens to be chemically similar to the neurotransmitter dopamine and has a relaxant, anti-spasm effect on the muscles lining the intestines. As a result, it's shown benefit for the treatment of cramping in irritable bowel syndrome.

1 tablespoon fennel seeds

350 ml boiling water

Sweetener (optional)

1. Crush the fennel seeds using a mortar and pestle or the back of a spoon or flat edge of a wide knife. You can also gently smash the seeds with a glass bottle or rolling pin.

2. Place in a large mug and cover with boiling water and let steep for 3 to 5 minutes. Strain using a fine-mesh strainer. Add sweetener, if desired.

SUMMERTIME COOLERS

How about an assortment of fun summertime refreshments that taste great and are also good for you. They're perfect to pour over large cubes of ice in a glass carafe or jar. Then, settle into a deck chair, turn on some summertime jams, take a deep breath, and just let go. What music are you turning on? I got Van Morrison—*Moondance*.

GINGER LEMONADE

Serves 2

60 ml freshly squeezed lemon juice

420 g fresh pineapple

1 cm piece fresh ginger, roughly chopped

In the base of blender, place the lemon juice, pineapple, ginger, and 240 ml cold water. Blend, then strain if desired, and serve over ice.

TURMERIC ORANGE COOLER

Serves 2

3 peeled medium oranges

65 g chopped carrot

1 teaspoon finely grated fresh ginger

¼ teaspoon ground turmeric

Pinch freshly ground black pepper

In the base of a blender, place the oranges, carrot, ginger, turmeric, and black pepper with 240 ml water. Blend, then strain as desired and serve over ice.

MATCHA HONEYDEW COOLER

Serves 2

1 teaspoon matcha powder

360 g honeydew melon, rind removed

2 tablespoons freshly squeezed lime juice

Pinch salt

1. In a small bowl, whisk together the matcha powder with 360 ml cold water, then add to the base of a blender along with the honeydew melon, lime juice, and salt.

2. Blend, strain if desired, and serve over ice.

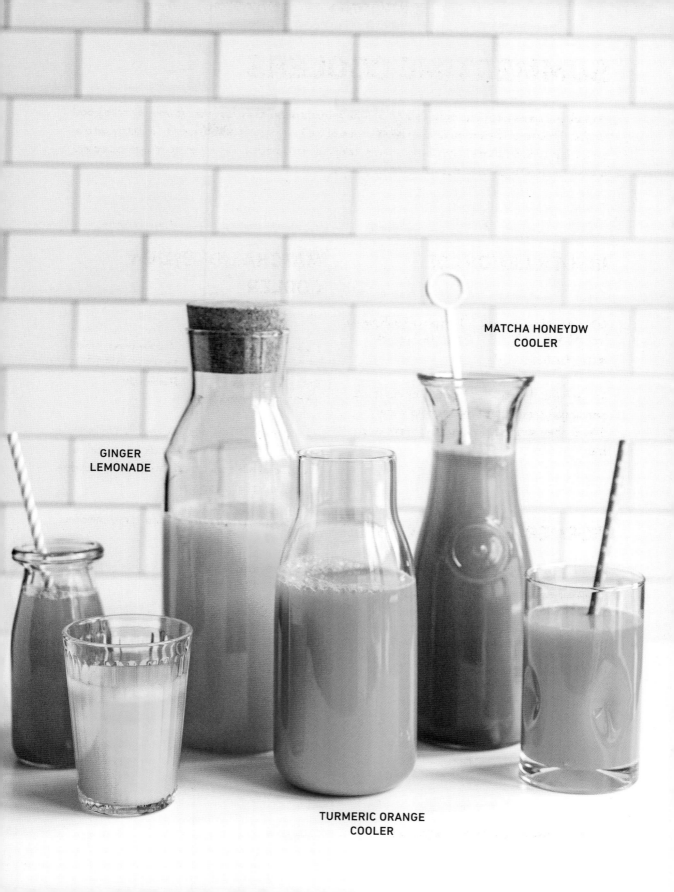

GINGER
LEMONADE

MATCHA HONEYDW
COOLER

TURMERIC ORANGE
COOLER

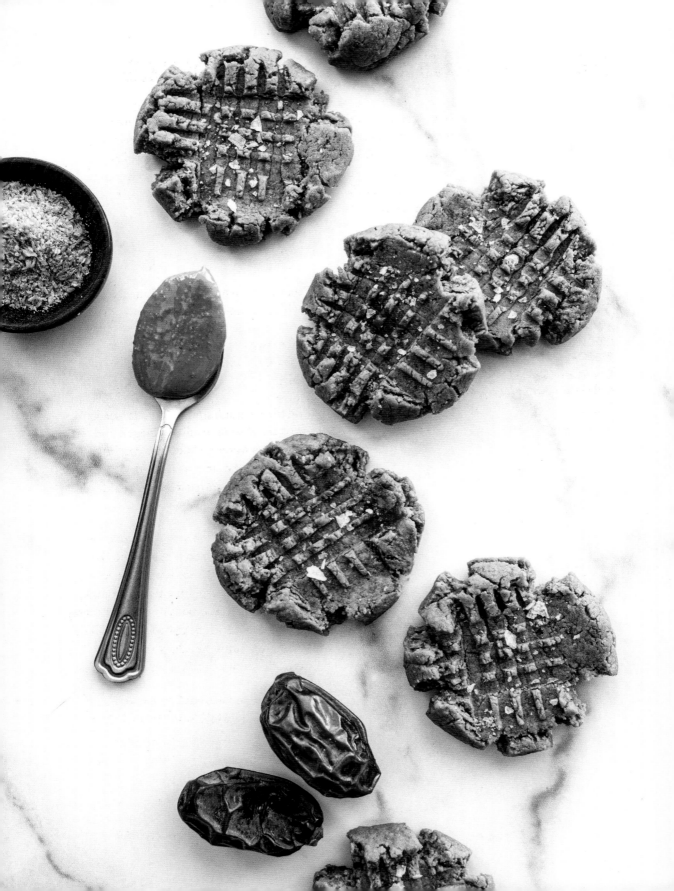

PEANUT BUTTER DATE COOKIES

3 Plant Points

Makes 9 cookies

Have you heard of the infamous "1-1-1" cookies? The idea is that just three ingredients—peanut butter, sugar, egg—can make you cookies. Shortcuts to delicious flavours are great, but not when they come at the expense of your health! How about we give you all that flavour but make it naturally sweetened and plant-based! This is a soft, chewy cookie.

120 g pitted Medjool dates

170 g smooth unsweetened peanut butter (stirred well)

2 teaspoons ground milled flaxseed

½ teaspoon bicarbonate of soda

½ teaspoon vanilla extract

½ teaspoon white or apple cider vinegar

Flaked sea salt, for topping

1. Preheat the oven to 175°C. Line a baking tray with parchment paper and set aside.

2. In the base of a food processor, place the dates and pulse until well chopped and crumbly.

3. Add the peanut butter, milled flaxseed, bicarbonate of soda, vanilla, vinegar, and 2 tablespoons water and pulse to combine, scraping down the sides as needed. The mixture should be fairly sticky and hold together when pressed.

4. Using a 2-tablespoon scoop, remove the dough, roll into a ball, then place onto the prepared baking tray. Repeat with the rest of the dough, then, using the tines of a fork, press down onto the cookies to make a hashtag pattern. Sprinkle with flaked sea salt and bake for 10 minutes, until the edges are just set. The cookies will continue to firm up as they cool.

5. Remove from the oven and let cool completely, then enjoy. Store in an airtight container in the fridge for up to 3 days.

MEXICAN HOT CHOCOLATE BROWNIES

4 Plant Points

Makes 12 brownies

Brownies made from black beans . . . sign me up immediately! Mexican hot chocolate is known for its spices. In this recipe, you get cinnamon and cayenne pairing with the cocoa powder for a fiesta in your mouth!

One 400 g can black beans, drained and rinsed

125 g peanut butter

55 g almond or oat flour

25 g cocoa powder

120 ml 100% maple syrup

1 tablespoon avocado oil or other neutral oil

1 tablespoon white or apple cider vinegar

1 teaspoon vanilla extract

1 teaspoon baking powder

½ teaspoon bicarbonate of soda

1 teaspoon ground cinnamon

¼ teaspoon cayenne pepper

¼ teaspoon salt

120 g chocolate chips

1. Preheat the oven to 175°C. Lightly oil an 20 × 20 cm pan (or line with baking parchment) and set aside.

2. In the base of a food processor, place the beans and pulse 5 or 6 times until well chopped.

3. Add the peanut butter, flour, cocoa powder, maple syrup, avocado oil, vinegar, vanilla, baking powder, bicarbonate of soda, cinnamon, cayenne, and salt. Process until creamy and smooth, stopping to scrape down the sides as needed.

4. Remove the lid and stir in 80 g chocolate chips. Pour into the prepared baking dish (the batter will be thick) and spread it out evenly. Top with the remaining 40 g chocolate chips.

5. Bake for 30 minutes, or until a toothpick inserted comes out clean.

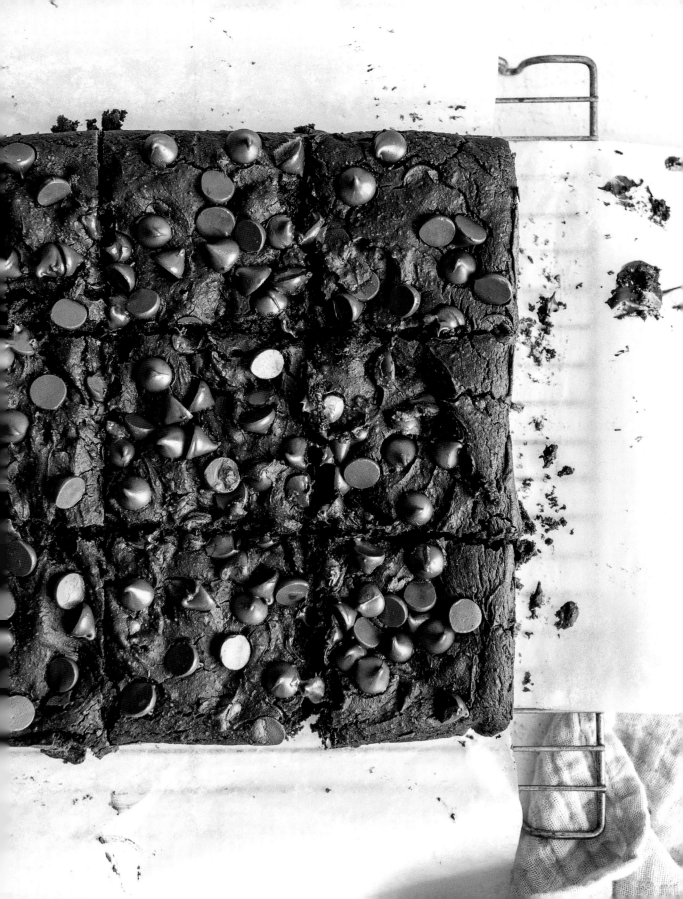

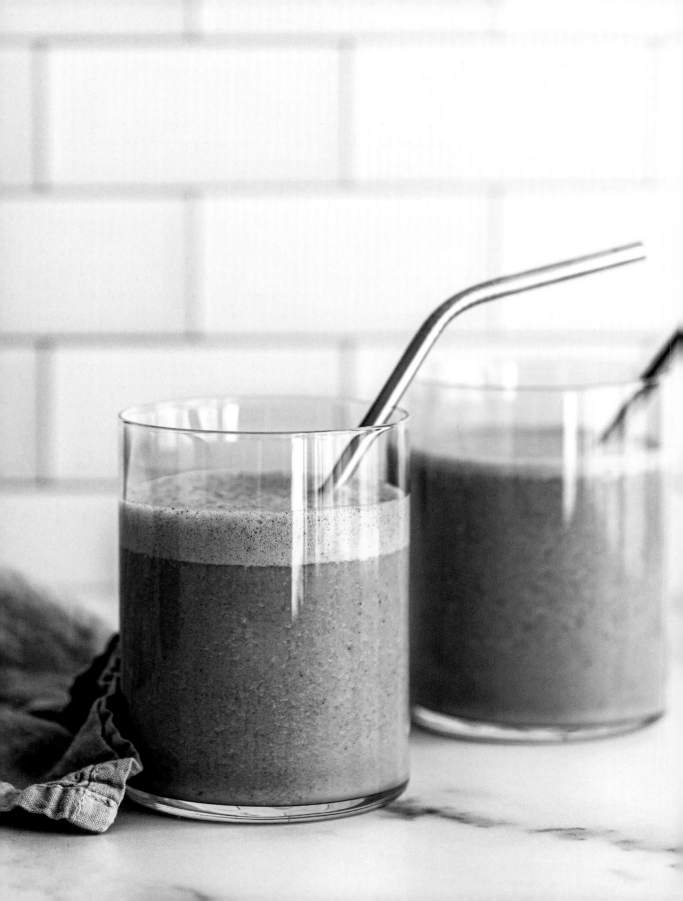

COOKIE MILK

1+ Plant Points

Serves 1

It's hard to beat cookies and milk. But if you could combine them into an ice-cold, refreshing beverage, this is what you would get—Cookie Milk! Simple, sweet, and delicious as a snack or dessert. This recipe serves one but is easily doubled, tripled, quadrupled, etc., for an extended remix worth sharing.

1 tablespoon almond butter

240 ml cold unsweetened oat milk (see Pro Tip)

¼ teaspoon ground cinnamon

¼ teaspoon vanilla extract

1 date, pitted and chopped

1. In the base of a blender, place the almond butter, oat milk, cinnamon, vanilla, and date and purée until creamy and smooth.

2. If it's not cold enough, shake with ice, strain, and enjoy.

PRO TIP:

To make oat milk at home, simply blend 240 ml water with 4 tablespoons organic jumbo oats in a blender for 30 to 45 seconds. Give yourself +1 Plant Point for your efforts. For a milkshake-like milk, add 1 chopped frozen banana before blending (another +1 Plant Point!).

CHOCOLATE COOKIE MILK

2+ Plant Points

Serves 1

Chocolate lovers, I haven't forgotten you! If it's chocolate cookies and milk you desire, then it's Chocolate Cookie Milk you will have! Use the oat milk recipe provided in the Pro Tip on page 297 for +1 Plant Point.

1 tablespoon almond butter

240 ml cold unsweetened oat milk

1 to 2 teaspoons cocoa powder

¼ teaspoon vanilla extract

Pinch ground cinnamon

Very small pinch salt

1 date, pitted and chopped

1. In the base of a blender, place the almond butter, oat milk, cocoa powder, vanilla, cinnamon, salt, and date and purée until creamy and smooth.

2. Enjoy at room temperature or, for a warm cocoa, place in a small saucepan and warm over medium heat.

PRO TIP:

For a delicious chocolate milkshake, add a frozen, chopped banana before blending (+1 Plant Point).

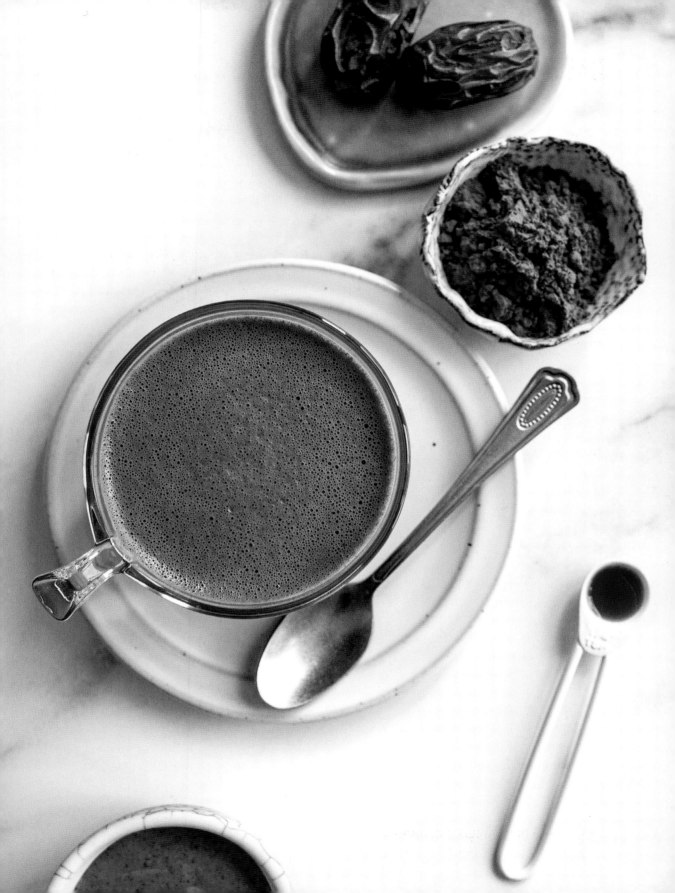

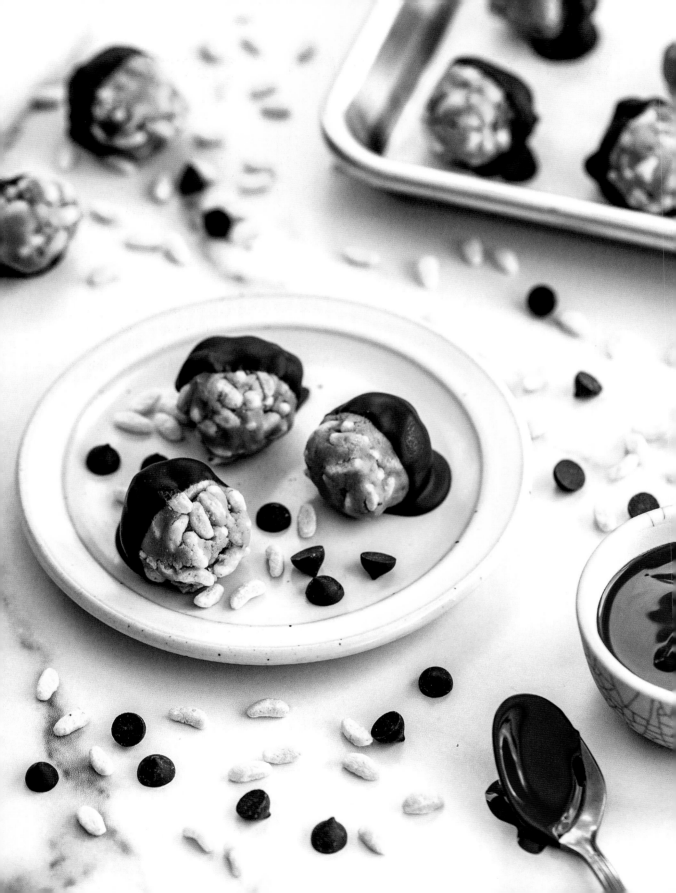

CRISPY DARK CHOCOLATE BITES

3 Plant Points

Makes about 12 balls

Polyphenols from cocoa have been shown to reach the colon, meet the microbes, and enhance the growth of some good guys—*Lactobacillus* and *Bifidobacterium*. Did you know that microbes are able to produce metabolites that make you desire, possibly seek out, chocolate? So when you reach for these Crispy Dark Chocolate Bites, you're not doing it for yourself. You're doing it for your microbes. It's a selfless act of love.

125 g cashew butter, at room temperature

1 teaspoon 100% maple syrup

20 g crispy brown rice cereal

170 g dark chocolate chips

1. Line a baking tray with parchment paper. In a large bowl, place the cashew butter and maple syrup and whisk until smooth. Add in the brown rice cereal and stir together until well combined.

2. Scoop out 1 tablespoon of the mixture at a time and roll into a ball, then place on the baking tray. Repeat with the rest of the mixture, then place in the freezer for 30 minutes to 1 hour, until hardened.

3. Melt the chocolate chips over low heat until creamy, taking care not to overheat them. Remove the balls from the freezer and dip or drizzle with the melted chocolate. Return to the freezer to allow the chocolate to harden.

4. Store in an airtight container in the freezer, letting sit at room temperature for a minute or two before eating.

THE SNICKERS BITES THAT MADE YOU FREAK OUT, SO NOW I'M QUADRUPLING DOWN

When you write a book with eighty recipes, you always wonder which ones people are going to freak out about and share left and right on their social media. I wasn't surprised the Biome Stock was a hit—that's my flagship recipe. But I really wasn't expecting such a powerful response to the Snickers Bites.

But it makes sense, too! Here's the thing . . . They're really, really good. And they're really, really easy to make. And you feel guilt-free when you're eating them. So they're the elusive win-win-win that we are all searching for. You shared them, and you let me know how much you adored them. I heard you! So we are coming back to you with more. Here they are, the Snickers Bites, but this time with four different variations. Bon appétit, my friends!

| SNICKERS BITES | SIMPLE AND SWEET DATE BITES | POMEGRANATE DATE BITES | SNICKERS ICE CREAM BITES |

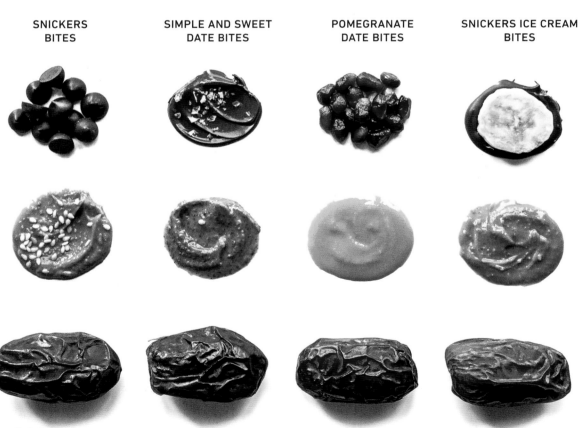

SNICKERS BITES

4 Plant Points

Serves 1

1 Medjool date, pitted

1 teaspoon peanut butter

4 to 5 chocolate chips

½ teaspoon sesame seeds

Transfer the teaspoon of peanut butter onto a halved date, add the chocolate chips liberally, and sprinkle with sesame seeds.

SIMPLE AND SWEET DATE BITES

3 Plant Points

Serves 1

1 date, pitted

1 teaspoon almond butter

2 teaspoons melted chocolate

Flaky sea salt

Stuff the date with almond butter, then dip into melted chocolate. Place on a parchment paper-lined plate or other non-stick surface. Sprinkle with flaky sea salt and let harden.

POMEGRANATE DATE BITES

3 Plant Points

Serves 1

1 Medjool date, pitted

1 teaspoon tahini

4 to 5 pomegranate seeds

Stuff the date with the tahini and pomegranate seeds.

SNICKERS ICE CREAM BITES

4 Plant Points

Makes 4

1 date, pitted

2 teaspoons peanut butter

4 slices banana

Melted dark chocolate

1. Line a small plate or baking tray with parchment paper. Pit the date and tear into 4 equal pieces. Place ½ teaspoon of peanut butter on the top of each banana slice, then press a piece of date onto the banana. Drizzle the dark chocolate onto the pieces (or dunk the banana into the dark chocolate), then place in the freezer for about 30 minutes, until hardened.

2. Keep in an airtight container in the freezer for up to 1 week.

>> To view the 23 scientific references cited in this chapter, please visit www.theplantfedgut.com/cookbook.

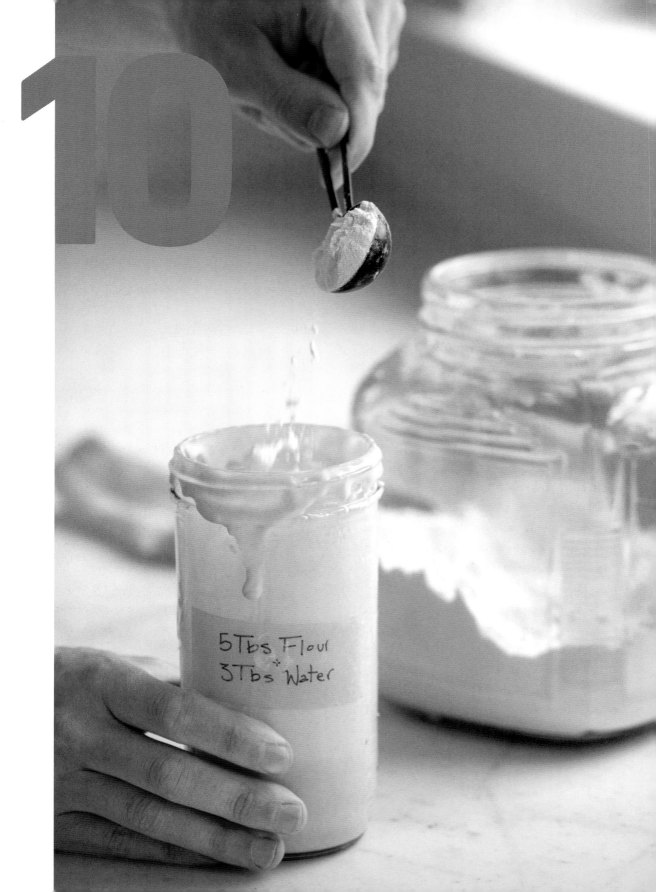

5Tbs Flour
3Tbs ✦ Water

Fermentation Nation Rising!

In *Fibre Fuelled*, I broke down fermentation in detail and discussed many of the health benefits of consuming fermented foods. But research continues to emerge and enhance our confidence that a healthy gut thrives with fermented foods as a part of the diet. Because it's such a game changer, this chapter is devoted to the science behind fermentation, along with recipes to get you excited to add more of these incredibly delicious foods to your *Fibre Fuelled* diet.

Let's back up a bit and talk more about the process of fermentation and how it is related to what I like to think of as the "microbiome code," or the way that microbes have connected and created life on Earth for billions of years. Essentially, microbes link and support all life on Earth, from soil to plants to animals to humans, even ecosystems and our planetary health. Consider this example: An apple tree bears fruit. You pick that apple and take a bite. About a hundred million microbes that were living as a part of the apple's microbiome become a part of your intestine, along with the apple's fibre, polyphenols, phytochemicals, vitamins, and minerals that provide benefits to the consumer. Then, say you throw part of the apple in the bushes. It slowly starts to decompose, shape-shifting from being luscious and fresh to being brown and mushy. But, as it "rots" it becomes nutrient-rich and full of carbon. Eventually, it is taken back to the ground and becomes a part of the soil. That soil is nourished by the apple compost. The apple seed gets taken into the cool, moist earth. It sprouts to life, emerges from the ground, and stretches towards the sun. It will soon grow to be a fruit-bearing apple tree.

Yes, the circle of life is indeed majestic. But it is important to acknowledge that everything that I just described was made possible by microbes, the stewards of life on this planet and the invisible workforce that tirelessly makes it all function seamlessly from one connection to the next.

Fermentation is a concrete way we can harness the power of these microbes even more for our own health. Historically, fermented foods were a part of every major food culture, largely due to the need for food preservation. But they were also celebrated for their unique flavour profile. Over time, many cuisines neglected these time-honoured ingredients and techniques, but now this ancient tradition is undergoing a resurgence. Using new laboratory technology that has been available only in the last few years, we now have a more complete picture of exactly why fermented foods are so beneficial.

When I think of fermentation, I think of transformation. During the fermentation process, a team of invisible microbes initiates a symphony of coordinated, timely enzymatic reactions that actually change the flavour and nutrition of the food. And just like an orchestra is never just one instrument or one band member, fermentation takes a collective effort to create something new and beautiful together. The right microbe steps in at the right time. Different microbes make unique contributions and call on new microbes to help. They transform the fibre in the ingredients into exopolysaccharides and create new bioactive peptides and polyphenols, along with healthy acids, vitamin K, and B vitamins. The process reduces gluten, phytic acid, FODMAPs, and even pesticide residues. The end product is more nutritious than the starting product. And the flavour becomes more pronounced and richer.

You've heard me refer to the American Gut Project, which is the largest study to date to connect the gut microbiome with our dietary choices. Run by Dr. Rob Knight, one of my heroes in clinical research, the American Gut Project first established the connection between the diversity of plants in our diet and diversity of microbes in our gut.

More recently, the American Gut Project released its results on the benefits of consuming fermented plants in our diet. Their research included 6,811 participants in a cross-sectional analysis followed by 115 people who did a more detailed longitudinal microbiome and fermented food study. In it, they discovered that there was a difference between the gut microbiome of those who consume fermented plants versus those who do not. The microbes being consumed in the fermented plants started showing up in the stool microbiome samples. They also found that those who consumed fermented foods had a stronger ability to produce conjugated linoleic acid, otherwise known as CLA. This is a healthy fat that's thought to be beneficial for weight control and prevention of cardiovascular disease.

In a different study, Drs. Erica Sonnenburg, Justin Sonnenburg, and Chris Gardner from Stanford University had a group of study participants add fermented food to their daily routine. They went from consuming less than half a serving of fermented food per day all the way up to six servings of fermented food per day. That's quite a bit! But the effort and addition of new foods to the diet paid off in a massive way. Over ten weeks, the microbial diversity within the participants' gut microbiomes increased significantly. The increase in microbiome diversity was more in those who consumed larger servings. Additionally, they found changes in the immune system with the consumption of fermented foods, with less activation of four types of immune cells and lower levels of nineteen inflammatory signalling proteins.

If that doesn't convince you to give fermenting a try, do it for the big pop of flavour! From savoury breads to kimchi and other pickled vegetables, these recipes offer bright, new tastes to enjoy on their own or as a side to liven up your meals. Each recipe has its own unique profile and health benefits, which we will share. While fermented foods are never going to be the backbone of your diet, I hope that you'll be inspired to eat them more routinely. They can give your gut function and cooking a great boost!

Tips for Fermenting Safely

The recipes in this chapter use lacto-fermentation techniques. No, this does not mean they involve using milk, but rather, this type of fermentation allows you to harness the power of lactic acid-producing bacteria (as well as a host of other beneficial bacteria). As your veggies ferment, you are not only preserving them but also enhancing the nutritional benefits.

The idea of eating live bacteria can be a bit scary, and when you are first starting out, it is difficult to know if you're "doing it right." In addition to getting over the fear of making and eating something fermented, you have the added challenge of learning to judge when your ferment is perfectly ripe and ready for consumption. But don't worry, it isn't as scary as it may seem. Remember, the microbes will be hard at work, even while you rest. They will be the ones doing most of the work; you just need to set them up for success.

Here are some tips to help you find your fermenting feet, so that you can ferment both safely and confidently.

Do

1. Always use pure salt. Not iodized salt or table salt or any salts with additives. The bacteria can only work with natural, rather than synthetic, ingredients.

2. Wash your veggies. Wash to remove dirt, but you do not need to scrub or peel them. The microbes are on the outside and on the inside of the veg, so you want to preserve as much of the bacteria as you can.

3. Weigh your vegetables and your salt accurately using a food scale. Salt acts as the key preserving agent here and helps to create a brine that is salty enough for the bacteria to begin working their magic. The veg-to-salt ratio is important, as too little salt can lead to your ferment going off and too much salt can slow down the fermentation process.

4. Look for the signs that fermentation is taking place. Bubbles, colour change, cloudy brine, and sediment in the bottom of your jar—these are all normal and are signs that the bacteria are working away at fermenting. You will also start to smell the distinctive "vinegary" smell that comes along with a maturing ferment. This is a good thing—it means the microbes are producing acid.

5. Keep your ferment submerged under the brine (a.k.a. the saltwater solution). Use a fermentation weight to help keep the vegetables submerged; anything poking out of the brine is likely to go off. Under the brine, all is fine.

6. Do give the bacteria enough time and warmth to work their fermenting magic. Ideal fermentation temperature is 20 to 22°C, and try to keep this consistent to ensure that the process runs smoothly. The process happens in stages and there are no shortcuts as far as time is concerned to achieving the nutritional and flavour benefits. We call this slow food, so give it time. Like a fine wine, you will often find that ferments get better with age. I love giving my sauerkraut extra time—it always seems to get better.

7. Always store your finished ferments somewhere cool. If you plan to eat them right away, store them in the fridge, but if your plan is to keep them for a later date, store them unopened in a cool cellar or basement. Keeping your ferment cool helps to keep the flavour consistent for longer and helps extend the shelf life.

8. Check the pH of your ferment, if this interests you. A finished ferment should have a pH of around 3.

9. Invest in some good-quality glassware. You want reinforced glass (to protect against cracks and breaks) if there is a big build-up of CO_2 (this is made during the fermentation process). And make sure they have strong, tightly fitting closures or lids.

Don't

1. Don't use dirty hands, utensils, or jars when preparing or serving from your ferments. And as tempting as it might be, never double-dip. If you do wish to sterilize your jars and tools, you can. Just be sure you follow the sterilization instructions.

2. Don't use jars with poorly fitting lids—the lacto-fermentation process is anaerobic, meaning it works best when there is an absence of or minimal oxygen inside the jar. So do invest in some good-quality glassware with nice, firmly closing lids.

3. Don't forget to "burp" or vent your ferments to release a build-up of carbon dioxide, which is produced as part of the fermentation process. Alternatively, you can make your life easier by buying self-regulating valves.

4. Don't use metal when fermenting, particularly if you aren't sure what type of metal you are working with. Stainless steel is fine, but other metals are not. So just get into the habit of using glass, ceramic, and plastic tools/utensils.

5. Never pour off the brine, particularly when your ferment is in its active phase (this will mean it's quite bubbly). If you avoid overfilling your jars, you should avoid leaks or overflow, but if a jar does start to overflow while you are fermenting, put it on a plate or in a bowl.

Now that we've established these general rules for success, you're ready to begin. In my experience, it takes a little time to gain your confidence. Once you do, you are going to be so glad that you've discovered this new, delicious hobby that also happens to be great for your gut!

Equipment

- Digital scale (capacity > 1 kilogram)
- Measuring spoons
- Large mixing bowl (ceramic, glass, or plastic)
- Knife and chopping board
- Wooden spoon/rolling pin
- Fermentation weights (alternatively, you can use a glass/ceramic ramekin or the cabbage cores)
- Fermentation airlocks (optional)
- 1 litre/2 litre/3 litre glass fermentation jars
- Swing-top pouring bottles
- Cast-iron enamelled casserole dish with lid (for sourdough)
- Sourdough banneton
- Bench knife
- Bread lame

Why Are the Fermentation Recipes in Grams and Why Do They Require a Kitchen Scale?

Kitchen chemistry requires precision for optimal results and safety. We are combining ingredients in specific proportions to elicit a chemical reaction, with the desired result being an explosion of flavour in your mouth. The problem with using volume-based measurements like tablespoons and cups is that the weight within the volume may vary depending on the ingredient you are using. For example, 1 teaspoon of salt may weigh very different amounts depending on whether it is coarse, fine, unrefined, etc. But 20 grams of salt is 20 grams of salt, no matter what type you purchase. Same goes for all the varieties of flour.

Let's Get This Sourdough Party Started!

In modern bread baking practices, you add baker's yeast to leaven bread, and though it may seem like just another ingredient, in reality it's a living organism called *Saccharomyces cerevisiae*. In ancient times, we didn't have packets of baker's yeast, but we did have microbes. They've always been there in and on our food, long before we crazy humans showed up. And eventually we had flour. Flour has microbes because everything has microbes unless you're intentionally sterilizing it. If you add water to the flour and keep it warm, those microbes will multiply. They'll feed on the carbohydrates in the flour. They'll release carbon dioxide gas and lactic acid. If you lean into this process and allow it to play out, you will eventually have bread—not just any bread, but bread with a slightly sour tang due to the lactic acid that the microbes contribute. Hence the term "sourdough."

The first evidence of bread making dates back 14,400 years ago to Jordan. But sourdough bread has its place throughout history. French bakers brought sourdough to Northern California during the 1849 gold rush, and it became the preferred food of gold prospectors. One of the bakeries opened in 1849 was the Boudin Bakery, and its legacy lives on. You can enjoy sourdough bread at the Boudin Bakery down by Fisherman's Wharf that is made with the same mother dough from the original 1849 bakery. There's even a specific bacteria found in San Francisco sourdough starters called *Fructilacto-bacillus sanfranciscensis*. Yes, a sourdough starter can live in perpetuity. The Boudin mother dough is the oldest dough in the United States.

Why do I love sourdough? Gosh, there's so much to love. I love the smell, the tangy flavour, the soft chewy centre, and the crispy, flaky crust. From a culinary perspective, it's my top choice among breads. There are also the health benefits of prolonged fermentation. Fermenting your bread increases the digestibility and availability of nutrients like magnesium while reducing the amount of gluten, phytic acid, trypsin inhibitors, and FODMAPs. The microbes transform insoluble fibre into soluble fibre and simultaneously create exopolysaccharides, both of which are prebiotics with added health benefits. They create bioactive peptides such as ACE inhibitory enzymes, which many people take to lower their blood pressure but which you can find naturally occurring in sourdough bread. They also increase the presence of antioxidants in the bread. And then there's the artisanal quality. This kind of bread baking takes time and requires an investment of effort and your attention. It helps you feel more connected to your food.

When you make a sourdough starter, you are creating a microbial ecosystem from water and flour. The microbes within that ecosystem are influenced by simple elements that you control: flour, water, and temperature. But let's face it, the bacteria create all the magic. Have fun with it. Find joy in creation, transformation, and the intelligence of nature. Making sourdough is a marriage of science and art that results in delicious food, but it's also the journey that makes it special.

Controlling the Elements within Your Sourdough Starter Ecosystem

The results of your sourdough will vary based upon the balance among three key elements: flour, water, and temperature. Let's explore each of these elements in more detail.

FLOUR

You have many options in choosing your flour. It should always be unbleached and unbromated and preferably organic, but in any event, the fewer chemicals and additives, the better. But you don't have to stick to just one flour throughout the process of creating your starter. Just bear in mind that whatever flour you feed your starter with will form a part of your bread. The reason to gravitate towards wholegrain varieties like wholewheat and rye is that they are less processed and therefore higher in fibre, micronutrients, and natural microbes and enzymes. This leads to healthier bread for humans. Here are a few options to choose from:

Plain Flour

Most readily available at your local store, but also the most processed. It is refined to remove the germ and bran of the wheat, reducing the fibre, protein, and micronutrient content.

Bread Flour

This flour is selected specifically for baking bread and rises higher than plain flour because it has more protein (gluten). Both white and wholewheat options are available.

Wholewheat Flour

Less processed, it contains the whole grain—bran, endosperm, and germ. It also has more microbes to jump-start fermentation, although the bran absorbs a lot of water and can impair the rise somewhat.

Wholewheat flour tends to result in a denser bread, but it has the advantage of having more fibre and micronutrients to feed both the starter and your gut microbes. The texture can be improved by using a combination of white and wholegrain flours, increasing the hydration, and letting the dough have a slightly longer fermentation period.

Heirloom Wholewheat Varieties

Modern wheat has been selectively bred by humans to have specific characteristics. Meanwhile, heritage wheat has remained largely unchanged through the years, making it appealing to those interested in consuming the ancient grains. Emmer wheat, known as "Pharaoh's wheat" for its history in Egypt, is high in fibre and great for baking. Spelt wheat is challenging to bake with but it's doable. Einkorn wheat doesn't make good bread and is better as a porridge.

Rye Flour

A very popular choice for starters! Rye flour is thought to create the most microbially diverse starters due to microbial density. You tend to see faster results with wholewheat and rye starters simply because they are less refined and therefore more microbe- and enzyme-rich. Rye is lower in protein (gluten) and holds more water than other grains.

Blended Flour

You can combine any of the above in different proportions based on your preferences and the availability of flour.

WATER

We want water that we use for fermentation to be free of chlorine and ideally also free of chloramines and fluoride so that they don't alter the balance of gut microbes that we need to make the fermentation process work. Distilled or bottled water from the shops accomplishes this, as does a home reverse osmosis filter. A charcoal filter or boiling the water and letting it cool will remove the chlorine.

TEMPERATURE

Temperature is also key when you are creating a thriving colony of microbes via your starter. When you are creating your starter and actively feeding/growing it, keep it somewhere warm. Warmth, but not too much, stimulates the process. Using warm or cold water can also speed up (in the case of warm water) or slow down (in the case of cold water) the rate of fermentation. Ideal temperature for sourdough is 23.8 to 26.6°C and for most other fermentation is 21.1 to 23.8°C. If the temperature is too cool, consider putting the starter on a baking tray inside the oven with the light on for a few hours (but not overnight, which may be too warm).

Fermentation Recipes

SOURDOUGH STARTER

780 g flour   Chlorine-free water

1. **Day 1:** In a small bowl or jar with tall sides, mix 60 g of any type of flour (or a 50/50 mix) along with 60 g room-temperature water. Stir well. Stirring helps to disrupt microbial activity and aerate the mixture, which both contribute to rapid yeast growth. The consistency should be thick and pasty. You can add a bit more water if needed to thin out the texture. Cover with a piece of muslin or paper towel and set in a warm space (ideally between 23.8 and 26.6°C).

2. **Day 2:** Leave your starter alone and let it rest. You may see bubbles, which are signs of microbial activity.

3. **Day 3:** Using a wooden spoon, remove and discard about half of your starter from your jar. Add in 60 g flour and 60 g tepid water in a 1:1 ratio, then mix it until smooth. The texture should resemble thick pancake batter. Cover the jar and leave it until the next feed the following day.

See page 321 for ideas on what you can do with discarded starter—Cheese-Its and Sourdough Pancakes, anyone?

4. **Day 4 and onward:** Repeat the same process as outlined on Day 3. As the yeast begins to develop, your starter will rise and bubbles will form throughout the culture. When the starter falls, it's time to feed it again. You can experiment with feeding once or twice per day; either can work. To easily measure growth, place a rubber band around the jar to gauge how much it grows after a feed.

5. When is your starter ready? When it's at its peak ripeness, it will be bubbly and double in size by 8 hours after feeding. It will smell yeasty and appear stringlike or weblike. You will also hear bubbles popping when you stir. At this point, it's ready to be used. Transfer it to a clean jar and give it a name. The entire process can take from 6 to 14 days, depending on the type of flour used and the temperature in your home. If you still don't have bubbles after 3 or 4 days, find a warmer spot.

What's That Brown Liquid on Top of My Starter?

This liquid is called "hooch" and is an indication that your starter needs to be fed. Simply pour the liquid off before feeding your starter.

Sourdough Starter Maintenance

Once your starter is bubbly, at some point each day, discard half of the mixture and add in 30 grams each of water and flour in a 1:1 ratio. Alternatively, if you keep your starter in the refrigerator, then you should feed it once per week. When active, the starter should double in size by 8 hours after feeding. If your starter hasn't been fed consistently, you may need to do this process every day for 2 to 4 days before it's ready to bake with. Remember, any discard can be repurposed using the recipes on pages 321-25.

Sourdough Starter FAQs

When is my starter ready?

Visually, the starter will have bubbles on the surface and throughout the entire culture. Try this test. Remove a scant teaspoon of starter and place it in a jar or small bowl of water. If it floats, it's ready to bake! If it sinks, then discard half of the starter and feed it again with 30 g each of water and flour and repeat this process each day until ready.

Can I stop feeding my starter?

The more frequently your starter is used, and therefore fed, the more vigorous it will be. You can start and stop the starter by covering and placing it in the fridge. A few days before you plan to use it, move it to a warm location and feed it again until bubbly and ready to use.

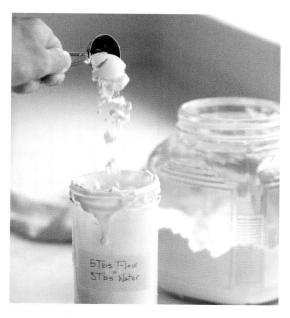
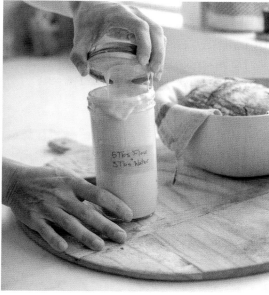

What happens if my starter goes bad in the fridge?

If you stop feeding your starter for a long period of time, it will become very acidic and putrid. If you notice any mould growing on it, then discard and start again. To revive an old, mould-free starter, pour off any of the often brown liquid (called hooch) and discard the entire top half of the starter.

Remove a few teaspoons of the starter from the bottom of the jar and place it in a new jar. Add in 60 g of flour and 60 g of water and stir well. Adding fresh flour and water will dilute any off-flavour and help to feed and awaken the dormant starter. Repeat this process daily, as you did in creating the original starter, until it is bubbly, doubles in size by 8 hours after feeding, smells yeasty, and appears stringlike or weblike.

What's the ideal feeding and baking schedule?

If you want to time your fed starter to use it in the Wholewheatish Sourdough Bread recipe (opposite), this is the schedule that we find works best:

8 a.m.: Discard half of the starter and feed. It should double in size and become active in 8 hours.

1:30 p.m.: Mix the bread dough and let rest for 1 hour.

3 p.m.: Stretch the dough and fold for the first time.

3:30 p.m.: Stretch the dough and fold for the second time.

4 p.m.: Stretch the dough and fold for the third time.

4:30 p.m.: Stretch the dough and fold for the fourth time.

5 p.m.: Let the dough rise (bulk rise) for 2 to 3 hours at 23.8 to 26.6°C.

8 p.m.: Cover and place in the fridge overnight.

The following morning, bring the dough back up to room temperature. Shape and bake the dough.

My house is very cold and draughty. How do I proof dough?

If you don't have a warm spot in your home, turn the oven on to the lowest setting for 2 minutes, then turn it off and place your bowl inside. You can also turn on the oven light and set your dough inside to proof. Dough that is too warm will become wet, sticky, and harder to work with.

WHOLEWHEATISH SOURDOUGH BREAD

1 Plant Point

Using 100% wholewheat flour produces a very tough sourdough. This recipe uses both traditional bread flour and 100% wholewheat flour. Bread flour contains more gluten than plain flour and, for best results, shouldn't be substituted with another flour.

50 g active sourdough starter

350 g warm water (about 29.4°C)

400 g bread flour, plus extra for dusting

100 g wholewheat flour

7 g fine sea salt

1. Place the sourdough starter and water in a large bowl and mix together.

2. Add in the flours and use your hand to mix and squeeze the dough in circular motions until no dry lumps remain. Cover and let rest for 20 minutes; this allows the flour to fully hydrate before proofing. Sprinkle the salt evenly over the surface, then mix well to combine. At this point, check on your dough. It should be fairly shaggy; if it's hard to mix and difficult to work inside the bowl, then add in more water in 20 g increments, thoroughly mixing until the dough feels supple and somewhat sticky. With wholegrain flour, there's the potential to need more water to achieve this consistency.

3. Cover with a damp tea towel and let rest for 1 hour in a warm place.

4. Do your first set of stretches and folds. Wet your hands so they don't stick, then gather a portion of the dough from the bowl and stretch it upwards and away from you, then fold it towards the centre of the bowl. Turn the bowl a quarter turn and do this again,

DR. B'S TIPS FOR SUCCESS:

YouTube has wonderful tutorials for the bread-shaping techniques if you are a visual learner.

You'll need a vessel with a tight-fitting lid to trap the steam; this is what produces the rise of the bread while baking. A cast-iron enamelled casserole with lid or cloche baker works best.

Sourdough is an art! If you don't succeed the first time, don't give up. You'll get better and better with your loaves the more you make!

Don't throw away your sourdough discard as you make your starter! Use it in the recipes on pages 321-25.

RECIPE CONTINUES

stretching and folding the dough towards the centre. Turn the bowl another quarter turn and repeat, then repeat again, performing four total stretches and folds around the entire bowl.

5. Let the dough rest for 30 minutes, then repeat another set of stretches and folds. Repeat this two more times for a total of four stretch-and-fold sessions.

6. After your last set of stretches and folds, cover the bowl and continue to let it bulk rise in a warm spot for 2 to 3 hours. It's ready when it's increased by at least a third of its size. At this point, cover the dough and place in the fridge overnight for baking the next morning.

7. In the morning, remove the dough from the fridge and place on a lightly floured surface. Let rest for 30 minutes to remove some of the chill from the fridge, then shape into a loose ball: Starting at the top of the dough, stretch and fold it towards the centre. Do the same with the bottom of the dough, then the left side of the dough and then the right like you are folding up an envelope.

8. Using a bench knife or a flat spatula, scoop the dough and flip it over so the smooth side is facing up. Cover and rest for another 30 minutes.

9. Prepare a banneton proofing basket sprinkled with flour. Alternatively, line a medium bowl with cotton or linen cloth, then sprinkle with flour. Set aside. Shape the dough again using the same envelope technique as described above. Flip it over,

then use your hands to gently cup the dough and pull it towards you in a circular shape. This will help to create tension in the dough and produce a rounded shape. Using the bench knife or spatula from before, scoop up the dough and place it in the prepared bowl with the smooth side facing up. Cover and rest again for 30 minutes to 1 hour. The dough is ready when it looks puffy and feels like an inflated water balloon when gently poked with your finger.

10. Towards the end of the final rise, preheat the oven to 230°C. Cut a sheet of parchment paper to fit the size of the casserole or other baking vessel (see Tips for Success), leaving enough space around the sides to easily remove the bread.

11. Place the parchment paper over the dough and invert the bowl to release. Sprinkle the dough with flour and gently rub into the bread with your hands. Using a bread lame, razor, or very sharp paring knife, make a few shallow cuts in the dough to allow for expansion. You can get as creative as you want here. For ease, make four shallow cuts at 12 o'clock, 3 o'clock, 6 o'clock, and 9 o'clock. Use the parchment paper overhang to transfer the dough to the baking pot.

12. Cover with a tight-fitting lid and place on a baking tray, then transfer to the preheated oven for 20 minutes. Remove the lid and continue to bake for 40 minutes, until golden brown on top.

13. Remove from the oven and let cool for at least 1 hour. The bread needs time to rest before slicing.

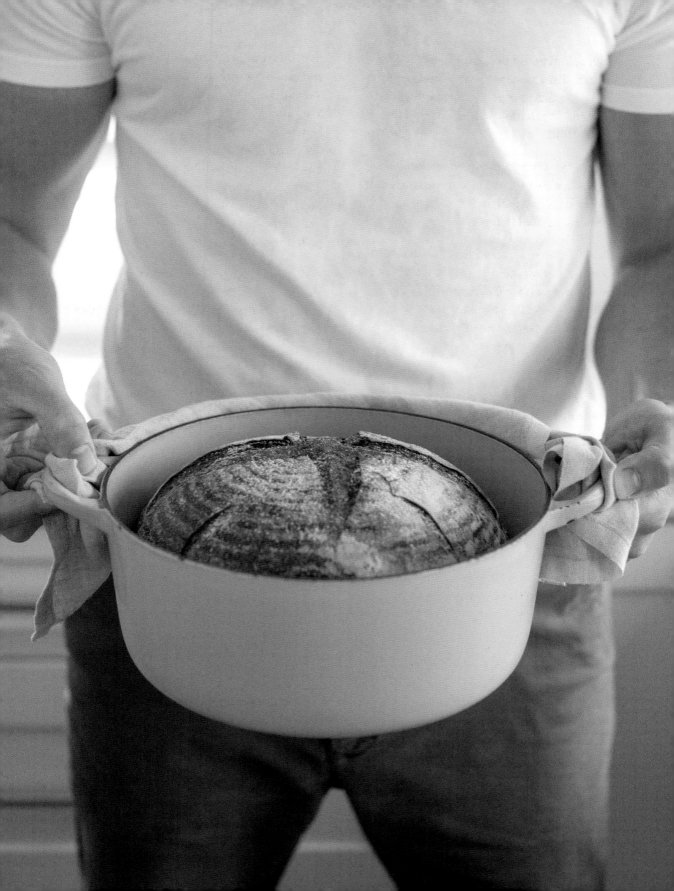

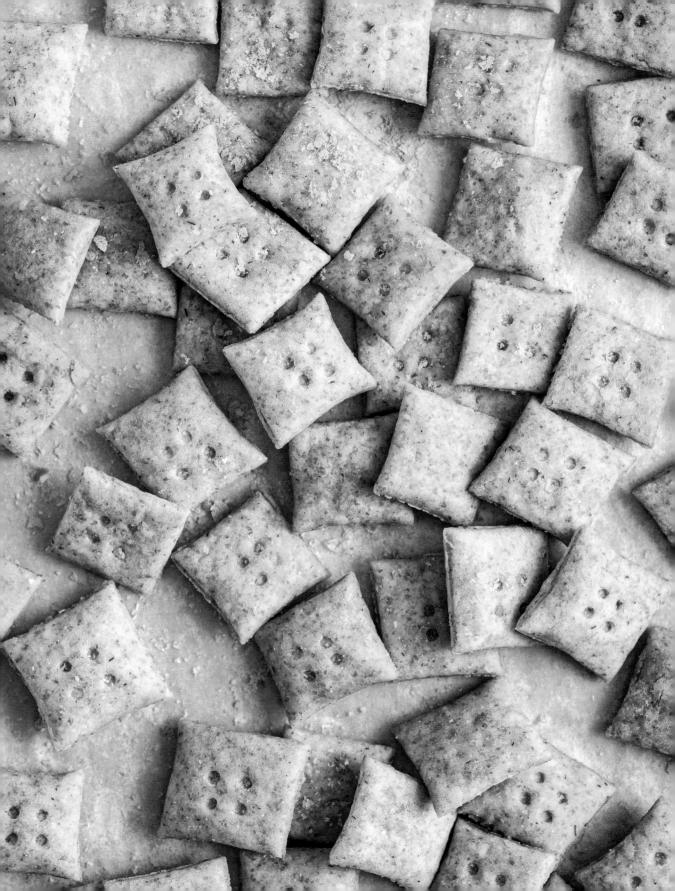

SOURDOUGH CHEESE-ITS

1 Plant Point

Makes 100 biscuits

In this recipe, we are repurposing the sourdough starter that you would otherwise discard and turning it into a fun snack.

150 g plain or white wholewheat flour

200 g sourdough starter discard (see page 314)

3 tablespoons olive oil

¾ teaspoon salt

3 tablespoons nutritional yeast

½ teaspoon garlic powder

1. In a large bowl, mix together the flour, sourdough starter, olive oil, salt, nutritional yeast, and garlic powder to create a smooth, not sticky, dough.

2. Divide the dough in half, then shape each section into a small rectangular slab. Cover with cling film, then place in the fridge for at least 30 minutes to help firm up the dough.

3. Preheat the oven to 160°C. Remove the dough from the fridge, then very lightly flour a piece of parchment paper, a rolling pin, and the top of the dough.

4. Place the dough on the parchment paper and roll until it is about 4 mm thick, about the same thickness as a pound coin. Transfer the parchment paper with the dough onto a baking tray, then lightly brush with more olive oil and sprinkle more salt on top.

5. Cut the dough into squares, then prick each square with the tines of a fork. Bake the biscuits for 17 to 20 minutes, until the squares are starting to brown around the edges. Midway through, rotate the baking tray from front to back to help the biscuits brown evenly.

6. Remove from the oven and let cool completely.

PRO TIP:

You need the olive oil here to keep the biscuits light and crispy. Using 100% wholewheat flour creates dense biscuits; use plain or white wholewheat for best results.

Store in an airtight container at room temperature for up to 1 week, or freeze for longer storage.

SOURDOUGH PANCAKES

2+ Plant Points

Makes 12 pancakes

Sourdough pancakes evolve this beloved breakfast to a higher frequency. Plus, they have a tanginess and fluffiness that you'll fall in love with. Add some fresh fruit on top for bonus Plant Points. Using wholewheat pastry flour will make lighter pancakes, while 100% wholewheat flour pancakes will have a denser texture. Note: You'll want to prepare this batter the night before to enjoy these pancakes in the morning.

240 ml almond milk or other non-dairy milk

1 teaspoon white or apple cider vinegar

100 g sourdough starter discard (see page 314)

150 g wholewheat pastry flour or white wholewheat flour

1 tablespoon 100% maple syrup (optional)

½ teaspoon salt

½ teaspoon bicarbonate of soda

1 tablespoon milled flaxseed mixed with 3 tablespoons water

½ teaspoon vanilla extract

1. In a large glass, mix the almond milk and vinegar together for 5 to 10 minutes, to slightly curdle.

2. In a large bowl, mix together the almond milk mixture with the sourdough starter, flour, and maple syrup, if using. Cover and place overnight in a warm place. In the winter, you can keep it in an unheated oven with the oven light turned on.

3. In the morning, uncover the batter and mix in the salt, bicarbonate of soda, flax mixture, and vanilla.

4. Heat a griddle or non-stick frying pan over medium heat. Pour the batter on the griddle, using 60 ml batter for each pancake. Cook until bubbles appear in the centre of the pancake, then flip and cook until the other side is set. Continue with the rest of the batter.

5. To keep the pancakes warm, place on a baking tray in a warm oven.

PRO TIP:

You can easily convert this recipe to make sourdough waffles! Simply increase the apple cider vinegar or white vinegar to 1 tablespoon. For extra crispy waffles, add a little olive oil or avocado oil.

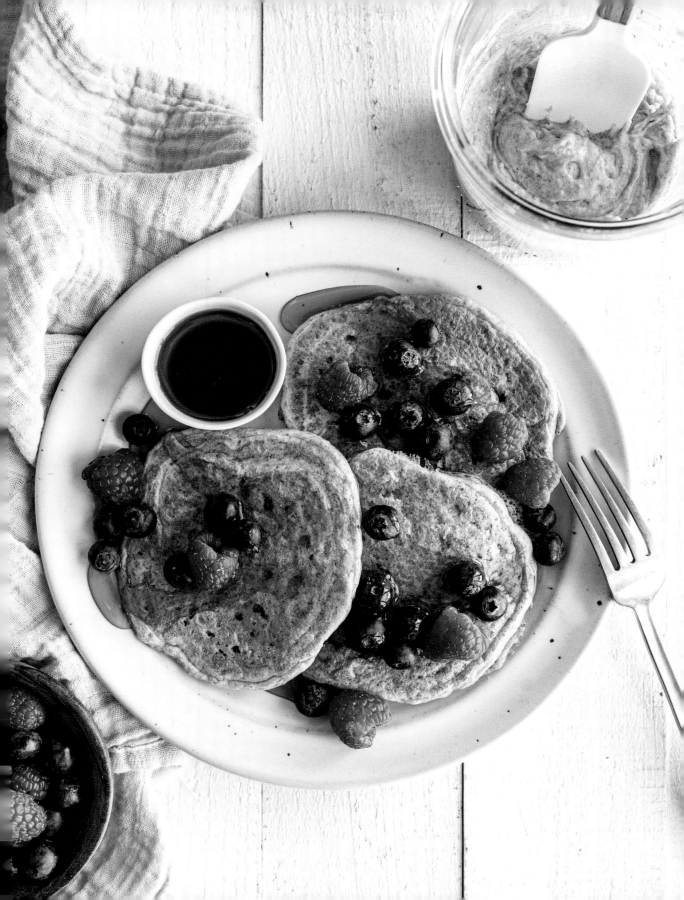

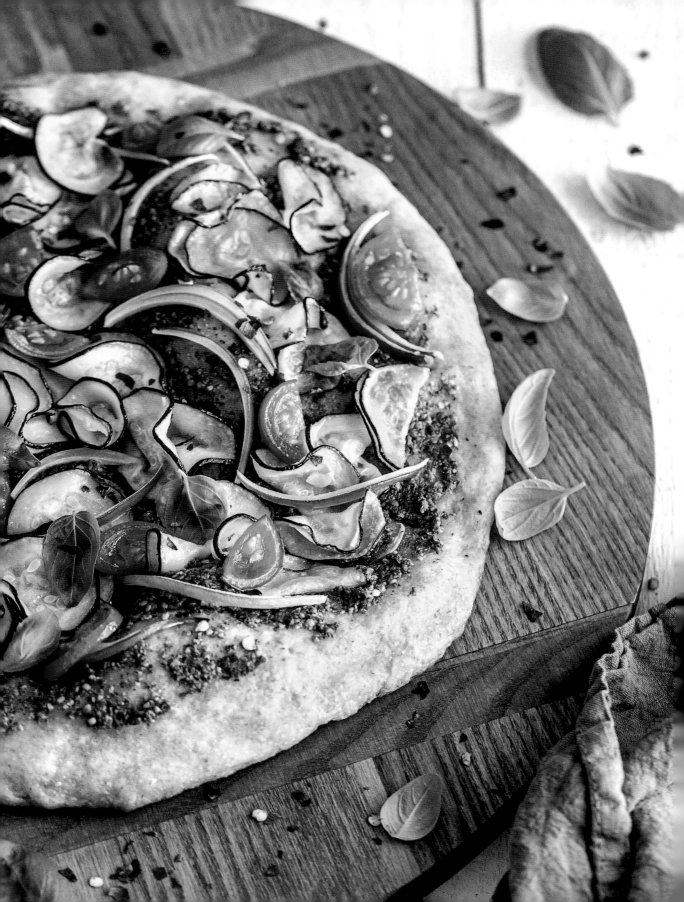

SOURDOUGH PIZZA CRUST

1 Plant Point

Makes 1 large pizza crust

Everyone loves pizza, but you will love it even more with a homemade sourdough pizza crust that you know has high-quality ingredients. This recipe is ideal to combine with Tuscan Flatbread (page 281).

50 g sourdough starter discard (see page 314)

40 g wholewheat flour

265 g plain flour

1 teaspoon coarse or fine sea salt

1 tablespoon olive oil

1. In a large bowl, place the sourdough starter, wholewheat and plain flours, salt, olive oil, and 180 ml water. Use your hands to mix until fully incorporated. It will be shaggy, though if the mixture is too wet, add a little more flour. If too dry, then add in a teaspoon or two of water at a time. Cover the bowl and place in a warm location to ferment for 10 to 12 hours or overnight.

2. When the batter has fermented, or the next morning, perform a series of stretches and folds. Lightly wet your hands to prevent the dough from sticking, then gently pull one side of the dough up and over itself, then turn the bowl and repeat with all four "corners" of the dough until you've completed the circle. At this point the dough is ready to bake, or you can place it in the fridge for up to 36 hours.

3. Remove the dough and place on a lightly floured surface and let rest for 30 minutes.

4. Using lightly floured hands, shape the dough into a ball. From here, shape into pizza crust (I prefer using a rolling pin) and use in your favourite recipe.

SIMPLIFIED DOSA CREPES

3 Plant Points

Makes 12 dosas

We've simplified traditional dosas—a fermented rice and lentil crepe with South Indian origin. The fermented dough has a tangy, sourdough-like taste that's delicious on its own, with a curried potato filling, or with your favourite Indian-inspired side dishes.

You may need to grab most ingredients from an international or Asian food shop, or buy them online. Enjoy them with Potato Dosa Filling (page 329) for a delicious meal!

330 g short-grain white rice

70 g skinned/split black urad dal (whole lentils)

2 tablespoons chana dal (optional), for a crispier dosa

½ teaspoon whole fenugreek seeds

½ teaspoon coarse or fine sea salt (iodine-free)

Avocado oil, for oiling the pan

1. In a fine-mesh strainer or large bowl, rinse the rice, urad dal, and chana dal, if using, then drain. Place in a large bowl along with the fenugreek seeds and cover the mixture with enough water to cover by at least 5 cm. Soak overnight.

2. The next morning, drain the water from the rice and dal mixture, then add to the base of a high-speed blender or food processor along with 300 ml cold water. Process until a smooth batter forms. Depending on the strength of your blender, you may need to add in an additional 60 ml or more water to get the desired consistency. The mixture should thinly coat the back of a spoon. Add the salt and cover the bowl, then place in a warm spot for 12 to 24 hours for bulk fermentation. In colder months, this will take closer to 24 hours, and in warmer months, the mixture may be ready in as little as 8 hours. The batter is ready when it has almost doubled in size, coats a spoon thickly when dipped, and has air bubbles throughout.

RECIPE CONTINUES

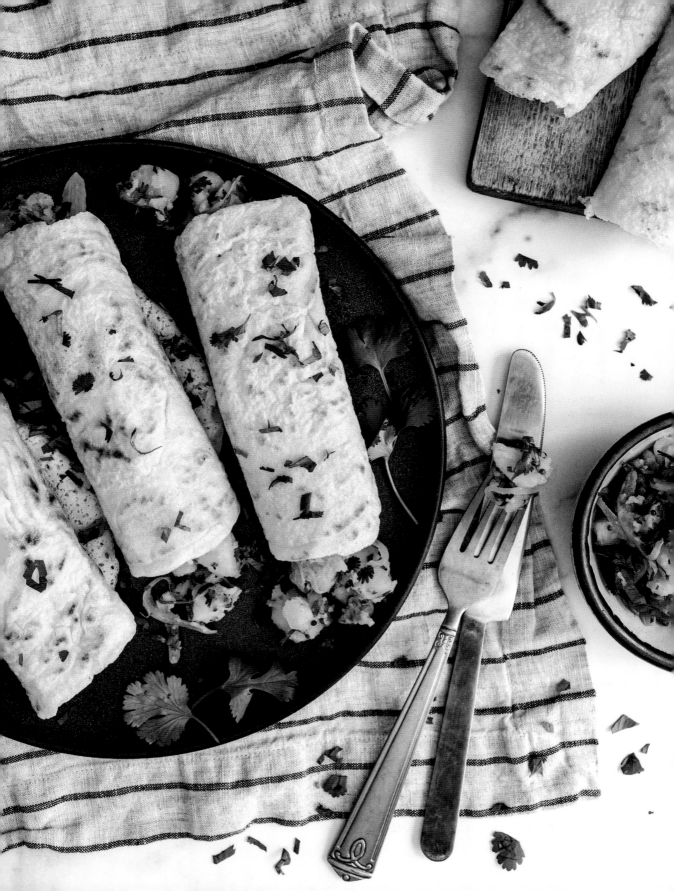

3. Now it's time to make the dosas! Heat a cast-iron frying pan or other flat frying pan over medium-low heat. If using a non-stick frying pan, you likely don't need to add additional oil. Lightly oil the pan with oil; I use a pastry brush dipped in oil to create a very thin coat. Too much oil on the pan and you won't be able to spread the batter. Ladle about 80 ml batter and swirl on the pan using the back of a ladle in a circular motion. It's normal if the batter develops small holes as you spread it. Raise the heat to medium, cover, and cook until the edges start to brown, then flip and cook an additional minute. Repeat with the rest of the batter.

DR. B'S TIPS FOR SUCCESS:

To get crispy dosas, you need the pan to be hot. However, because the batter is thick, if the pan is too hot, then you won't be able to spread the batter evenly and you will get fluffy dosas instead of crisp crepes. If your pan gets too hot, sprinkle ice water on the pan, then wipe it to quickly bring down the temperature. I use a well-seasoned cast-iron pan to make dosas. If you use a non-stick pan, then as soon as one dosa is done, reduce the heat to medium-low, then spread the batter on the pan and raise the heat and let the dosa cook.

For faster proofing, you can use an Instant Pot on the yoghurt setting for 8 to 12 hours or place the covered bowl in an oven with the light on.

I recommend using a blender over a food processor to grind the batter. You don't want to add more water than needed, and a high-speed blender will produce smoother results than a food processor.

Any leftover batter can be tightly covered and refrigerated for up to 3 days. If you place the dosa batter in the fridge after fermenting, then let it stand at room temperature for 30 minutes before cooking.

These are best straight from the pan. To store already-made dosas, stack and place the dosas in a lidded dish to keep warm. They will lose their crispness as they sit but will still taste delicious.

POTATO DOSA FILLING

5 Plant Points

Makes enough
for 12 dosas

The dosas were never meant to be a stand-alone meal. But when you combine them with this filling, you will experience the full glory that comes from teaming up with the microbes to create this delicious pairing.

1½ teaspoons avocado or olive oil

½ teaspoon mustard seeds

150 g thinly sliced white onions

1 teaspoon finely chopped fresh ginger

1 green chilli, seeded and finely chopped (keep seeds in for spicier filling)

¼ teaspoon ground turmeric

¼ teaspoon yellow curry powder

400 g boiled and roughly chopped potatoes

Salt and freshly ground black pepper

10 g finely chopped coriander

1. In a medium saucepan over medium heat, heat the avocado oil. Add the mustard seeds and allow them to bloom and sputter, about 1 minute, then add in the onions and cook for about 10 minutes, until soft and translucent, stirring often.

2. Add the ginger and green chilli and cook for another 5 minutes, then add the turmeric and curry powder. Add 60 ml water and allow the mixture to thicken, then add the potatoes and a pinch of salt. Simmer for 5 minutes, stirring occasionally, until the mixture is thick and reduced.

3. Season to taste, adding in more salt and pepper as needed. When ready to serve, remove from heat and stir in the coriander.

PINK SAUERKRAUT

2+ Plant Points

Makes 1 litre

This recipe is for a gorgeously vibrant pink sauerkraut. It is pink due to the mix of red and green cabbage, which when it ferments undergoes a pretty spectacular colour transformation from a deep indigo to fuchsia pink. Sauerkraut can be enjoyed several ways: as a garnish, on a salad or a sandwich, or in a soup. It is easy to make and can be stored in your refrigerator and enjoyed for several months. Once you get the hang of it, feel free to experiment with different spices and flavours. A few vegetable and spice combinations to consider are listed below! Use whatever vegetable combination you like alongside your cabbage. Just make sure that you maintain the proportion of 1 kg of vegetables to 20 g of salt to achieve the desired 2 per cent salt concentration.

1 red cabbage

1 green cabbage

5 to 7 garlic cloves

20 g pure salt
(no iodine)

1 tablespoon cumin
seeds (optional)

1 teaspoon chilli flakes
(optional)

**Supercharge It!
(optional toppings):**

Carrot

Ginger

Beetroot

Apple

Caraway seeds

Celery + onion

Turmeric + black
mustard seeds

Apple + onion

Dried fruits
(e.g. juniper berries,
cranberries, or raisins)

Turnip

Horseradish

1. Remove and save 1 or 2 outer cabbage leaves. Cut the cabbages in half through the centre to reveal the core. Make a triangular cut on either side of the core and remove it. Keep the leaves and core for packing your sauerkraut.

2. Finely shred or grate the cabbage (or any other vegetable you wish to use). Weigh as you shred. You'll need in total 1 kg. This can be 50:50 red and green, or whatever ratio you like.

3. Place the cabbage in a large plastic bowl once chopped. Sprinkle the salt on the cabbage and mix it through. Let the cabbage sit for 10 to 15 minutes. The salt will draw the water out of the cabbage to create the brine.

4. Once the cabbage has rested, use your hands to "massage" and squeeze it for 5 to 10 minutes to release more brine, which will begin to collect in the bottom of the bowl.

5. When you have a little pool of brine in the bottom of your bowl, add the cumin seeds and chilli flakes, if using, and mix.

6. Once mixed, start packing the cabbage into a 1 litre wide-mouth preserving jar (kilner jar is ideal). As you pack, press it down hard using your fists (if they fit into the jar), a rolling pin, or a muddling stick. You want to leave about a 2 cm gap at the top of the jar.

7. Make sure the cabbage is submerged in liquid. Cover the cabbage with a few of the leftover leaves (you may have to tear these to fit).

8. Place a clean weight (a ramekin, fermentation weight, sterilized stone, or the core of the cabbage) on top of the cabbage.

9. Seal the jar and allow the sauerkraut to ferment on the kitchen worktop or in a cool, dry place (ideally 18 to 22°C). Burp the jar daily for the first week by removing the lid briefly (you may need to burp it twice a day, depending on the temperature). Alternatively, you can use a fermentation airlock so that it vents pressure on its own when it builds up.

10. Once it has fermented for a week, open and taste it using a wooden or plastic spoon. Seal it up and transfer it to a cool place to continue to ferment for another 1 to 6 weeks, depending on your personal preference. I find it gets better with age.

11. Once you are happy with the flavour, you can transfer the sauerkraut into smaller jars and store it in the fridge.

CUCUMBER AND SPRING ONION KIMCHI

6 Plant Points

Makes about
3 litres

Packed with antioxidants, and hydrating, there is little more satisfying than crunching into a cucumber. Enter kimchi-style cucumbers—they are crunchy, spicy, and highly addictive. I promise you'll want to eat these straight from the jar! (See photo, page 335.)

600 g cucumbers, chopped into half moons

4 chopped spring onions (white and green parts)

35 g pure salt (no iodine)

5 garlic cloves, roughly chopped

40 g fresh ginger, roughly chopped

1 tablespoon Korean chilli flakes

2 tablespoons gochujang chilli paste

1 tablespoon brown or red miso paste (preferably live miso)

1 teaspoon coconut sugar or 1 date, finely chopped

2 teaspoons raw apple cider vinegar (with the mother)

3 g dried seaweed (I use dried hijiki, but nori would also work) (optional)

1. In a large bowl, add the chopped cucumbers and spring onions and sprinkle with the salt. Let this sit while you make the paste.

2. To make the paste, in the base of a blender, place the garlic, ginger, chilli flakes, chilli paste, miso, sugar, and vinegar and blend into a smooth paste (you can also place the ingredients in a bowl and use an immersion blender).

3. Add the paste to the cucumbers along with the dried seaweed, if using, and mix. Let the mixture stand for 5 minutes, then place in a 1 litre wide-mouth preserving jar, pressing it down to pack it tightly using a wooden spoon or the flat end of a rolling pin. Use a fermentation weight to weigh down the cucumbers. Seal and leave to ferment for 1 to 2 weeks, burping/venting daily to release the build-up of carbon dioxide gas. Alternatively, you can use a fermentation airlock.

4. Refrigerate when ready and eat within 2 months.

GARLICKY DILL PICKLES

2 Plant Points

Makes 2 litres

Lacto-fermented gherkins take 1 to 2 weeks depending on how you like them—super crunchy or softer in the middle. You may want to give them less initial fermentation time if you like them on the crunchy side, as they will soften slightly with age—but they are just as delicious! Adding the bay leaves also helps them to stay crunchier.

650 g pickling cucumbers, whole

10 garlic cloves, whole or sliced

1½ tablespoons yellow mustard seeds

1 teaspoon black peppercorns

6 bay leaves (ideally fresh)

5 or 6 sprigs dill (optional)

45 g Himalayan pink salt

1 litre filtered water

1. Thoroughly wash the cucumbers to remove dirt. Slice the cucumbers if you prefer or leave them whole. Leaving them whole will help keep them firm.

2. Place the cucumbers, garlic, mustard seeds, peppercorns, bay leaves, and dill, if using, into a clean or sterilized 2 litre jar or two 1 litre jars.

3. Make the brine by dissolving the salt in about 200 ml freshly boiled filtered water. Pour the remaining 800 ml cold filtered water into the salt water. Check the temperature using your finger to ensure that the water is about room temperature.

4. Pour the brine over the cucumbers and spices. Fill to just over the shoulder of the jar.

5. Ensure that the cucumbers are submerged in the brine. You can use a cabbage leaf or fermentation weight to keep them submerged.

6. Ferment at room temperature for 1 to 2 weeks. When you are ready to eat these, transfer them to the fridge, where they will keep for 4 to 6 months.

PRO TIP:

The key to making really good pickles is to use the darker green, knobby, thick-skinned pickling cucumbers. If you can't find these, try using baby cucumbers and increase the salt to 50 g for best results.

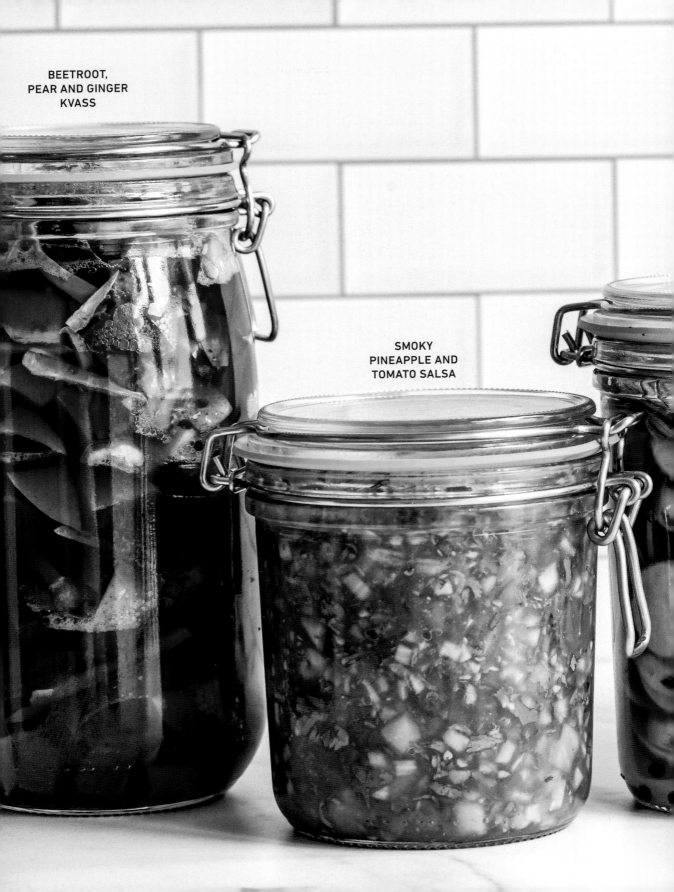

BEETROOT,
PEAR AND GINGER
KVASS

SMOKY
PINEAPPLE AND
TOMATO SALSA

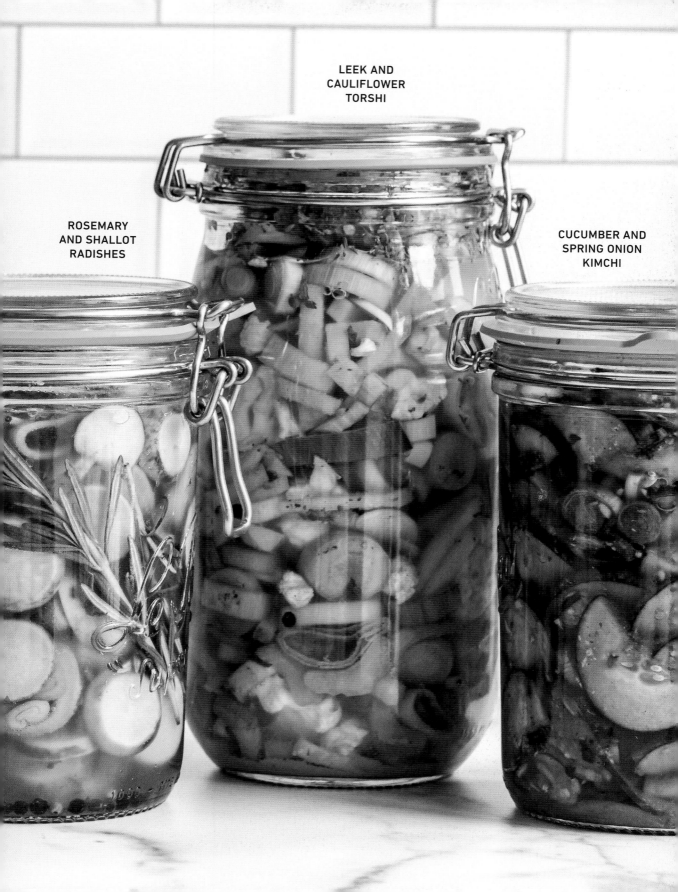

ROSEMARY
AND SHALLOT
RADISHES

LEEK AND
CAULIFLOWER
TORSHI

CUCUMBER AND
SPRING ONION
KIMCHI

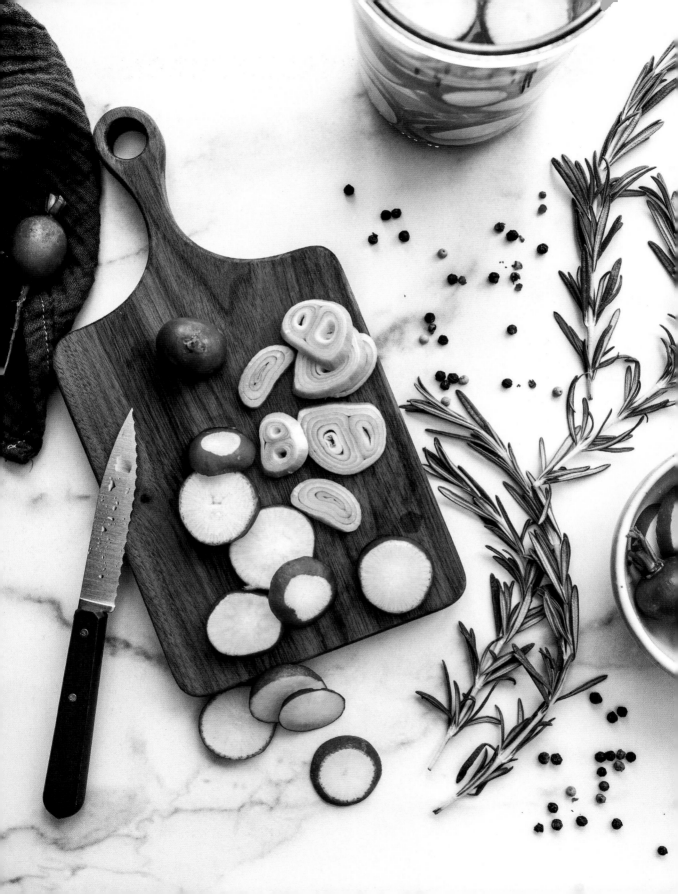

ROSEMARY AND SHALLOT RADISHES

2 Plant Points

Makes 1 litre

I am obsessed with fermented radishes! Even if you don't dig radishes, you have to give these a look. The high fibre content translates into a crunchy ferment. The pepperiness mellows when fermented, but the added black peppercorns ramp it back up. The red coat of the radish gets shed and the white heart turns a shade of pink. The end result is a fermented treat. Adding in rosemary contributes anti-inflammatory and antifungal benefits. Enjoy the crisp punchiness of these radishes on a sandwich, in a salad, as a little snack, or as a flavour-packed garnish. (See photo, page 335.)

400 g radishes, sliced

1 shallot, sliced into rounds

4 sprigs rosemary

10 to 15 peppercorns (whole)

500 ml 3% brine (15 g salt plus 500 ml water)

1. Add all of the ingredients to a 1 litre wide-mouth preserving jar.

2. Make the brine by dissolving the salt in just enough boiled water, then topping up with cool water to the full amount.

3. Pour the cooled brine over the mixture in the jar and top with a fermentation weight.

4. Seal the jar and set it on the kitchen worktop to ferment for 1 to 2 weeks. The ferment will become bubbly and slightly cloudy, but when the fizziness settles and the brine is clear, it's ready to eat.

5. Store the finished ferment in the fridge, where it will stay crunchy and delicious for about 2 months.

PRO TIP:

You can use the brine to flavour other dishes like hummus or a pesto, or use as a salad dressing. Not only is it delicious, but once fermented, it's also probiotic-rich.

LEEK AND CAULIFLOWER TORSHI

7 Plant Points

Makes 3 litres

This recipe is inspired by traditional torshi, a popular Persian, Middle Eastern, Turkish, and Balkan ferment. Torshi is eaten with most meals, and this version adds a few extra prebiotic twists—leeks and apples. As well as being fibre-rich, this ferment is packed with a host of micronutrients, including vitamins C, A, K, B_6, B_9, copper, and iron—just to name a few.

1 medium cauliflower, broken into florets (be sure to save any leaves)

1 large leek, sliced into rounds

2 medium carrots, cut into rounds

1 apple, sliced into matchsticks

2 celery sticks, sliced

6 garlic cloves, sliced

1 chilli (I use red), sliced

2 teaspoons dried parsley

1 teaspoon dried mint

2 teaspoons dried oregano

1 tablespoon coriander seeds

2 teaspoons ground turmeric

10 black peppercorns

1.25 litres 2.5% brine (31 g pure salt + 1.25 litres filtered water)

1. Add the cauliflower, leek, carrots, apple, celery, garlic, and chilli to a large mixing bowl along with the parsley, mint, oregano, coriander, turmeric, and peppercorns. Mix to combine.

2. Add the mixture into three 1 litre preserving jars, pressing down as you go.

3. Next, make the brine by dissolving the salt in just enough boiled water, then topping up to the full amount with cold water.

4. Pour the brine over the mixture and weigh it down with leftover cauliflower leaves or a fermentation weight.

5. Seal the jar(s) and ferment for 10 days to 2 weeks. Burp/vent the jars occasionally to check the progress and release the built-up CO_2. Alternatively, you can use a fermentation airlock to release the pressure that builds up.

6. When your torshi is ready, transfer into smaller jars and store in the fridge. This should keep for 4 to 6 months.

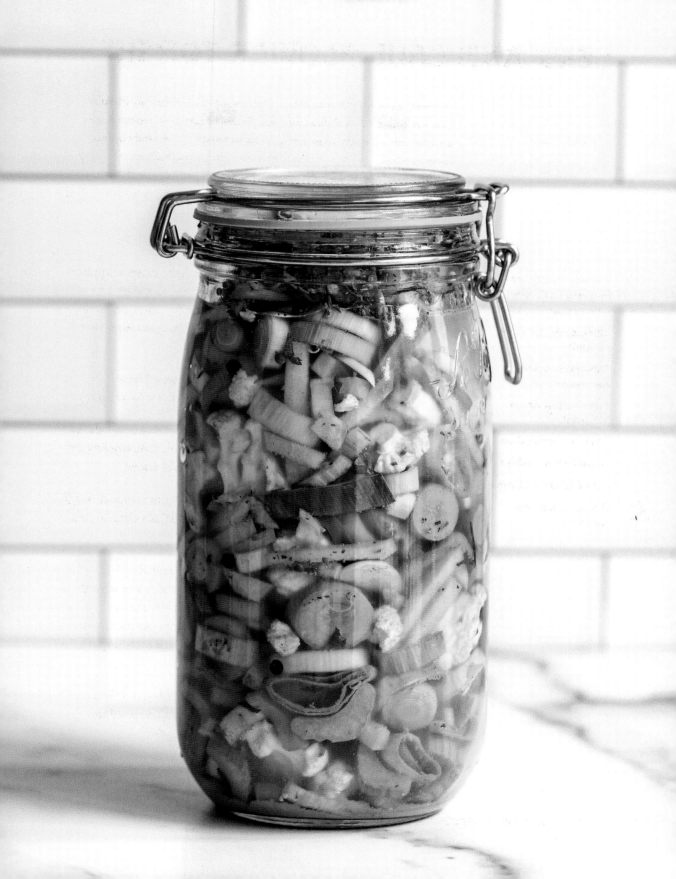

FERMENTED VEG STICKS

2 Plant Points

Makes two litre jars

These aren't just veg sticks, but supercharged, probiotic ones. This recipe is great for using up a glut of carrots or that never-ending bunch of celery. These make great additions to snack boards and work as a treat in packed lunches. So whether you're taking these to a picnic to share or snacking on your own at home, these are sure to become a fermented staple.

400 g carrots unpeeled, cut into batons

2 cardamom pods, cracked

400 g celery, cut into batons

1 teaspoon cumin seeds

1 litre 2% salt brine (20 g pure salt + 1 litre filtered water)

1. Put the carrot sticks and cardamom in one jar and the celery and cumin seeds in another. Be sure to pack them in tightly, side by side, as this will help them stay under the brine while fermenting.

2. Next, make your brine solution by dissolving the salt in just enough boiling water and top up to 1 litre with cold filtered water.

3. Pour the cooled brine over the vegetables and use a fermentation weight to keep them submerged. Seal the jar(s).

4. Allow the veggies to ferment for 10 to 14 days. The brine will go cloudy and fizzy as the veg ferments, but don't worry— this will clear up.

5. Once the carrots and celery are ready to eat, store them in the fridge and consume within about 4 to 6 months. They will keep for longer if left unopened.

SMOKY PINEAPPLE AND TOMATO SALSA

8 Plant Points

Makes 1 litre

A delicious, fresh, and zingy salsa that pairs well with just about everything—from tacos to tofu scrambles! Use a mixture of colours and shapes of tomatoes to make it more flavourful and eye-catching! If you grow your own tomatoes, it is a great way to preserve any extras. Adding the pineapple imparts more colour, flavour, and a hint of sweetness, not to mention more vitamin C. (See photo, page 334.)

400 g mixed tomatoes, roughly chopped

200 g fresh pineapple, chopped

1 medium red onion, finely diced

1 to 2 jalapeños or chilli peppers, finely chopped (leave the seeds in if you want the heat)

1 dried chipotle or ancho chili, crumbled

7 garlic cloves, finely chopped

20 g fresh coriander, chopped

14 g pure salt

Juice of 1 lime

2 teaspoons raw apple cider vinegar (with the mother) or ½ tablespoon unflavoured kombucha

1. In a large plastic or ceramic bowl, place the tomatoes, pineapple, onion, chillies, garlic, and coriander.

2. Add the salt and mix until the salt is well combined and the ingredients are mixed.

3. Next, add the lime juice and vinegar and stir.

4. Remove about a quarter of the salsa and blend; add this back into the bowl.

5. Pack the salsa into a 1 litre preserving jar, pressing down so that the brine rises above the veg.

6. Close the jar and allow it to sit out for 3 to 5 days. You will see bubbles form and rise in the jar or hear a pop or burping sound when you release the lid or latch.

7. Taste the salsa. It should be tangy and slightly fizzy. If the fizziness hasn't developed or it is still salty, give it another day or so. When you are ready to eat it, store it in the fridge and use within 1 month.

FERMENTED PUMPKIN, APPLE AND MAPLE SODA

Makes about
1.2 litres

Packed with fibre, including gut-loving prebiotic fibre thanks to the apples, this soda is unlike any you can buy because it's not only great for supporting your gut but also a delicious way to get key immune-supporting micronutrients like vitamins A and C, with a dose of antioxidants thanks to its gingery kick.

250 g pumpkin or butternut squash, skin on and grated

200 g apple, grated (I use the sweeter varieties)

50 g fresh ginger, grated

2 tablespoons 100% maple syrup plus 2 teaspoons for bottling

2 cinnamon sticks

2 teaspoons pure vanilla paste or 1 vanilla pod, split

1 teaspoon raw apple cider vinegar (with the mother)

1.2 to 1.4 litres filtered water

1. Add the pumpkin, apple, ginger, maple syrup, cinnamon, and vanilla into the fermenting jar. Next, add the vinegar and top up with filtered water to the neck (or just at the shoulder if you're using a 2 litre jar).

2. Allow the mixture to ferment for 3 to 5 days, swilling every day to mix. You should start seeing bubbles and hearing a release of CO_2 when you flip the latch.

3. After 3 to 5 days, check for flavour and fizziness before straining off the liquid using a sieve. Be sure to squeeze out as much liquid as you can.

4. Transfer the liquid and the 2 remaining teaspoons of the maple syrup into a pouring bottle before closing.

5. Set the bottle back on the kitchen worktop to ferment for an additional day, taking care when you open it, as it will be fizzy.

6. Serve chilled and store in the fridge. It should keep for 1 week, but do remember to open it daily to release any built-up CO_2.

BEETROOT, PEAR AND GINGER KVASS

Makes just
under 1 litre

Kvass is traditionally a Russian fermented beverage often made from beetroot. It is touted as a general health tonic. This recipe is inspired by the Russian version but adds additional spices and sweetness that comes with the added pear, a great source of gut-loving fibre, dates, and spices. There's no need for a starter culture with a kvass, as the skins of the beetroot, ginger, and pear are a plentiful source of *Lactobacillus*, so keep those skins on! Nature prepared the plants with fermenting bugs in tow. (See photo, page 334.)

300 g beetroot, chopped (washed and skin on)

2 large ripe pears, chopped (washed and skin on)

50 g fresh ginger, sliced into matchsticks (skin on)

6 dates or dried figs, chopped

¼ teaspoon pure salt

2 star anise

1 litre filtered water

1. Add the beetroot, pears, ginger, and dates to a 1.5 litre or 2 litre fermenting jar. Next, add the salt and star anise.

2. Fill the jar with the water, leaving a 3 cm gap at the top. Seal the jar.

3. Ferment at room temperature for 3 to 4 days, giving it a gentle shake every day. Taste and check the flavour; it should be slightly fizzy. You may want to ferment it for an additional 1 to 2 days for the flavours to further develop.

4. Strain the liquid into a jug using a plastic sieve. Using a funnel, pour the liquid into a swing-top drinks bottle. You can enjoy it right away or store at room temperature for 2 to 3 days to generate additional fizz. Make sure that you let the gases escape from the drink daily by releasing the lid on the bottle for a few seconds. Once you are happy with the fizziness, transfer to the refrigerator and use within 10 days.

>> *To view the 14 scientific references cited in this chapter, please visit www.theplantfedgut.com/cookbook.*

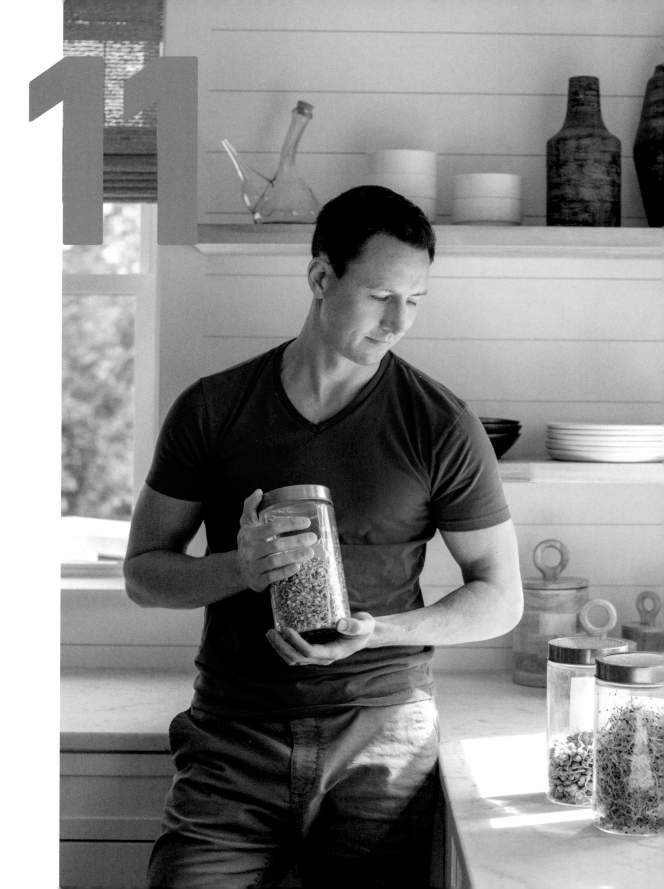

You Know You Make Me Want to Sprout!

Unlock the magic of nature and enjoy the benefits

When something seems too good to be true, it usually proves to be just that. Hype elevates expectations and ultimately leads to disappointments. We've all been there too many times. But every once in a while, you come across something that perhaps you've heard whispers about but you haven't yet taken the time to really look into. And when you finally do—holy moly! It turns out to be a game changer, and you wish you had found it sooner.

I discovered sprouts just a few years ago, but they have quickly become a big part of my diet. In *Fibre Fuelled*, I explained the wonders of broccoli sprouts—they are a foundational food with a very high concentration of sulforaphane, a phytochemical with anti-cancer, anti-inflammatory, and anti-microbial effects. At that time my wife and I were routinely adding broccoli sprouts to our smoothies and smoothie bowls. It wasn't until I met Doug Evans, author of *The Sprout Book*, that I grew to fully understand the power that exists in these little seeds. Not just broccoli seeds, but *all* of them. I now view them as having an almost mystical quality.

In order to really appreciate sprouts, we have to take it from the top. Seeds are baby plants in their earliest stages of development. They're dormant, enjoying the comforts and safety of their protective outer covering, waiting for their opportunity. Sprouting is a process initiated by soaking seeds in water, which is nature's way of opening the window blinds to reveal a bright light. Suddenly the seed comes out of its slumber in what's called germination. At this point, the baby plant soaks up water and swells to the point of splitting its hard shell. It's time for this baby plant to grow beyond the confines of the seed.

Like fermentation, sprouting is a natural transformation process. Hydration activates the plant metabolism and gene transcription. Storage reserves saved for this moment get activated. Enzymes turn on and start breaking down and simplifying proteins, fats, and starches. These simplified compounds are, in a way, predigested. But they also form the building blocks of a rapidly growing young plant that gets reassembled. Organelles are being created. Multiple biochemical reactions lead to the production of essential amino acids, protein, fibre, healthy fats, vitamin C, B-group vitamins. Simultaneously, the antinutrients like phytic acid, lectins, and protease inhibitors start to disappear.

Let's pause for a moment to ponder nature's power and intelligence. A dormant seed discovers the proper conditions that activate a symphony of synchronized, synergistic enzymatic reactions that facilitate biotransformation and growth from a speck to a full-size plant. This isn't only marvellous in isolation—there are also potential synergies and connections within the surrounding biological network. In nutrition, we're really good at identifying macro- and micronutrients, but we struggle to identify the biochemical powerhouses, the progenitors of transformation—the enzymes. They may be fleeting and transient, but they are powerful and, if consumed, have the possibility to contribute to our digestive process and enhance our health as they do the young sproutling.

Sprouting makes food more digestible. Soaking and sprouting are the most efficient way to reduce alpha-galactosides from pulses, which are the flatulence-promoting FODMAPs that kids and guys like me are referring to when we sing, "Beans, beans, good for the heart . . ." Sprouting reduces phytic acid, which is the antinutrient known to inhibit mineral absorption, particularly calcium, and impair digestive enzyme activity.

There's more. The biochemical transformations occurring during early plant life often create superhero foods with medicinal qualities. Germinating seeds could contain from two to ten times more phytochemicals as compared with adult plants, or potentially even more. Broccoli sprouts can produce ten to one hundred times more sulforaphane than mature broccoli. Sulforaphane is thought to activate cellular defence and have anti-inflammatory and antimicrobial properties with far-reaching benefits throughout the body. Some of the other phytochemicals you'll find in sprouts include chlorophyll, flavonoids, hydroxycinnamic acids, glucosinolates, and carotenoids. These phytochemicals are thought to have anti-inflammatory and antioxidant properties that help protect the human body against our all-too-common latent diseases like cardiovascular diseases, diabetes, and cancer.

In the histamine chapter, we discussed the importance of diamine oxidase (DAO) for regulating histamine balance in the body. Legume sprouts produce DAO! Sprouted lentils have 165 times more DAO than their unsprouted counterpart. Similarly, sprouted alfalfa has 280 times more DAO! We're coming in hot, folks. If you have histamine intolerance, you absolutely should be incorporating sprouted legumes routinely into your meals. Sprouted peas, lentils, chickpeas, and soybeans have the highest levels of DAO.

Dr. B's Advice

If you want to really crank up your DAO activity, sprout your peas and other legumes in the dark. The stress of darkness actually brings out the best in your sprouts and increases the DAO activity even more!

And then there are the implicit benefits of growing your own food. You are maximizing nutrient density by consuming it at the time of harvest, its freshest state. You have control over what goes into and nurtures your food (and ultimately you). You don't have to trust the assurances of someone you don't know; you know for a fact that your food was grown pesticide-free in ideal conditions. And the beauty of sprouting is that you don't need to have a green thumb to enjoy the benefits of a garden. You can have a garden sitting right there on your kitchen worktop. It's simple, quick, inexpensive, and hypernourishing. What's not to love?

In a world where healthy food is inaccessible to some due to cost and availability, sprouting offers one solution. Start with vegetable seeds or pulses. They are relatively inexpensive even in organic form because a little goes a long way. They also have a long shelf life, and as a result can be purchased in bulk off the internet. Bulk purchases reduce costs and protect against food scarcity. And there is also the radical expansion that occurs when you sprout your seeds. Think of how far a kilo of broccoli seeds goes when 2 tablespoons becomes several large handfuls of sprouts in just a few days. If you want to witness nature's jaw-dropping power, in just three days 80 g of dry lentils will become a large punnet of lentil sprouts. So what are you waiting for? Let's sprout this thing!

"Cool, Doc, but How Do You Eat Sprouts?"

However you want. I love them as a garnish. They're awesome in soups, stews, salads, and sandwiches. I also love sprouts in smoothies. Legume or chickpea sprouts make a nice addition to spaghetti sauce. It seems like sprouts only pair with S words, so let me throw you a curveball to keep you on your toes—avocado toast. It's glorious.

"Can I Just Go to the Shop and Buy Whatever Is on the Shelf, Doc?"

People often wonder what type of seeds to purchase. Generally, you're best off purchasing your seeds from an online purveyor that specializes in sprouting. There are three qualities that you want: organic, so that they haven't been treated with chemical desiccants; pathogen negative, meaning they've been tested for pathogenic microbes and tested negative; and high germination, indicating that we expect a high per centage to turn into sprouts.

Your Step-by-Step Guide to Sprouting

What You'll Need

1 to 2 litre jar with a wide, open mouth (a wide-mouthed kilner jar will do)
A mesh sprouting screen or muslin
Raw, organic seeds or legumes

Sprouting is all about firing up the engine and then maintaining a nice rhythm until you hit the finish line. By firing up the engine, I mean that nature has created an ignition sequence that you can activate by soaking your seeds or legumes for 12 hours. This is the secret code that nature has created to let the seed or legume know that it's time to come into this world. Once you fire up the engine, you want to maintain a consistent rhythm by rinsing and draining your sprouts twice daily until they are ready. If you follow these simple steps, you will have delicious, nutritious food that's organic and inexpensive and created right there in your kitchen garden.

The formula for the seeds and legumes is the same. The only thing that varies is how much seed or legume you place in the jar at the beginning and how long you have to maintain the rinse-and-drain rhythm.

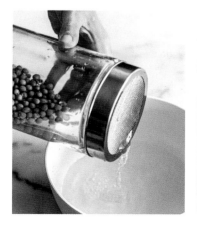
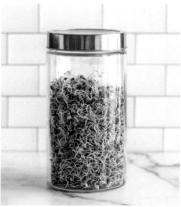
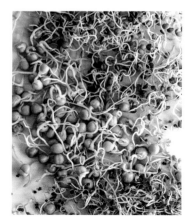

Seed	Starting Amount	Yield	Harvest
Alfalfa	2 tablespoons	100 g	5 to 6 days
Broccoli	2 tablespoons	180 g	3 to 6 days
Kale	2 tablespoons	170 g	3 to 6 days
Onion	2 tablespoons	170 g	10 to 15 days
Radish	2 tablespoons	100 g	3 to 6 days

Legume	Starting Amount	Yield	Harvest
Chickpeas	80 g	280 g	2 to 4 days
Lentils	40 g	160 g	2 to 3 days
Mung bean	50 g	400 g	2 to 5 days
Peas	60 g	360 g	2 to 3 days

Here's how to do it:

1. Add the starting amount of your desired seed or legume to a jar.

2. Cover with at least 3 times the amount of cool, filtered water than you have seeds. No need to measure—just make sure you're generous.

3. Place the sprouting lid of your choice on the jar. If you're using muslin, make sure to secure it using a rubber band.

4. Keep the jar upright and allow to soak for 12 hours on the kitchen worktop, out of direct sunlight.

5. Using the lid to keep the sprouts inside your jar, pour off the water. You will not soak your sprouts again. The engine has officially been fired up. From this point forward, we will have a twice-daily rinse-and-drain rhythm.

6. Rinse your sprouts with cool, clean water and swish around gently.

7. Pour off the water, trying to keep the seeds or legumes evenly distributed within the jar and not clumped up by the lid.

8. With the water poured off, place the jar on a 30- to 60-degree slant upside-down. This can be done with a bowl, in your sink drain. I personally use a dish drying rack with a flat tray below it to catch the water that drips out.

9. Twice a day, repeat steps 6 to 8.

10. Upon completion, rinse the sprouts one last time and drain, then remove the lid and dump all the sprouts out onto a clean, absorbent tea towel. Spread them all out into one layer and let them air-dry for 30 to 60 minutes. This can be done with some added gentle sunlight, which will allow the sprouts to generate some chlorophyll for added nutrition. Store them in a glass food container with a clean, unbleached paper towel. They will keep in the refrigerator for up to 1 week.

"If You Were Me, Doc, Where Would You Start?"

Personally, if I were sprouting for the first time, I would start with lentil sprouts. They are quick, pretty darn easy to do, and produce a large volume of sprouts. Once you master lentils, then you should have a handle on the basic principles of sprouting and may want to move toward broccoli sprouts. They take an intermediate amount of time, but the reward is perhaps the most medicinal of all foods.

On the Safety of Sprouting

You've probably heard that sprouts are a microbial biohazard with an excessively high risk for foodborne illness. There is some truth to this, but it is not the whole truth, so we might as well take it head-on and also establish some rules for optimal safety.

Here's the breakdown: Seeds can potentially become contaminated with pathogenic microbes during production. There are a number of reasons this can happen: the anatomy of the seed, the water supply, exposure to animal waste products, unsanitary practices by workers or during storage or transport, or the way the seeds are processed to increase germination. Sprouting is higher risk because if pathogenic microbes are present, they can multiply during the sprouting process.

In 1999, there were multiple outbreaks of salmonella poisoning across the United States. All involved alfalfa sprouts. The Food and Drug Administration did an investigation and discovered poor sanitation practices on multiple levels in the production of the alfalfa sprouts at commercial facilities. This resulted in the FDA releasing a guidance document to improve food safety laws for raw sprouts.

The process has improved; however, caution is still advised. From 1998 to 2018, there were fifty-seven foodborne outbreaks and 1,940 illnesses reported in association with various types of sprouts. Certainly, that's more than we wish to see, but as a matter of context it's worth mentioning that according to the Centers for Disease Control and Prevention's most recent report on foodborne illness, 48 per cent of foodborne illnesses and 50 per cent of deaths are due to animal product consumption. The death rate is substantially higher than the 23 per cent attributable to plant produce.

Should we be cautious? Of course. Should we throw all sprouts in the rubbish and miss out on the amazing nutrition that they provide? Of course not. Let's just follow some simple rules.

If you purchase sprouts from a commercial supplier:

- Make sure they have tested negative for pathogenic bacteria.
- Buy only sprouts that are kept refrigerated.
- Purchase and consume sprouts prior to their "best by" date.
- Do not purchase sprouts that look slimy, have a musty smell, or are a dark colour.

When growing your own sprouts at home:

- Purchase seeds from a commercial source, produced for sprouting specifically, pretested for pathogenic microbes, and organic when possible.
- Wash sprouting containers thoroughly with hot water and soap prior to use.
- Similarly, always wash your hands with hot water and soap prior to interacting with your sprouts.
- Use a clean, fresh source of drinking water to rinse your sprouts.
- Each time you rinse the sprouts, give particular attention to removing as much water as possible after the rinse.
- Grow your sprouts in an area that is temperature controlled, where they will not be disturbed by direct sunlight or contact with other foods or pets.

How to handle your sprouts, whether purchased or grown:

- Keep your sprouts refrigerated at 5°C or cooler.
- Store sprouts in clean containers.
- Sprouts should smell fresh and clean at the time of consumption.
- Wash your hands with hot running water and soap each time before handling sprouts.
- Wash raw sprouts thoroughly with cool running water immediately before use.

Dr. B's Tips for Success

When I first started sprouting, I was a total disaster. I just couldn't figure it out. Honestly, I'm writing this chapter hoping that I can spare you the humiliation of the multiple failed sprouting attempts that I had to face. My wife was questioning her decision to marry me. Thankfully, I eventually got on track. So even if your sprouting dreams don't come true, the first time, just know that you are probably closer than I was, and now here I am writing a book heralding the benefits of sprouting.

Here are a few tips I wish I had known when I was getting started:

· *Don't overthink it! Sprouting is a simple formula—soak for 12 hours, then rinse and drain twice a day until ready. If you stick to this, you will likely be successful. If you panic and deviate, there's a high probability of things going awry.*

· *Make sure to get the water out. It's important to really drain the jar because excess moisture creates an environment for funky stuff to grow.*

· *Let your sprouts breathe! It's important to have a wide-mouthed sprouting jar and to maintain the sprouts upside down at an angle so air can get in there.*

· *If you want chlorophyll, expose them to sunlight. This can be done in the last few hours before you harvest your sprouts.*

· *Recycle your water! It's totally fair game to pour the water from one jar into the next. Then, when you're on your last jar, you can use it to water your houseplants. They love it!*

Now you are ready to embark on your sprout-enhanced Fibre Fuelled journey. I hope you find it as delicious, nutritious, and fun as I have!

>> *To view the 9 scientific references cited in this chapter, please visit www.theplantfedgut.com/cookbook.*

Epilogue

Imagine for a moment that you're holding in your hand a photo of yourself from the future. You look down at it and see yourself at a dinner party, surrounded by people whom you love. There's joy on your face and comfort in your body language. In front of you sits a delicious meal, filled with a colourful diversity of plants. Right smack dab in the middle is a heaping serving of that plant that you *never* thought you were capable of eating. But quite clearly from the photo, there you are, not just eating it but enjoying it. Your foe has become your friend.

How did you get there? You took this book to heart and implemented the GROWTH strategy. You identified the root, or genesis, of your symptoms. You used the Restrict—Observe—Work It Back In method to identify your food intolerances, then you Trained Your Gut like exercising a muscle at the gym. Low and slow is the tempo. It grew stronger than ever. You healed your relationship with food and addressed the wounds of trauma from the past as part of Holistic Healing. You set realistic goals, accomplished them, and celebrated the victories—no matter how small. You let go of perfection, allowed grace for your imperfect self, and placed your focus on progress. Above all, you never quit or backed down. There were challenges, but your unyielding commitment to the process made it not a question of whether you would accomplish your goal and overcome those challenges; it was simply a question of when. And here you are . . . You've done it.

So, what's next? There's a reason I chose GROWTH as the name for our approach. Beyond the eponymous strategy, "growth" is a word that eloquently describes our relationship with food. It's imperfect, but it's constantly evolving and we are helping to shape it so that it flourishes. It is an abundance mindset where restriction is temporary and plant-based diversity is always the ultimate goal. Progress over perfection.

The word "growth" also vividly articulates our mindset for life. Remember the 2 hour 15 minute barefoot marathon, the 18-plus-minute breath hold, the 2,750 free throws in a row, and the 4.5-second Rubik's cube mastery? What incredible feats or amazing things do you want to accomplish during your lifetime? With effort, grit, and knowledge, you can accomplish anything that you set your mind to. I never thought I could write a book and be a full-time doctor at the same time. I'm on call 24 out of every 72 hours! But I *really* wanted to share what I had learned with you, and now here we are wishing one another a fond adieu for the second time.

I often read Dr. Seuss's *Oh, the Places You'll Go!* to my children before tucking them in for bed. As a father, I can't help but get a little choked up with love and enthusiasm as I optimistically ponder the limitless possibilities of their future life. The world is their oyster. I just want them to be happy and feel satisfied. This is what I want for you. I want to be your cheerleader and supporter as you continue to grow and manifest the best version of yourself in a life filled with an abundance of love and satisfaction.

Until we meet again.

HIGH FODMAP FOODS AND POTENTIAL LOW FODMAP SUBSTITUTIONS

Adapted from Nanayakkara et al., *Clin Exp Gastroenterology* 2016.[1]

	High FODMAP foods	Low FODMAP substitutions
Oligosaccharides–Fructans	**Grains:** wheat-, rye-, and barley-based products **Vegetables:** onion, garlic, artichokes, leeks, beetroot, and savoy cabbage **Fruits:** watermelon, peaches, persimmon, prunes, nectarines, and most dried fruits	**Fruits:** banana, most berries (except boysenberries and blackberries), grapes, lemon, lime, mandarin, orange, kiwi, pineapple, passion fruit, and rhubarb **Vegetables:** chives, spring onion tops, sweet peppers, pak choi, green beans, parsnip, Swiss chard, cucumber, carrots, celery, aubergine, lettuce, potatoes, yams, kabocha squash, tomatoes, and courgettes
Oligosaccharides–Galactans (or GOS)	**Legumes:** red kidney beans, baked beans, split peas, silken tofu, and soybeans **Vegetables:** butternut squash, beetroot, and peas **Nuts:** cashews, almonds, pistachios	**Grains:** wheat-free grains/flour, gluten-free bread or cereal products, and quinoa **Legumes:** canned lentils or chickpeas, tempeh, firm tofu **Nuts:** walnuts, pecans, macadamias, pine nuts, pumpkin seeds, peanuts and peanut butter
Disaccharides–Lactose	**Dairy products:** cow's/goat's milk and derivatives like ice cream, soft cheeses and yoghurt, sweetened condensed milk, evaporated milk, soya milk	**Dairy products:** lactose-free, almond, or rice-based milk, yoghurt, and ice cream. Hard cheese, feta, and cottage cheese
Monosaccharides–Fructose	**Fruits:** apples, pears, watermelon, mango, cherries, boysenberries, and fruit juice from high-fructose foods **Honey** **Sweeteners:** high-fructose corn syrup **Vegetable:** asparagus and sugar snap peas	**Fruits:** banana, grapes, honeydew, melon, kiwi, lemon, lime, mandarin, orange, passion fruit, and most berries (except boysenberries and blackberries) **Sweeteners:** maple syrup and golden syrup
Polyols–Sorbitol	**Fruits:** apples, pears, avocado, apricots, blackberries, nectarines, peaches, plums, prunes, and watermelon	**Sweeteners:** Maple syrup and table sugar (sucrose) **Fruits:** banana, grape, honeydew, melon, kiwi, lemon, mandarin, orange, and passion fruit
Polyols–Mannitol	**Vegetables:** sweet potato, mushrooms, cauliflower, and mangetout	

Note that for each of these foods the portion size is important. Low FODMAP foods can be made high FODMAP if consumed in large amounts, and high FODMAP foods can be made low FODMAP if consumed in a small enough portion size. How that interacts with your body will be entirely unique to you. This is why "low and slow is the tempo." But to learn more about the relative thresholds for each of these foods, please refer to the Monash University Low FODMAP app.

1 Wathsala S. Nanayakkara et al., "Efficacy of the Low FODMAP Diet for Treating Irritable Bowel Syndrome: The Evidence to Date," *Clinical and Experimental Gastroenterology* 9 (June 17, 2016): 131–42, https://doi.org/10.2147/CEG.S86798.

FOODS TO AVOID DURING A HISTAMINE RESTRICTION PHASE

Adapted from Comas-Baste et al., 2020, and Maintz et al., 2007.[2]

Plants		Animal products
Alcohol	Teas: black, green, maté	Cheese
Aubergine	Tomatoes	Eggs
Avocado	Vinegar and vinegar-containing foods (pickles, olives)	Fish, canned or preserved fish, fish derivatives like sauces
Banana		
Chickpeas (canned)		Ham
Chocolate, cocoa, cacao		Milk, fermented milk
Citrus foods		Pork
Coffee (caffeinated)		Sausages, deli meats, hot dogs, and other processed meats
Dried fruit: apricots, prunes, dates, figs, raisins		Shellfish
Energy drinks		
Fermented plant foods like sauerkraut, kimchi, tempeh, miso, etc.		
Fruit juices		
Kiwi		
Lentils (canned)		
Liquorice		
Mushrooms		
Nuts and nut milks, walnuts, cashews		
Papaya		
Peanuts		
Pineapple		
Plum		
Spinach		
Spices		
Soybeans (canned), soya milk, fermented and unfermented soy derivatives		
Strawberries		

2 Comas-Basté et al.; Maintz and Novak, "Histamine and Histamine Intolerance."

ADDITIONAL RESOURCES

It is impossible to write a book that covers all things for all people. Consider this book your foundation, and with these additional resources you can continue to expand your knowledge on the subject of gut health.

Remember, you can also find the resources I've discussed in the book and a few extras at www.theplantfedgut.com/cookbook for free!

Books

Fibre Fuelled
Dr. Will Bulsiewicz (a.k.a. me!)
My first book, *Fibre Fuelled*, is jam-packed with science, actionable steps for optimal health, and more than seventy recipes. Now's the time to grab your copy if you haven't yet!

The Sprout Book
Doug Evans
This is *the* book about sprouts! Low-cost and accessible, sprouts are an ultra-food for health, weight loss, and optimum nutrition. Plus, they're fun as heck to grow!

The Proof Is in the Plants
Simon Hill
One of my all-time-favourite books. Simon lays out the argument for why eating a plant-predominant diet is best for you and for the planet.

Re-challenging and Reintroducing FODMAPs
Lee Martin
This book will further your knowledge on FODMAPs and how to rechallenge individual FODMAPs.

The Plant-Based Baby and Toddler
Alexandra Caspero and Whitney English
This book is a must-read for parents and families, co-authored by Alex Caspero, the recipe developer for both *Fibre Fuelled* books.

Courses

The Plant Fed Gut Masterclass
This is my signature course, a seven-week comprehensive educational programme designed to deliver the transformational knowledge that you seek in a format that's fun, engaging, and collaborative. The course includes structured video lessons, audio lessons, journal article breakdowns, case studies, a 100-plus-page guidebook, exclusive recipes, Q&A sessions, and a private Facebook group.

I also routinely offer other topical webinars and online trainings such as Conversations About Constipation and Going Head-to-Head with Heartburn. Learn more at www.theplantfedgut.com/course, and make sure to sign up for my newsletter so you can stay up to date on new studies, recipes, events, and courses!

Apps & Tech

ZOE At-Home Test Kit
We are all unique individuals with a completely distinct gut microbiome. There can be no "one-size-fits-all" diet. Introducing ZOE, a personalized nutrition company using science and technology to help you understand your unique biology. Learn more at www.joinzoe.com/drb, where you'll also find my checkout code to save on your At-Home Test Kit purchase.

Nibble
Nibble is a fun and easy way to track your plant diversity to improve your overall health. You can compete with friends and users on the Plant Point leaderboard and discover meals made by other people around the world. Learn more at nibble.health.

Low FODMAP Diet App by Monash University
With the largest FODMAP food database available, the Monash FODMAP App provides an easy guide to which foods are low and high in FODMAPs. Learn more at www.monashfodmap.com/.

ACKNOWLEDGEMENTS

It's one thing to have an idea. But it is a much bigger thing to bring that idea fully to life.

This book was once an idea. Every day I would meet people suffering from food intolerances. Food is supposed to be a source of great pleasure. It certainly is for me. But these people sitting before me would experience pain rather than pleasure from their food. Further, they would be forced to subject themselves to that pain several times daily, like it or not, because we all need to eat in order to live. I care deeply about my patients. They are real people, not just diagnoses or codes. Witnessing their suffering and their need became my motivation. I needed a way to help them.

So I set out to create a book that would provide a solution to this problem. That would lay out a path to identify the source of the problem and then offer a solution that addresses the root cause and facilitates healing. In order to do this, it had to involve food. Lots and lots of recipes. And so, this became *The Fibre Fuelled Cookbook*.

I couldn't have brought this idea to life without the help of some amazing people, and I want to thank them for their contribution to this book.

First off, thank you to the people whose work you are seeing in these pages. Alex Caspero created most of the delicious recipes in this book, including the sourdough recipes. Nena Foster contributed many incredible recipes to the fermentation chapter. Ashley McLaughlin prepared every one of the recipes, styled them, and took the brilliant food photographs that you see. She was assisted by Chef Kathleen Casanova. Margaret Wright did all the lifestyle photography, which I'm obsessed with. Cynthia Groseclose is my talented chef friend who styled the food for our lifestyle shoot. Colleen Martell was my brilliant co-author for the book and helped me transform my ideas into words on paper. I owe a debt of gratitude to these incredibly talented people who are able to elevate this work and make it so much more than I could have ever dreamed of. I am so proud of what we have done together.

This work was made possible by my publishing team. I can't thank my editor, Lucia Watson, enough. This is our second book together. She is talented, smart, but also very thoughtful in helping me shape these books. Love ya, Lucia! I must also thank Suzy Swartz, my awesome assistant editor and fellow Northwestern grad. I'm grateful for the leadership at Avery Publishing who support my work, specifically Megan Newman and Lindsay Gordon, as well as the marketing and publicity legends Farin Schlussel, Anne Kosmoski, and Carla Iannone. The opportunity to write books that change people's lives began when I met my literary agent, Stephanie Tade, and her team, which includes Gretchen van Nuys and Colleen Martell. Colleen, you're everywhere. Stephanie, I'm eternally grateful.

I have an incredible team that works really hard behind the scenes to support me and help me spread my message through social media, podcasts, courses, webinars, emails, and blog posts. Thank you to Christina Roberto, Caitlin Hornik, Lindsay Marder, Jonathan Jacobs, Liora Mann, Kelly Ziv, Bryan Trindade, Allison Lovrin, Katie Karas, and Ana Bartel. It's been a rocket ship thanks to your help, and a lot of fun. You are all amazing, and I am so grateful. Let's keep it rolling.

I clearly couldn't have done this without my family—Noreen, Susan, Larry, and of course my wife, Valarie. Your love and support mean the world to me, and I also thank you for all the times that you stepped up to help with extra work so that I could pursue this project.

I must thank my mentors through the years who have given their time and energy to my professional development and helped me to become the person that I am today—Drs. Nick Shaheen, John Pandolfino, Balfour Sartor, Doug Drossman, Peter Kahrilas, William Li, and Tim Spector.

I'd like to give a special shout-out to my brother from Down Under, Simon Hill. The internet drives me nuts, but one of the great things about it is that it allows us to find friends literally on the other side of the planet.

I'd like to thank all of the podcast hosts who took a chance on me; my friends on social media and in "real life" who support me; my trainer, Eli; my partners, Jeff and Josh; our PA, Gina; and our entire staff. Thank you, thank you, thank you!

Finally, I want to acknowledge my father, Bill Bulsiewicz, who passed away unexpectedly in January 2020. I think about you all the time, Dad, and I'm pretty sure you know that.

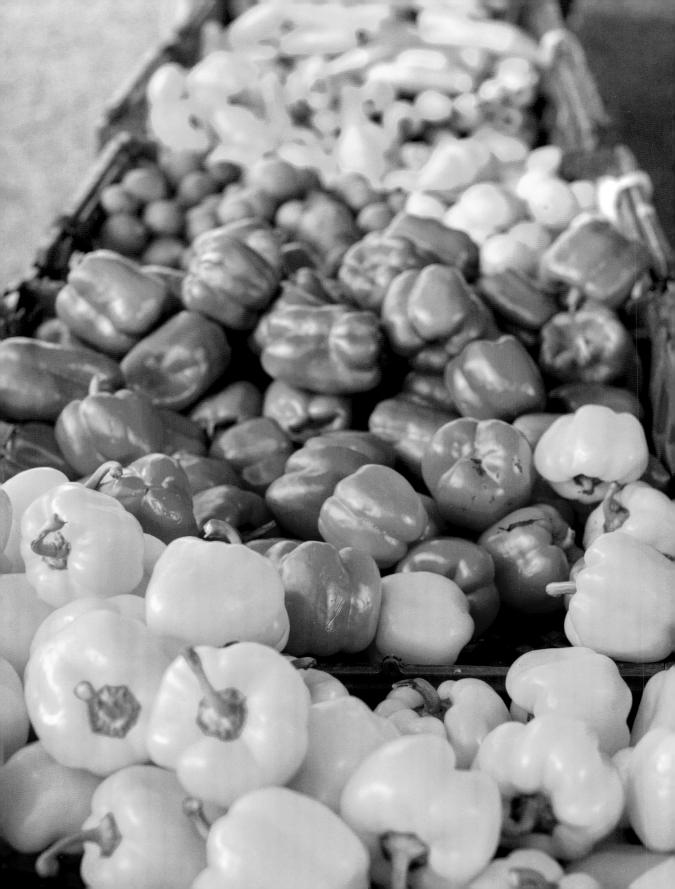

INDEX

Note: *Italicized* page numbers indicate material in tables or illustrations.

tips for success with, 351–52
standard American diet (SAD), 21–22
stool, blood in, 26
strawberries, 133, 356
Streptococcus thermophilus, 129
stretches, 219
strokes, 17, 203
Stuffed Sweet Potatoes, 190–91, 282–85
sucrose intolerance, 196–98
sugar alcohols, 48
sugar snap peas, 355
sugars, dietary recommendations for, 21
sulphites, *201*
Sunburst Summer Salad, 148–49
supplements, 30, 37, 214
Sweet and Spicy Peanut Tempeh Wraps, 106–7
Sweetcorn and Pepper Gazpacho, 162–63
Sweet Potato and Black Bean Tacos, 169–71
Sweet Potato and Okra Bowl, 277–79
Sweet Potato Bar, *283*, 284–85
Sweet Potato Burritos, 172–73
sweet potatoes, *53*, 355
Sweet Potato Hummus Wraps, 166–67
Sweet Potato Shawarma Bowl, 185–87
Sweet Potato Waffles, 142–43
sweets and treats
Chocolate Cookie Milk, 298–99
Cookie Milk, 296–97
Crispy Dark Chocolate Bites, 300–301
Mexican Hot Chocolate Brownies, 294–95
Peanut Butter Date Cookies, 292–93
Snickers Bites (variations), 302–3
symptoms
associated with damaged gut, 26

associated with FODMAPs, 52, 54
of constipation, 36
delay in onset of, 29
heart-related, 124, *125*
of histamine intolerance, 124, 125
identifying the cause of, 26 (*see also* GROWTH Strategy)
neurologic, 26
of salicylate intolerance, 198
tracking, in food diaries, 29

T
tartrazine (yellow #5), *201*
T cells, 18
tea, 198, 356
teff, 131
tempeh, 356
Tempeh Bacon BLTA with Celeriac Fries, 256–57
Tempeh Stir-Fry with Saffron Rice, 114–16
Tex-Mex Sweet Potatoes, *283*, 285
ticks and alpha-gal syndrome, 200
timing of meals, 218
tofu, silken, 355
Tofu Bánh Mì, 252–53
Tofu Peanut Satay, 254–55
tomatoes, 133, 198, 356
training your gut, 205–15
adaptability of microbiome, 206
contraindications for, 210
experiencing discomfort while, 208
setbacks in, 209
six tools to help with, 210–14
starting low and going slow, 207–9
See also GROWTH Strategy
trauma, dealing with, 220–21
Trinity Overnight Oats, 60–61
Turmeric Orange Cooler, 290–91
Tuscan Biome Stock, 240
Tuscan Flatbread, 280–81

U
ulcerative colitis, 16, 43, 130

V
Vanilla Berry Overnight Oats, 62–63
Vegetable Ceviche, 250–51
vegetables
average consumption of, 21
and FODMAPs, 48, 355
reintroduction of, *53*
Veggie Scramble and Sourdough Toast, 66–67
Very Vegetable Soup, 164–65
Very Veggie Indian Curry, 272–73
vinegar, 127, 134, 356
visualization, 211–12
Vitamin B6, 135–36
vitamins, 30
vomiting, 26, *125*

W
walking after meals, 214
walnuts, 356
Warm Apple Pie Porridge, 146–47
watermelon, 50, 355
Weeknight Minestrone Soup, 86–87
weight loss/control, 17, 26, 39, 306
wheat, 27, 48, 50, 51, 355
wheat allergies, 51
wheezing, 124
Where's the Beef? Steak Plate, 264–67
White Bean Hummus Toast, 168
wholefoods, 200
wholegrains, 21, 131
wholewheat flour, 312
Wholewheatish Sourdough Bread, 317–19
wounds, emotional, 220–21

X
xylitol, 48

Y
yoga, 218–19

Z
Zippy Coriander Bowl, 98–100